Foundations of Nutrition Science for Health and Performance

Updated, revised and edited by Cliff Harvey
Based on the FNDH FlexBook by Brian Lindshield

Cliff Harvey PhD, DipFit, DipNat, MNMHNZ, FCNA is a naturopath, registered clinical nutritionist, author and researcher. He is the founder of the Holistic Performance Institute. His areas of research and expertise are in metabolic adaptations to diet, especially lower-carbohydrate diets, keto-induction, 'carbohydrate appropriate diets' and symptoms of carbohydrate withdrawal. He is a former world champion and world record holder in All-Round Weightlifting and is the author of several best-selling books.

Published by Katoa Health Publishing, a division of Holistic Performance Ltd.

7 Ascension Place, Rosedale, Auckland 0632, NZ

www.katoahealth.com

ISBN 978-1719463591

This textbook is based on material from The Kansas State University Human Nutrition (FNDH 400) Flexbook by Brian Lindshield, as allowed by a CC-by licence. It has been extensively modified, updated and expanded by Cliff Harvey.
We thank Brian Lindshield for providing such a valuable resource.

The original FNDH 400 textbook is available free of charge here: goo.gl/vOAnR

Table of Contents

1 Nutrition Basics

The field of nutrition is incredibly dynamic, and our understanding and practices are constantly evolving.

The dynamic nature of the study of nutrition may be in part because nutrition, as a discipline, is relatively young compared to other scientific fields. Innovative research is constantly being conducted around the world by research labs and universities, with the findings continuously being reported to the public, albeit sometimes by well-meaning science reporters who misinterpret the results and conclusions!

However, it can take time for new findings to be validated by being replicated in other studies so that there is a sufficient body of evidence from which to draw firm conclusions and to become part of the dietary guidelines that we use in clinical practice.

With so much emerging information, discernment must be exercised, most especially by practitioners and allied health professionals who are at the 'coal face' of delivering guidelines to members of the public.

There needs to be a thorough understanding of nutrition science, an understanding of how research is conducted, what the data *actually* shows,

and whether the analysis and reporting is accurate. There also needs to be an evaluation of any new evidence considering the totality of evidence in the field. For example, several of the early randomised controlled trials (RCTs) for a popular joint health supplement, glucosamine, hinted at positive benefits for conditions like osteoarthritis.[1] However, later studies showed little or no effect.[2, 3] If we were to only look at the early studies, we could draw an incomplete conclusion and quite a different one than if we had evaluated the evidence in its totality.

Nutrition is such a fascinating area of science because everyone must eat to survive! Moreover, people are constantly facing nutrition choices and challenges, and these inevitably lead to many questions and, I must say, much confusion. This section will introduce the study of nutrition and provide you with a better understanding of the different forms of nutrition research and how to evaluate them relative to one another.

1.1 Defining Nutrition

Nutrition is defined as "the act or process of nourishing or being nourished". Alternatively, *the sum of the processes by which an animal or plant takes in and utilises food substances.*[4] So, for our purposes, we could say that nutrition is the science of how we utilise food for the nourishment of the body. This nourishment includes the functions of growth, repair and fuelling. The nutrients that allow these processes are classified according to the amounts required by the body.

1.1.1 What's a nutrient?

Simply put, a 'nutrient' is a chemical that we ingest which provides nourishment. In other words, it's any of the substances we eat that help us to maintain life. Some definitions refer only to essential nutrients (i.e. those that cannot be created within the body and so must be derived from the diet directly), but we will use the broader definition which includes the non-essential nutrients that help the body to function optimally.

1.1.2 Essential vs. non-*essential* in the nutritional sciences

People often confuse 'essential' with necessary. In the nutritional sciences when we refer to something as 'essential' we mean that we cannot create it within the body, and so, we need to eat it. A notable example of this is the essential amino acids. We cannot create them within the body, and so we need to regularly eat protein-containing foods that, in turn, contain these essential amino acids. On the other hand, certain substances like the simplest sugar 'glucose' that we derive from the carbohydrate foods we eat, can be created easily within the body, and so, although it can be beneficial for us to eat in the form of carbohydrate-containing foods, it is not strictly 'essential'.

1.2 Macro- and micronutrients

Macronutrients (macro = big) are the nutrients needed in larger amounts; carbohydrate, protein and fat (lipids). These can also provide energy to the body. Micronutrients (micro = small), on the other hand, are just as important but are required in much smaller amounts, i.e. vitamins and minerals. Micronutrients do not provide energy to the body (i.e. they are not calorie-containing), but they can help us to liberate energy from the macronutrients.

1.2.1 Carbohydrates

The name carbohydrate means 'hydrated carbon', or carbon with water. Thus, it isn't a surprise that carbohydrates are made up of carbon, hydrogen, and oxygen. Examples of foods high in dietary carbohydrates are table sugar, bread, pasta, grains, tubers and fruit.

1.2.2 Proteins

Proteins are also made up of carbon, hydrogen, and oxygen, but they also contain nitrogen. Dietary sources of protein include nuts, beans and legumes, milk, cheese and yoghurt, eggs, and meat.

1.2.3 Lipids

Lipids or 'fats' are fatty acids, triglycerides, phospholipids, and sterols (i.e. cholesterol). Lipids are also composed of carbon, hydrogen, and oxygen. Some dietary sources of lipids include oils, nuts and seeds, butter, and egg yolks.

1.2.4 Water

Water is made up of hydrogen and oxygen (H_2O) and is the only macronutrient that doesn't provide energy.

1.2.5 Vitamins

Vitamins are organic compounds ('organic' meaning related to or created by living organisms) that are essential for normal growth and development and that can't be created within the body.

1.2.6 Minerals

Inorganic substances (elements) that are essential for normal physiologic processes in the body.

1.3 Epidemiology

Epidemiology is defined as the study of human populations. These studies are also called 'population' or 'observational' research, in which the relationship between dietary consumption and disease development, or health or performance, is monitored and recorded. An observational study differs from an intervention study because there is no intervention being applied by researchers during the study. Thus, they are observational in nature. There are three main types of epidemiological studies: cross-sectional, case-control, and prospective cohort studies.

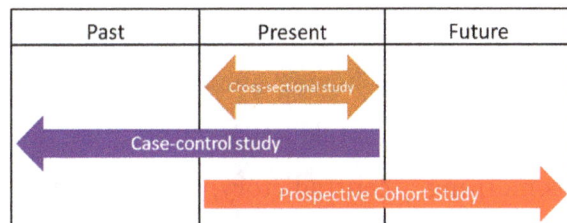

Figure 1. Types of epidemiological studies

1.3.1 Cross-Sectional Studies

Cross-sectional studies compare different populations at the same point in time. It is as if you take a snapshot of the two different populations to compare them to one another. An example of a cross-sectional study led to a phenomenon known as the "French Paradox". Cholesterol and saturated fat intake were associated with increased risk of coronary heart disease (CHD) across some countries. However, within the study, they noticed a surprising result. European countries with corresponding levels of cholesterol and saturated fat intakes had lower rates of mortality from CHD.

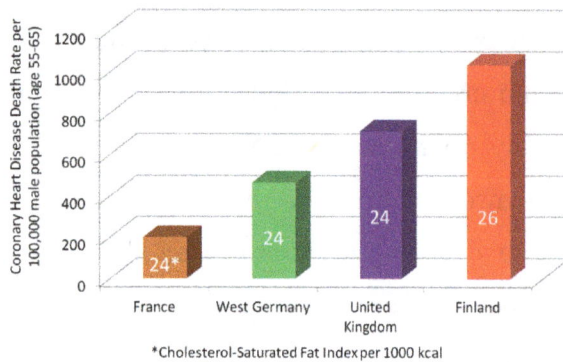

Figure 2. An example of a cross-sectional study, showing the 'French Paradox'

The French had a five-fold lower risk of dying from coronary heart disease than the Finns, despite having similar cholesterol-saturated fat intakes.[5] A paradox means something contradictory, which this finding seemed to be based on the prevailing theory that saturated fat was a causative factor in the development of heart disease. The 'French Paradox' led to research on red wine, and one of its active components, resveratrol (because the French consume much wine). Now, with a better understanding of the limitations of using saturated fat intake, cholesterol and LDL cholesterol as proxy measures for the likelihood of developing heart disease, we know that there are likely to be many other factors linked to these apparent 'paradoxes'.

Cross-sectional studies are considered the weakest type of epidemiology because they are based only on group outcomes. There are typically many confounders, and there can be invalid correlations drawn. They can also lead people to believe that members of a group have certain characteristics, which as individuals they do not. This is known as an ecologic (another name that is used to refer to this type of study) fallacy and is a further limitation of cross-sectional studies.[6]

1.3.1.1 What is a confounder?

In simple terms, a confounder is a variable that confuses an outcome. A more accurate statistical definition is an extraneous variable in a statistical model that correlates (directly or inversely) with both the dependent variable and the independent variable. Although for many non-statisticians this is confusing!

A confounder is something within a study that leads to people making a 'spurious' (incorrect) correlation (such as the incorrect link between vaccination rates and autism) or something that alters the outcome (such as smoking or exercise in a study of nutrition). This is known as 'causal confounding'. An example of a spurious correlation is shown in Figure 3.

Divorce rate in Maine
correlates with
Per capita consumption of margarine

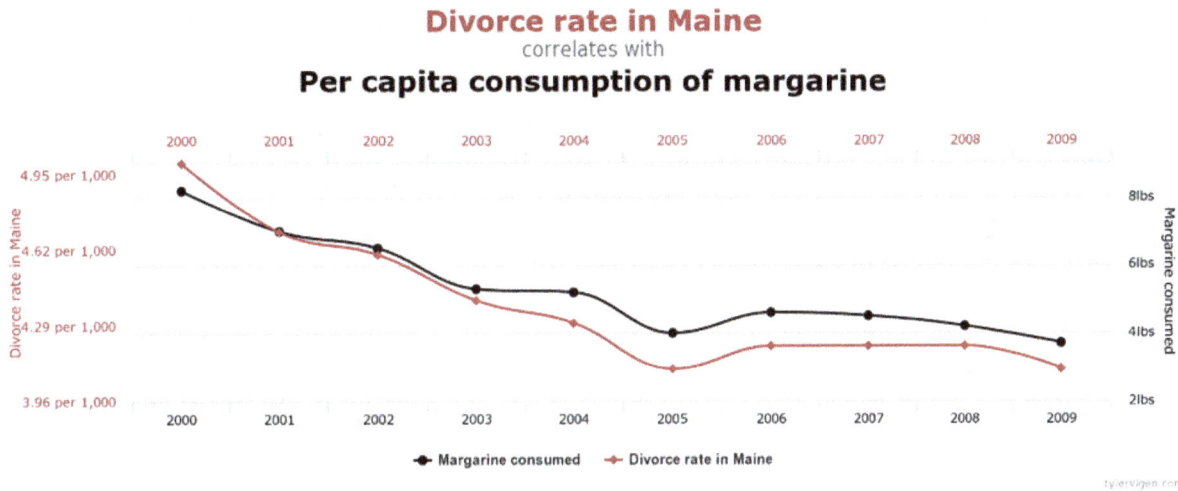

Figure 3. An example of a spurious correlation. Common-sense would tell us that margarine has no relationship with divorce rates![i]

1.3.2   Case-Control Studies

Case-control studies look at a group of cases (people with a disease) vs. controls (people without the same disease). Most case-control studies are retrospective (looking back in time or looking at the past). These studies try to determine if there were differences in the diets of the cases compared to controls in the past. Cases and controls are matched on characteristics such as age, sex, body mass index (BMI), familial, medical or dietary history, or disease, among others. To reduce the likelihood of confounders and provide a more meaningful outcome, researchers attempt to choose a control group that has similar characteristics to the case group. The researchers then compare the exposure levels between the cases and controls as shown below. In this example, a greater proportion of diseased (cases) individuals than disease-free individuals (controls) are exposed to a treatment.

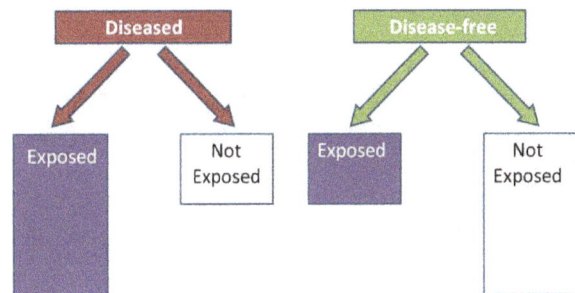

Figure 4. An example of a case-control study in which the diseased were more likely to have been exposed that those who were disease free

Using trans-fat intake as the exposure, and cardiovascular disease as the disease,

[i] Vigen T. Divorce Rates in Maine Correlate with Margarine Consumption. In: correlation.png s, editor. http://www.tylervigen.com/spurious-correlations: Own work; 2015.

the figure would be expected to look like this:

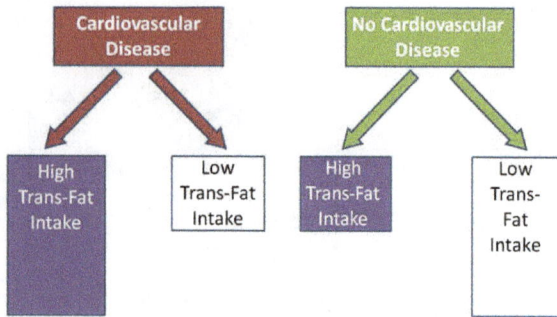

Figure 5. An example of a case-control study that indicates that more cases had high trans-fat intake, compared to controls

Food frequency questionnaires are oftne used in research to determine dietary intake. As the name suggests, a food frequency questionnaire is a series of questions that determine how frequently you consume a certain food. An example of a question on a food frequency questionnaire is shown below:

"Over the past 12 months, how often did you drink milk?"

Never
1 time/month
2-3 times/month
1-2 times/week
3-4 times/week
5-6 times/week

less 1 time/day
2-3 times/day
4-5 times/day
6 or more times/day

1.3.3 Prospective Cohort Studies

A cohort is a group of subjects. Most cohort studies are prospective. Initial information is collected (usually by food frequency questionnaires) on the intake of a cohort of people at baseline, or the beginning. This

cohort is then followed over time (normally many years) to quantify health outcomes of the individuals within it. Cohort studies more robust than case-control studies, because these studies do not start with diseased people and normally do not require people to remember their dietary habits in the distant past or before they develop disease. An example of a prospective cohort study would be if you filled out a questionnaire on your current dietary habits and are then followed into the future to see if you develop osteoporosis. As shown below, instead of separating based on disease versus disease-free, individuals are separated based on exposure. In this example, those who are exposed are more likely to be diseased than those who were not exposed.

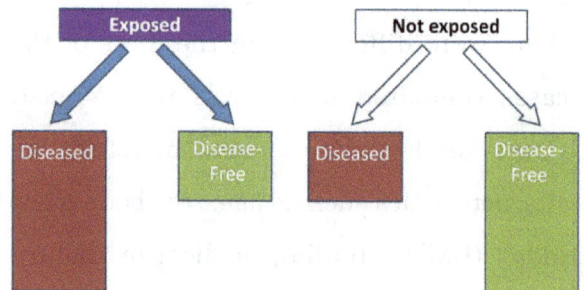

Figure 6. An example of a cohort study in which those exposed are more likely to develop the disease

Using trans-fat intake again as the exposure and cardiovascular disease as the disease, the figure would be expected to look like this:

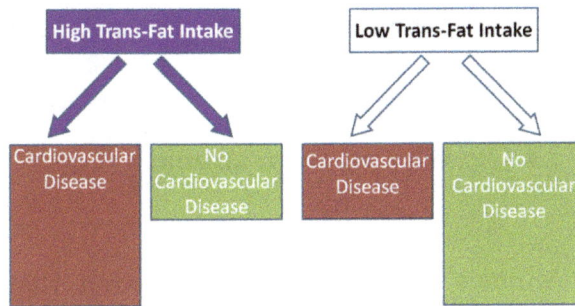

Figure 7. An example of a cohort study where higher trans-fat intake is associated with a higher incidence of cardiovascular disease

There are several well-known examples of prospective cohorts' studies.

1.3.3.1 Framingham Heart Study

The Framingham Heart Study started in 1948 and has been following the residents of Framingham, Massachusetts to identify risk factors for heart disease. This cohort has been very fruitful in finding some principal factors associated with CHD. In 2002, the third generation of participants was enrolled.

1.3.3.2 Nurses' Health Study

The Nurses' Health Study started in 1976 and enrolled 122,000 female nurses. Every four years they received a food frequency questionnaire to assess their dietary habits.

1.3.3.3 Health Professionals Follow-Up Study

The Health Professionals Follow-Up Study started in 1986 and enrolled 51,529 male health professionals (dentists, pharmacists, optometrists, osteopathic physicians, podiatrists, and veterinarians). Every four years they received a food frequency questionnaire to assess their dietary habits.

The Health Professionals Follow-Up Study is a good example of how cohort studies can be important in nutrition research. We will consider one example in which the researchers administered food frequency questionnaires that contained 131 food and beverage items to determine whether their intake was associated with increased or decreased risk of developing prostate cancer. Of these items, intake of four foods (tomatoes, tomato sauce, pizza, and strawberries) were associated with decreased incidence of prostate cancer.

The three tomato-based foods are red due to the presence of the carotenoid lycopene. Strawberries don't contain lycopene (their red colour is due to anthocyanins which may also be protective). This finding has led to interest in the potential of tomatoes/lycopene to decrease the risk of prostate cancer.[7]

1.4 *In Vitro* & Animal Studies

In vitro research is conducted outside an organism. In simple terms, it is research carried out in living tissue, or non-living

7

solutions in the lab. In vitro research is commonly referred to as 'test-tube' or 'petri-dish' research, as much of it involves growing cell-cultures in flasks and dishes and observing them under conditions (such as exposing them to interventions). Most of these cells are isolated from specific tissue, such as breast cancer cells or macrophages. Some cells are then treated with a dietary compound to compare the growth of the treated cells versus the untreated (control). For cells to grow they require a nutrient source. In cell cultures, the nutrient source is referred to as *media*. Media supplies nutrients to the cells in vitro in a comparable way to blood providing nutrients to cells within the body. Most cells adhere to the bottom of the flask and are so small that a microscope is needed to see them.

Cells are grown inside an incubator, which is a device that provides the optimal temperature, humidity, and carbon dioxide (CO_2) concentrations for cells and microorganisms. By imitating the body's temperature and CO_2 levels (37° C, 5% CO_2), the incubator allows cells to grow even though they are outside the body.

1.4.1 Animal Studies

Animal studies are one form of *in vivo* research, which translates to "within the living". Rats and mice are the most common animals used in nutrition research.

1.4.1.1 Why perform animal research?

Animals can be used in research that would be unethical to conduct in humans. While many people disagree with animal research, it is commonly conducted because researchers can make sure that a certain regimen is safe before it is researched in humans. One advantage of animal dietary studies is that researchers can control the animals' consumption of food and liquid.

In human studies, researchers can ask and provide participants with foods and liquids to consume. However, this does not necessarily guarantee that they are going to adhere to the researchers' instructions. Typically, people are not great at estimating, recording, or reporting how much or what they eat/ate.[8] Animal studies are also often far less expensive than human studies.

There are some principal factors to keep in mind when interpreting animal research. Firstly, an animal's metabolism and physiology are different to a human's. As a result, animals' absorption and metabolism of dietary compounds can differ markedly from humans. For example, we would not expect that rabbits (being obligate herbivores) will respond in the same way to a diet suitable for the omnivorous, human animal. Furthermore, animal models of disease (such as cancer and cardiovascular disease), although similar, are different from the human disease. So, these factors must be considered when interpreting results from this type of research. Nevertheless, animal studies have been, and continue to be, important for nutrition research.

1.4.1.2 The problem with 'chow'

As mentioned, an advantage of animal studies is that food intake can be controlled. However, the food supplied in animal studies (often referred to as 'chow') is typically controlled for its macronutrient content but is generally of poor overall quality when compared to even a poor human diet.

1.5 Human Intervention Studies and Clinical Trials

There are a variety of human intervention study designs in nutrition research, but the most common, especially in pharmaceutical, medical and nutritional research, is the clinical trial. A clinical trial is a scientifically controlled study using consenting volunteers to find the safety and effectiveness of different treatments or regimens. Clinical trials are the "gold standard" research method. Their findings carry the most weight when making decisions about a certain research area because they are the most rigorous scientific studies. Every pharmaceutical must go through a series of clinical trials (specifically randomised, single-, double- or even triple-blind, placebo-controlled experiments) before being approved for market by the US FDA and similar organisations around the world.

As shown in the figure below, human intervention studies/clinical trials are normally prospective. By the end of this section, you should understand what randomised, double-blind, and placebo-controlled means.

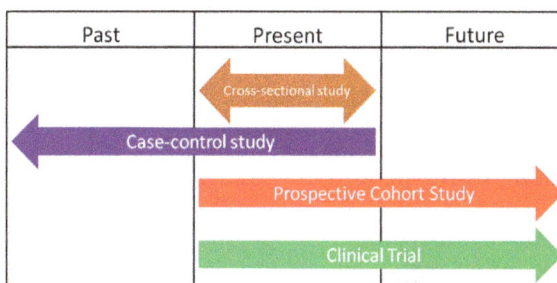

Figure 8. Clinical trials are prospective

1.5.1 Placebo and the Placebo Effect

A placebo is an inactive treatment that serves as a comparison to an active treatment. The use of a placebo is necessary in medical research because of a phenomenon known as the "placebo effect". The placebo effect results from a subject's belief in a treatment, even though there is no treatment being administered. An example would be an athlete who consumes a sports drink and runs the a 100-meter sprint in 11.00 seconds. The athlete then, under the exact same conditions, drinks what she is told is 'Super Duper Sports Drink' and runs the 100-meter sprint in 10.50 seconds. But what the athlete didn't know was that Super-Duper Sports Drink was just the Sports Drink with food colouring added. There was nothing different between the drinks, but the athlete believed that the 'Super Duper Sports Drink' was going to help her run faster, so she did. This improvement is the placebo effect.

1.5.2   The Nocebo Effect

A similar phenomenon can be observed when an inert (i.e. no active ingredient) compound promotes negative side-effects. In this case there is no physiological reason why the inert substance results in adverse effects, but like the placebo effect it is a psychogenic phenomenon resulting from the belief that there 'will' be negative effects.

1.5.3   Active placebo effect

In the active placebo effect phenomenon, an active drug or compound which elicits some negative side effects has a positive effect that is either greater than expected or provides beneficial effects for an outcome that is at odds with its physiological mechanism of action. This is believed to be due to the belief that results from the negative effects themselves. For example, you take a medication for depression and begin to experience nausea and headaches. You believe that 'it must be working' because you are experiencing side effects, and thus, a placebo effect is initiated. So, in this case, you have a nocebo + placebo effect occurring within an active treatment!

1.5.4   Randomisation

Randomisation is the process of randomly assigning participants to experimental groups to decrease bias. Bias can occur in assigning participants to these groups in a way that will influence the results. An example of bias in a study of an antidepressant drug is shown below. In this nonrandomized antidepressant drug example, researchers (who know what the participants are receiving) put depressed participants into the placebo group, while "less depressed" participants are put into the antidepressant drug group. As a result, even if the drug isn't effective, the group assignment may make the drug appear effective, thus biasing the results. This is a bit of an extreme example, but even if the researchers are trying to prevent bias, sometimes bias can still occur. However, if the participants are randomised, the sick and the healthy people will ideally be equally distributed between the groups. Thus, the trial will be unbiased and a true test of whether the drug is effective.

1.5.5 Blinding

Blinding is a technique to prevent bias in human intervention studies. A study without blinding is referred to as 'open label' because both the subject and the researchers know what treatment the subject is receiving (i.e. placebo or drug). This can lead to bias, so these types of trials are used less frequently.

In a single-blind study, the researcher knows what treatment the subject is receiving, but the subject does not. If the participants are randomised, these types of trials should produce robust results, but it is still possible that the researcher can bias the results.

Blinding can also occur at certain time-points within a research study. For example, in many nutrition trials the researcher (and participants) might know the dietary allocation being studied because it is often impossible to blind people to a 'diet', but the researcher is blinded to the group allocations during the

analysis of results to reduce the chance of bias.

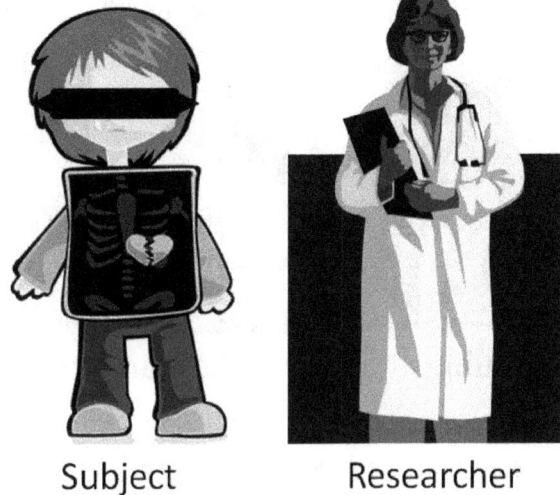

Subject   Researcher

Figure 9. In a single-blind study the researcher knows what treatment the subject is receiving, but the subject does not

Finally, there is the double-blind study, where neither the researcher nor the subject knows what treatment the subject is receiving. A separate board reviews the collected results and decides the fate of the trial. This is the 'gold-standard' because it prevents observer bias from occurring.

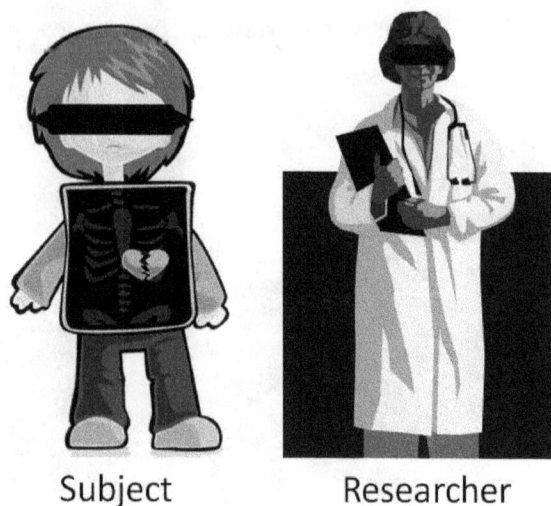

Subject   Researcher

Figure 10. In a double-blind study, neither the subject nor the researcher knows what treatment the subject is receiving

1.6 Statistics in Nutrition Research

To be able to interpret research one must have a basic understanding of statistical significance. Statistical significance means that there is sufficient statistical evidence to suggest that the results are most likely *not* due to chance.

In most statistical research, significance is represented by *p*-values. The *p*-value is an estimate of whether the difference is a statistical accident or due to random chance. A *p*-value of less than 0.05 (commonly written *p*-value <0.05 or $p < 0.05$) is used in most cases to indicate 'statistical significance'. This value means that 5% of the time the statistical results are likely to be accidental or not true. It is a convention that researchers accept this level of uncertainty.

Epidemiological researchers often use different statistics to analyse the results. Epidemiological results are commonly reported as odds ratios (ORs), relative risks (RRs), or hazard ratios (HRs). These values can be interpreted similarly regardless of which is used. For example, the odds ratio represents the odds of a certain event occurring (often a disease) in response to a certain exposure (in nutrition this is often a food or dietary compound). In a paper, it is common to see one of these measures in this form: OR = 2.0.

1.6.1.1 What do odds and hazards ratios mean?

As shown in figure 1.51, an OR, RR, or HR of 1 means that exposure is associated with neither increased nor decreased risk (in other words the effect is neutral). If an OR, RR or HR is less than 1, that exposure is associated with a decreased risk. If an OR, RR, or HR is greater than 1, that exposure is associated with an increased risk. An OR, RR, or HR of 2 means there is twice the risk, while an OR, RR, or HR of 0.5 means there is half the risk of the exposure versus the comparison group.

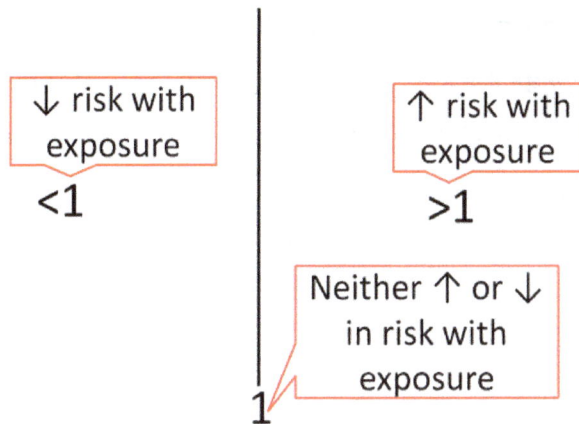

Figure 11. Risk in relation to exposure for OR, RR, or HR

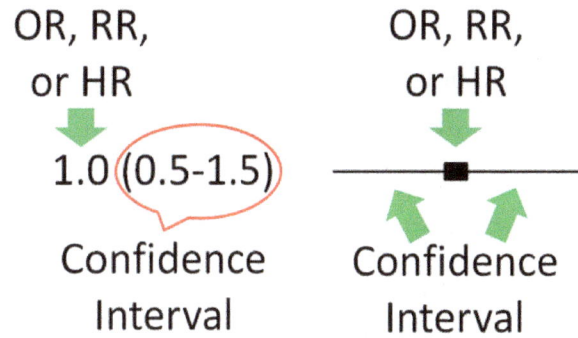

Figure 12. Confidence Intervals for OR, RR, or HRs in text form (left) and figure form (right)

To determine whether OR, RR, and HR are significantly different for a given exposure, most epidemiological research uses 95% confidence intervals. Confidence intervals indicate the estimated range that the measure is calculated to include. They go below and above the OR, RR, and HR itself. It is a calculation of how confident the researchers are that the OR, RR, and HR value is correct. Thus:

Large Confidence Intervals = Less Confidence in Value

Small Confidence Intervals = More Confidence in Value

Thus, 95% confidence intervals indicate that researchers are 95% confident that the true value is within the confidence intervals. A confidence interval is normally written in parenthesis or brackets following the OR, RR, or HR or represented as bars in a figure as shown below.

If the 95% confidence intervals of the OR, RR, or HR does not include or overlap 1, then the value is significant. If the 95% confidence intervals include or overlap 1, then the OR, RR, or HR is non-significant.

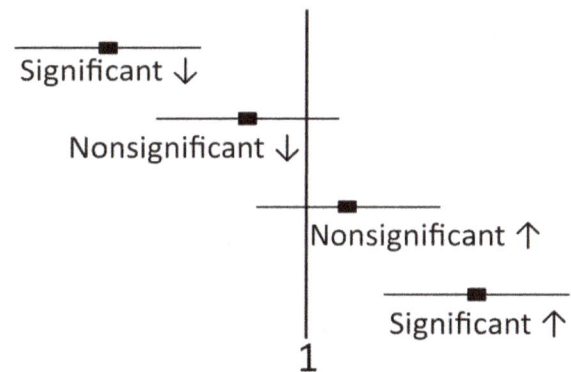

Figure 13. Confidence intervals (95%) that include 1 indicate that the value is not significantly different. Confidence intervals above or below 1 without including it indicate that the value is significantly different.

1.6.2 Clinical Significance

Compared with statistical significance, clinical significance is a more ambiguous concept. Whereas statistical significance tells us whether something is likely to be significant and *not due to chance*, clinical significance tells us whether something will have a meaningful relationship with a clinical outcome. A good example of this is the surrogate relationship between sodium, blood pressure and perceived cardiovascular risk. Reduction of dietary sodium intake has the *statistically significant* effect of reducing blood pressure. So, if one eats less salt they are almost certain to reduce blood pressure. However, this reduction is a very small one (approximately a 1-3.5% reduction[9]) that would not be considered clinically meaningful.

Statistical analysis techniques such as 'Magnitudes Based Inference' (MBI) analysis have been developed to try to better show the likely clinical effect of an intervention. Irrespective of the type of analysis used (and MBI has been heavily criticised) it is important for researchers to provide not just statistical significance but inferences as to the 'meaningfulness' of results in the real world.

1.7 Publishing Research

After nutrition researchers have completed the collection and analysis of data and written about their findings, the next step is to disseminate them, or let people know what they found. The primary method for dissemination is by publishing their results in scientific peer-reviewed journals The researchers put together a paper explaining their experiment and findings in a journal article. An article's primary components are normally an introduction, abstract, methods, results, and discussion/conclusion. They submit the paper to a chosen journal and the journal editor then selects expert researchers who will critically review the article. These reviewers make sure that research published in journals will be adding to the current subject literature, is of a robust nature, superior quality and of interest to readers. In more rigorous journals the article might also need to meet a certain theme of an issue that a journal wants to publish.

To give you an idea of how rigorous this process is, let's consider some major nutrition journals.

- Journal of Nutrition (JN)
- American Journal of Clinical Nutrition (AJCN)
- Journal of the Academy of Nutrition and Dietetics (formerly Journal of the American Dietetic Association)
- Nutrition and Metabolism
- Nutrition Reviews
- Annual Reviews of Nutrition
- British Journal of Nutrition

- European Journal of Clinical Nutrition

There are two major nutrition societies in the US: The American Society for Nutrition (ASN) (www.nutrition.org) and the Academy of Nutrition and Dietetics (AND, formerly the American Dietetic Association) (www.eatright.org).

ASN publishes the Journal of Nutrition and the American Journal of Clinical Nutrition, while AND publishes the Journal of the Academy of Nutrition and Dietetics.

The following table contains two measures, impact factor and acceptance rate for these journals. The impact factor is a measure of influence of the journal. This measure indicates how many people read the articles that are published in that journal. The acceptance rate is the percentage of articles that are submitted that are accepted for publication.

Table 1. Selected nutrition journals, impact factors, and acceptance rates

Journal	Impact Factor	Acceptance Rate
Annual Reviews of Nutrition	9.2	
American Journal of Clinical Nutrition	6.5	25%
Journal of Nutrition	4.2	25%
Nutrition Reviews	4.6	
Journal of the Academy of Nutrition and Dietetics	3.8	
British Journal of Nutrition	3.3	
European Journal of Clinical Nutrition	3.1	40%

The acceptance rate for three of these journals ranged from 25-40%. Thus, the majority of submitted articles are rejected and sent back to the researchers. To put nutrition journals in perspective, some of the top medical and science journals with a broad following have impact factors as high as 75 and an acceptance rate of 5-10%. Hopefully this helps you to understand that peer review is a rigorous process and a valuable one to preserve the integrity of research published in credible, reputable journals.

There are often extensive revisions to make (maybe even multiple times) before the paper can be published. Generally, the more difficult it is to get a paper accepted into a journal, the more solid the research must be. Thus, most of the information on the internet (which has not gone through peer review) should be explored with some caution. It might be useful information...but equally it could be BS! And it is extremely unlikely to have had the level of scrutiny of a peer-reviewed article.

1.8 Interpreting Research

A systematic literature review does what the name implies; it systematically reviews the literature related to a certain research question. For example, the research question might be, "Does dietary sodium increase blood pressure?" There is a method for performing the review established ahead of time that details answers to questions such as:

- How will journal articles be identified?
- Which databases will be searched?
- What search terms will be used?

The end-product is a conclusion based on the evidence in the identified journal articles.

Because they synthesize the findings from multiple trials, systematic literature reviews are considered the highest level of nutrition research evidence and are therefore shown at the top of the strength of nutrition research pyramid below. *In vitro* studies are shown at the bottom of the pyramid because they are the weakest form of evidence overall. Most systematic literature reviews only consider epidemiological studies and clinical trials and do not include animal studies or *in vitro* evidence. While these studies aren't as strong, they should still be considered.

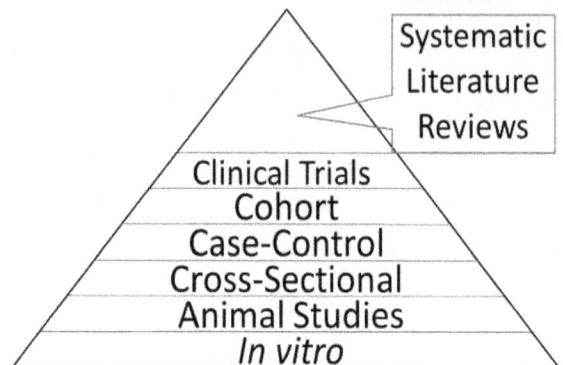

Figure 14. Strength of scientific research, a higher position on the pyramid mean greater strength of that form of evidence

There are a couple of other factors to consider relating to the different forms of research. First, epidemiological studies cannot show causality (i.e. smoking causes lung cancer), but instead identify relationships or associations (i.e. smoking is associated with lung cancer occurrence). Clinical trials/human studies are the best form of primary research because their findings should be directly translatable to patients. So why use other forms of research? The description below should help explain why the other forms of research are also important.

In general, a certain sequence of studies in nutrition research is often followed as shown in the figure below.

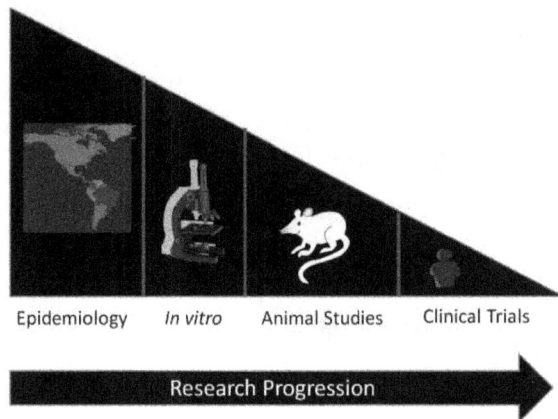

Figure 15. The progression of nutrition research.

Epidemiological nutrition studies find relationships between food/food components and (a) specific health outcome/s. This relationship is then investigated by *in vitro* studies and then, some of the most promising move to animal studies. Then the most promising and safe food/food components are moved into clinical trials/human studies. If it is an individual compound, there will be smaller trials designed to see if the compound is safe before it is moved into larger clinical trials to determine whether the food/food component results in beneficial health outcomes. The overall effect of this process is to select the most promising and safe food/food components for the clinical trials/human studies. This allows time and money to be used more efficiently, because while clinical trials/human studies are the best form of research, they are also normally the most expensive and time-consuming. Researchers nevertheless have been tempted to skip directly to clinical trials in the past rather than following the research progression. To illustrate what happens in these situations, the following describes a couple of examples when "normal" research progression hasn't been followed.

1.8.1 Beta-Carotene and Lung Cancer

In the early 1980s there was a lot of excitement among researchers over the epidemiological evidence showing that higher dietary consumption of the carotenoid, beta-carotene, decreased lung cancer risk.[10] By the mid 1980's, two large, randomized, placebo-controlled trials began to determine whether high-dose ß-carotene supplementation (far higher than dietary intake) could decrease lung cancer incidence in high-risk populations before *in vitro* or animal studies had investigated this relationship. The research community was shocked when these two studies were terminated early in the mid-1990s because of significant increases in lung cancer incidence among smokers receiving ß-carotene supplements. *In vitro* and animal studies completed after the clinical trial found that as ß-carotene intake shifts from normal dietary levels to high, supplement-type levels, the effect on lung cancer development also shifts from beneficial to detrimental in combination with smoke or carcinogen exposure.[11] Thus, if the normal research progression had been followed, it is likely that a lower dose of beta-carotene would have been used or trials wouldn't have been undertaken at all.

In addition to the lessons learned about the sequence of research in nutrition, these studies add to growing evidence that suggests that single-agent interventions, even in combination, may not be an effective strategy for improving health. The common nutrition research approach, after epidemiology finds an association or relationship, is to use *in vitro* and animal studies to identify the specific compound in a certain food that is responsible. This has been termed the reductionist approach because it takes something complex (food) and reduces it down to its simpler components. However, there is growing evidence that this may be a flawed approach. Some nutrition researchers feel that more focus should be on the food itself, rather than trying to discern exactly what is responsible for the beneficial health outcomes. Because it may not be one or two compounds alone that are responsible for the effect, it might be difficult to determine from the multitude of nutrients in foods which are responsible for the beneficial effect. This will mean changes in the overall research approach, especially at the human intervention studies/clinical trials level, because in most cases there is not a way to give a placebo food.

1.8.2 Traditional Use, Traditional Medicine and Case Histories

Another type of evidence for nutritional, supplemental, and especially herbal medicine interventions is the case evidence provided by the long history of foods, supplements (such as mineral salts) and herbs being used for both culinary purposes and as medicine. For example, in the traditions of Ayurvedic medicine and Traditional Chinese Medicine (TCM) we have consistent and long-term use of many medicinal herbs. This can give researchers a 'head-start' for formulating hypotheses to test in clinical trials. The uses of herbs and other medicines in traditional systems also gives clinicians an additional layer of evidence for the use of interventions for conditions. The widespread use of many herbs in cooking also provides an additional layer of safety data too. We would expect for example, that due to the common use of herbs such as rosemary, thyme, basil and oregano, that in the amounts suggested for cooking, they are safe. Finally, long term use of dietary types (such as lower-carbohydrate diets) by certain population groups, without concomitant disorders associated with diet, also provides additional evidence for the safety of these diet types.

1.8.3   Calories (Food Energy)

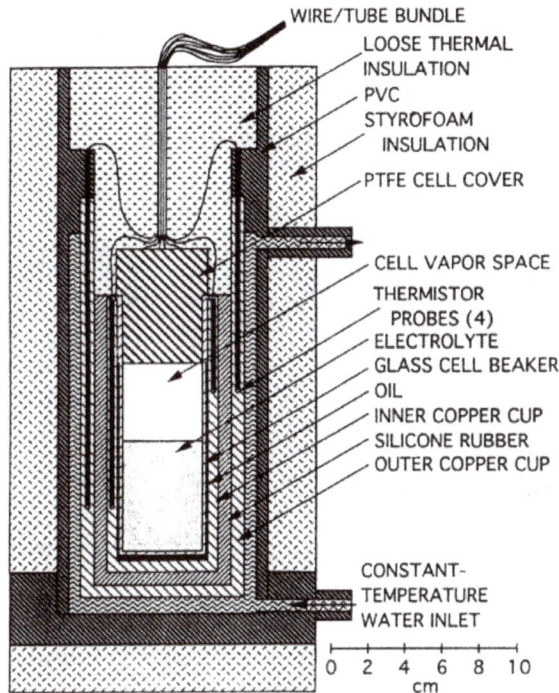

Figure 16. Diagram of a bomb calorimeter[ii]

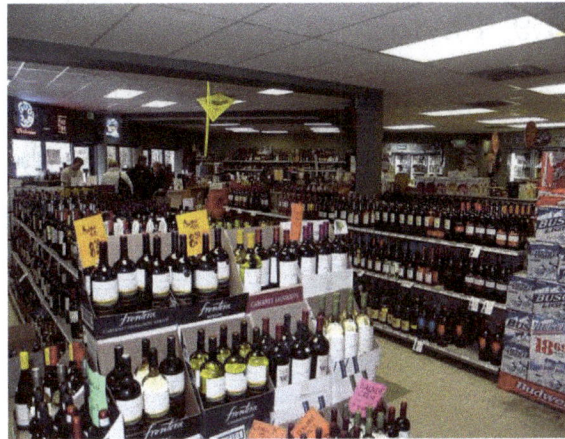

Figure 17. Alcoholic beverages can be a significant source of calories[iii]

As can be seen, only carbohydrates, protein, and lipids provide energy directly, although vitamins and minerals allow for co-factors that enable the release of (usable) energy. Alcohol is also another source of energy in the diet. It is not technically a nutrient, but it does provide a considerable number of calories.

The following table lists the energy sources in the diet from lowest calories per gram to the highest calories per gram. Note that we have listed protein first because although it has the same number of calories as carbohydrates, there is a greater thermic effect elicited by protein, meaning that it has less calorific effects (especially with respect to gaining excess fat). Knowing these numbers allows you to estimate the amount of calories food contains, assuming you know the grams of the different macronutrients.

Energy Sources (kcal/g)

- Protein (4)
- Carbohydrates (4)
- Alcohol (7)
- Lipids (9)

ii Shkedi Z. Heat Loss Calorimeter. In: Heat-loss_calorimeter.gif, editor. http://commons.wikimedia.org/wiki/File:Heat-loss_calorimeter.gif: Own work; 2008.

iii 24.   Shankbone D. Liquor store in Breckenridge Colorado. In: Liquor_store_in_Breckenridge_Colorado.jpg, editor. http://commons.wikimedia.org/wiki/File:Liquor_store_in_Breckenridge_Colorado.jpg: Own work; 2009.

1.9 Phytochemicals, Zoochemicals & Functional Foods

1.9.1 Phytochemicals

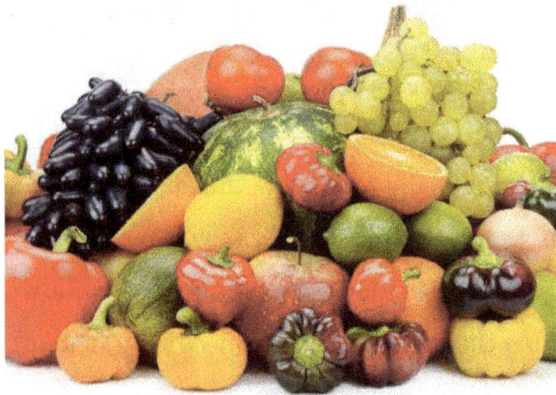

Figure 18. Vegetables, fruits and berries contain phytochemicals that play a role in nutrition

Phytochemicals (phyto = plant) are compounds in plants that are believed to provide health benefits beyond that provided by the essential nutrients. An example is lycopene in tomatoes, which is thought to decrease the risk of prostate cancer. Diets rich in fruits and vegetables have been associated with decreased risk of chronic diseases. For example Pooled data from 12 studies (n=200,000+) show that increased consumption of fruit and vegetables from less than three to more than five servings/day is related to a 17%

reduction in CHD risk [12] others show a 4% reduction in risk per serve of vegetable or fruit added per day.[13] Many fruits and vegetables are rich in phytochemicals, leading some to hypothesize that phytochemicals are responsible for the decreased risk of chronic diseases. The role that phytochemicals play in health is still not fully understood relative to other areas of nutrition such as the macro- and micronutrients.

1.9.2 Zoochemicals

In biology and the medical sciences (including nutrition) the prefix 'zoo' simply means 'animal'. This should be easy to remember because animals can be found at the zoo. So, zoochemicals are other chemicals from animal foods that may influence health. They are the animal equivalent of phytochemicals in plants. Some compounds can be both phytochemicals and zoochemicals. An example of compounds that can be classified as both are the yellow carotenoids lutein and zeaxanthin. Kale, spinach, and corn (phytochemicals) are useful sources of lutein and zeaxanthin. However, egg yolks are also a good source of these carotenoids (zoochemicals).

1.9.3   Functional Foods

Functional foods are generally understood to be a food, or a food ingredient, that may provide a health benefit beyond the traditional nutrients (macro- and micronutrients) it contains. Functional foods often contain phytochemicals or zoochemicals or contain more of a traditional nutrient or nutrients than a normal food.

2 The Macronutrients

The macronutrients are the 'big' (macro) nutrients. In other words, they are required in multiple gram quantities and perhaps more importantly, the 'energy-yielding' macronutrients are the parts of the diet that provide fuel for us to function, along with important structural building-blocks of tissue.

2.1 Carbohydrates

In recent years the amount of carbohydrate required for health and performance in humans has become incredibly controversial. While some swear that carbohydrates should make up most of our energy intake, others suggest that we need very little. Therefore, it is important to understand the roles and functions of carbohydrates (or any other macro- or micronutrient) and the role that biochemical individuality plays.

Carbohydrates are named as such because they are hydrated (as in water, H_2O) carbon. Below is the formula showing how carbon dioxide (CO_2) and water (H_2O) are used to make carbohydrates $(CH_2O)_n$ and oxygen (O_2). The "n" after the carbohydrate in the formula indicates that the chemical formula is repeated an unknown number of times, but that for every carbon and oxygen, there will always be two hydrogens.

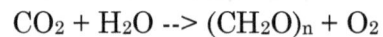

$$CO_2 + H_2O \rightarrow (CH_2O)_n + O_2$$

Carbohydrates are produced by plants through a process known as photosynthesis. In this process, plants use the energy from photons of light to synthesize carbohydrates. The formula for this reaction looks like this:

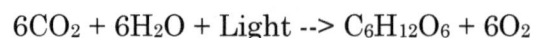

$$6CO_2 + 6H_2O + Light \rightarrow C_6H_{12}O_6 + 6O_2$$

There are many types of carbohydrates as shown in the figure below. The primary classification method is by the number of sugar units the carbohydrate contains. The unit classification uses three terms 'simple, complex, and sugar alcohols' to define carbohydrates structure, Complex carbohydrates contain more sugar units, while simple carbohydrates contain either one or two sugars. In the next sections, you will learn more about the different forms of carbohydrates.

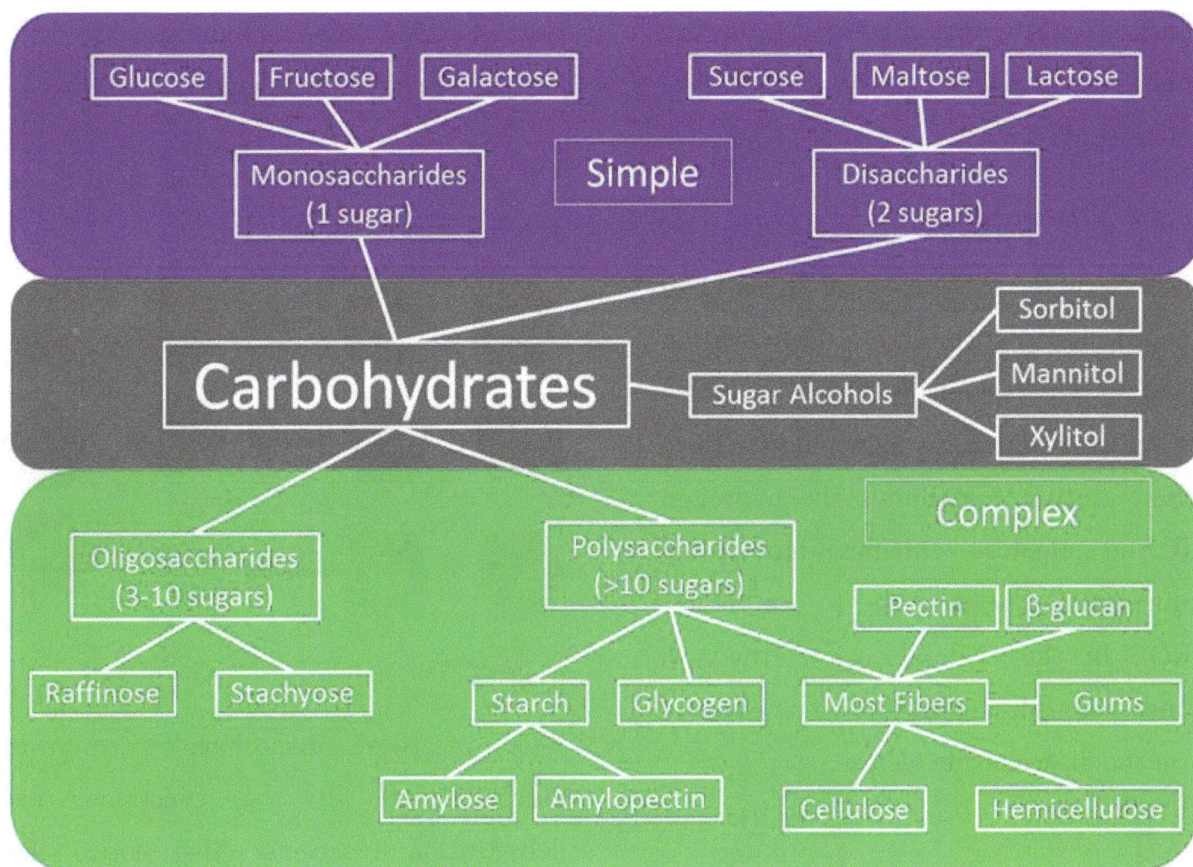

Figure 19. The different forms of carbohydrates

2.1.1 Simple Carbohydrates

As shown in the figure X, simple carbohydrates can be further divided into monosaccharides and disaccharides. Mono- means one, thus monosaccharides contain one sugar. Di- means two, thus disaccharides contain two sugar units.

2.1.1.1 Monosaccharides

The three monosaccharides are: glucose, fructose and galactose. Notice that all are 6-carbon sugars (hexoses). However, fructose has a five-member ring, while glucose and galactose have six-member rings. Also notice that the only structural difference between glucose and galactose is the position of the alcohol (OH) group.

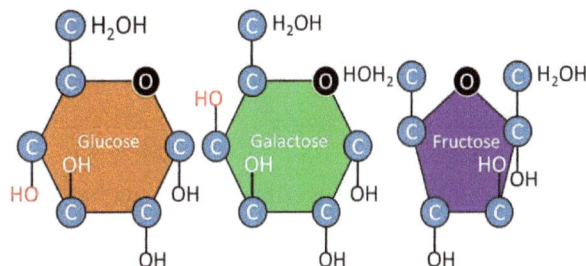

Figure 20. The monosaccharides

Glucose – Product of photosynthesis, major source of energy in our bodies

Fructose – Commonly found in fruits and used commercially in many beverages

23

Galactose – Not normally found in nature alone, normally found in the disaccharide lactose (milk sugar)

2.1.1.2 Disaccharides

Disaccharides are produced from two monosaccharides through a dehydration reaction. This means water is produced during the reaction. As shown in the figure below, glucose contributes the hydrogen (H), and galactose contributes an alcohol group (OH). Together these form water (H_2O). In the example below, the two monosaccharides galactose and glucose form the disaccharide lactose.

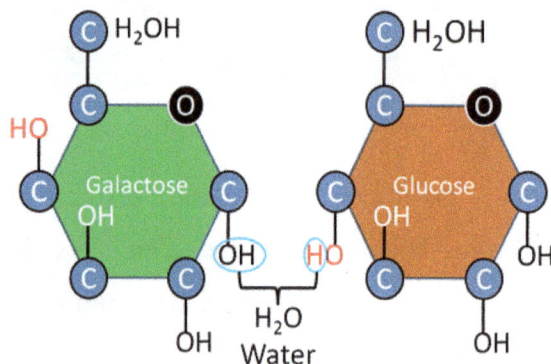

Figure 21. Dehydration reaction between galactose and glucose to form lactose

The commonly occurring disaccharides are:

Maltose (glucose + glucose, aka malt sugar) – seldom found in foods, present in alcoholic beverages and barley

Sucrose (glucose + fructose, aka table sugar) – only made by plants

Lactose (galactose + glucose, aka milk sugar) – primary milk sugar

The formation of each disaccharide is shown below:

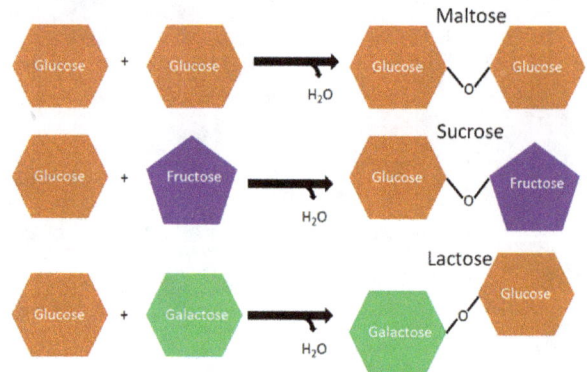

Figure 22. The formation of disaccharides

Each of these disaccharides contains glucose and all the reactions are dehydration reactions. Also notice the difference in the bond structures. Maltose and sucrose have alpha-bonds, which are depicted as v-shaped above. You might hear the term glycosidic used in some places to describe bonds between sugars. A glycoside is a sugar, so glycosidic is referring to a sugar bond. Lactose, on the other hand, contains a beta-bond. We need a special enzyme, lactase, to break this bond, and this leads to a problem of lactose intolerance.

2.1.1.3 High-Fructose Corn Syrup

Food manufacturers seeking to find a cheaper replacement for sugar from cane or sugar beets were able to begin using a (mainly) corn derived sugar-like compound called High-Fructose Corn Syrup (HFCS) due to the economies provided by the US Governments support of corn manufacturing for food security. High-fructose corn syrup contains around 42-55% fructose, which is similar to sucrose.[14] Nevertheless, because an increase in high-fructose corn syrup consumption (see figure below) has coincided with the increase in obesity in the U.S., there is a lot of controversy surrounding its use.

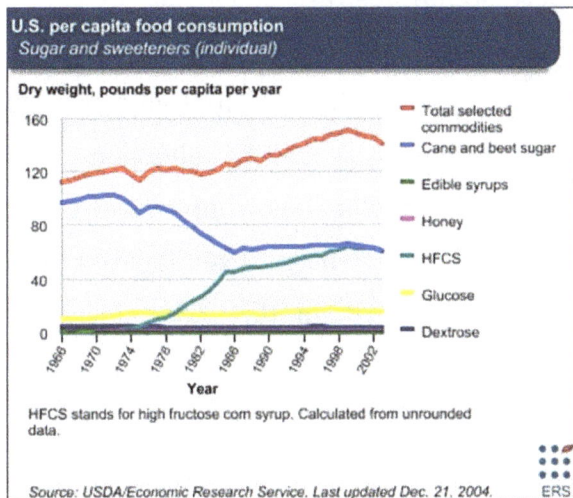

Figure 23. US per capita sugar and sweetener consumption

Opponents of high-fructose corn syrup claim that it is contributing to the rise in obesity rates. As a result, some manufactures have started releasing products made with natural sugars as alternatives, although these are often just as high in fructose (or higher in the case of some 'natural' alternatives such as Agave syrup) than HFCS.

Some manufacturers have also rebranded high-fructose corn syrup as 'corn sugar' to get around the negative perception associated with the name. But the United States FDA has rejected the Corn Refiners Association request to change the name officially to corn sugar.

2.2 Alternative Sweeteners

Alternative sweeteners are simply alternatives to sucrose and other mono- and disaccharides that provide sweetness. The first subsection will first describe the sugar alcohols (aka sugar replacers) and then the next subsection will describe other commonly used alternative sweeteners.

2.3 Oligosaccharides

Within complex carbohydrates, there are oligosaccharides and polysaccharides. Oligosaccharides (oligo means few) are composed of 3-10 sugar units and polysaccharides contain greater than 10 sugar units [15]

Raffinose and stachyose are the most common oligosaccharides. They are found in legumes, onions, broccoli, cabbage, and whole wheat.[16] The table below shows the raffinose and stachyose content of some plant foods.

Table 2. Raffinose and stachyose content of selected foods

Food	Raffinose content	Stachyose Content
Soy beans (raw)	0.7	3.2
Chickpeas (raw)	0.7	2.4
Onions (raw)	1.4	0.7
Broccoli (raw)	0.1	0.2
Cabbage (raw)	0.1	0.1
Adzuki beans (raw)	0.2	3.9
Whole wheat flour	0.2	/
Cottonseed flour (defatted)	9.2	0.8

The structures of the two oligosaccharides are shown below.

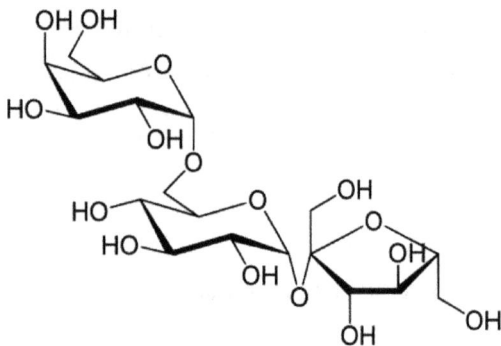

Figure 24. Structure of raffinose

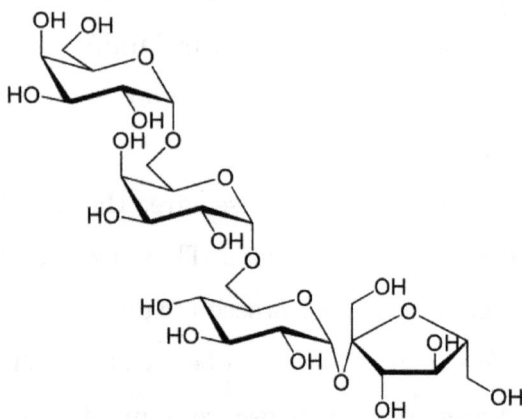

Figure 25. Structure of stachyose

Our digestive system lacks the enzymes necessary to digest these alpha 1-6 glycosidic bonds found in oligosaccharides. As a result, the oligosaccharides are not digested and reach the colon where they are fermented by the bacteria there. Gas is produced as a by-product of this bacteria fermentation that can lead to flatulence.

2.4 Polysaccharides

Poly means "many" and thus polysaccharides are made up of many monosaccharides (>10 monosaccharides). There are 3 main classes of polysaccharides: starch, glycogen, and most fibres. The following sections will describe the structural similarities and differences between the three classes of polysaccharides.

2.5 Sugar Alcohols (Sugar Replacers)

Sugar(s) can provide a lot of calories and contribute to tooth decay. Thus, there are many other compounds that are used as alternatives to sugar that have been developed or discovered. We will first talk about sugar alcohols and then the alternative sweeteners.

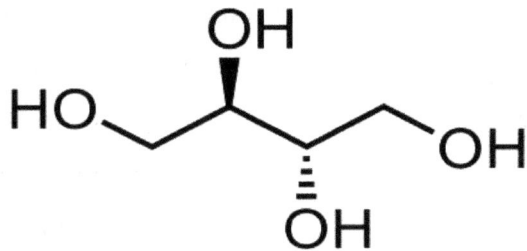

Figure 26. Erythritol, an example of a commonly used sugar alcohol

Remember that alcohol subgroups are (OH), and you can see many of them in these structures.

Sugar alcohols are also known as "sugar replacers", because some in the public might get confused by the name sugar alcohol. Some might think a sugar alcohol is a sweet alcoholic beverage. Another name for them is nutritive sweeteners, which indicates that they do provide calories. Sugar alcohols are nearly as sweet as sucrose but only provide approximately half the calories as shown below.

Table 3. Relative sweetness of various sweeteners[17, 18]

Sweetener	Relative Sweetness	Energy (kcal/g)
Lactose	0.2	4.0*
Maltose	0.4	4.0
Glucose	0.7	4.0
Sucrose	1.0	4.0
Fructose	1.2-1.8	4.0
Erythritol	0.7	0.4
Isomalt	0.5	2.0
Lactitol	0.4	2.0

Differs based on an individual's lactase activity

Sugars are fermented by bacteria on the surfaces of teeth. This results in a decreased pH (higher acidity) that leads to tooth decay and, potentially, cavity formation. The major advantage of sugar alcohols over sugars is that sugar alcohols are not fermented by bacteria on the tooth surface. Certain sugar alcohols such as xylitol have even been shown to inhibit cavities and reduce bacteria and bacterial biofilms associated with cavity formation.

2.5.1 Sugar Alcohols and the Human Gut Microbiome

There is a relative paucity of evidence on the effects of sugar alcohols on the microbiome, however, a 2012 review published in *Obesity Reviews* summarises available research suggesting that sorbitol may be metabolised by E. coli, Salmonella and Shigella, mannitol by lactobacillus and Streptococcus and that Xylitol is generally unfavourable for metabolism by gut bacteria.[19]

2.6 Other Alternative Sweeteners

Other alternative sweeteners have been developed to provide zero-calorie or low-calorie sweetening for foods and drinks. The sweeteners that are approved by the FDA in the United States are saccharin, aspartame, neotame, acesulfame potassium (K), sucralose, tagatose.[18] Other natural low- or non-calorific sweeteners such as stevia and thaumatin are also in common use. In late 2008 the FDA first decided that it would allow the use of "highly purified stevia preparations in food products,"[2] essentially allowing the natural sweetener to begin to be used. Thaumatin conversely is not yet recognised as a sweetener and is labelled as a flavour or flavour modifier (due to its masking effect on some flavour profiles.) Because many of these provide little to no calories, these sweeteners are also referred to as non-nutritive sweeteners. Aside from tagatose, all the sweeteners on the list below meet these criteria. Aspartame does provide calories, but because it is far sweeter than sugar, the small amount used does not contribute any meaningful calories to a person's diet. Until the FDA allowed the use of stevia, this collection of sweeteners was known as artificial sweeteners because they were synthetically or artificially produced. However, with stevia, the descriptor artificial can no longer be used to describe these sweeteners. The table below summarizes the characteristics of some common alternative sweeteners.

Table 4. Alternative sweeteners

Scientific Name	Trade Name	kcal/g	Approximate Relative Sweetness[a]	Heat-Stable
Saccharin	Sweet & Low, Sweet Twin, Sweet 'N Low Brown, Necta Sweet	0	200-700	
Aspartame	Nutrasweet, Equal, Sugar Twin	4	160-220	
Neotame		0	8000	X
Acesulfame-K	Sunett, Sweet & Safe, Sweet One	0	200	X
Sucralose	Splenda	0	600	X
Tagatose	Nutralose	1.5	0.75-0.92	X
Stevia	Truvia, PureVia, SweetLeaf	0	150-300	X
Thaumatin	Thaumatin	4	500-2000	X

[a] Relative to Sucrose =1

Aspartame is perhaps the most common sweetener currently in use. It is made up of two amino acids (phenylalanine and aspartate) and a methyl (CH_3) group. The compound is broken down during digestion into the individual amino acids. This is why it provides 4 kcal/g, just like protein.[15] Because it can be broken down to phenylalanine, products that contain aspartame contain the following message; "Phenylketonurics—contains phenylalanine." Phenylketonuria (PKU) will be covered in greater detail in section 2.25. When heated, aspartame breaks down and thus loses its sweet flavor.[18]

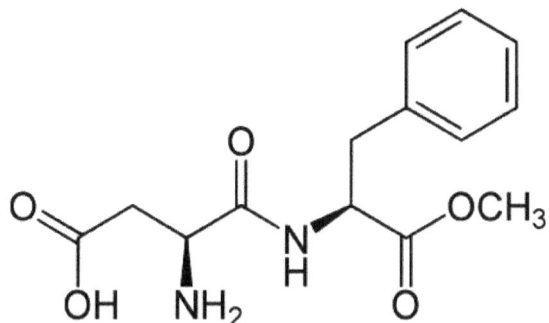

Figure 27. Structure of aspartame

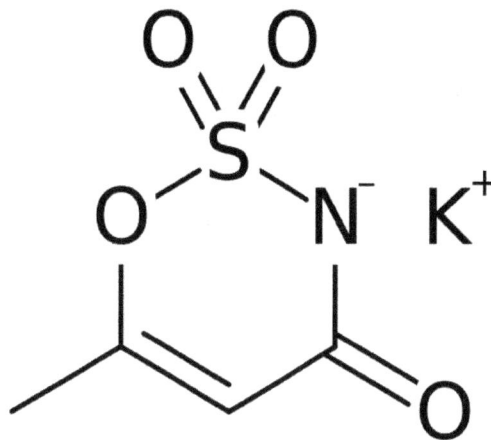

Figure 28. Structure of acesulfame potassium[iv]

Neotame is an updated version of aspartame. Neotame is structurally identical to aspartame except that it contains an additional side group (bottom of figure below, which is flipped backwards to make it easier to compare their structures). While this looks like a minor difference, it has profound effects on the properties of neotame. Neotame is much sweeter than aspartame, is heat-stable, and is not broken down into the individual amino acids during digestion. As a result, it is not considered a concern for those with PKU.[15, 18]

Acesulfame-potassium (K) is not digested or absorbed, therefore it provides no energy or potassium to the body.[18]

Sucralose is structurally identical to sucrose except that three of the alcohol groups (OH) are replaced by chlorine molecules (Cl). This small change causes sucralose to not be digested and as such is excreted in faeces.[15, 18]

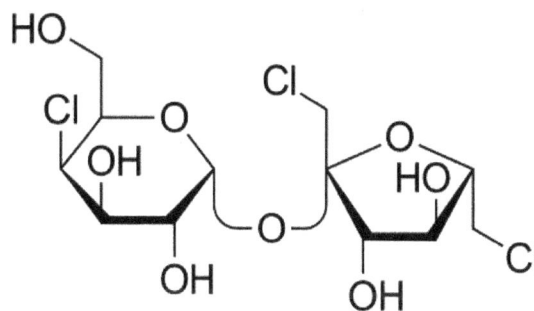

Figure 29. Structure of sucralose

Tagatose is an isomer of fructose that provides a small amount of energy (1.5 kcal/g). 80% of tagatose reaches the large intestine, where it is fermented by bacteria, meaning it has a prebiotic-type effect.[18] Notice the similarity in structure of tagatose to sugar alcohols, the only difference being a ketone (=O) instead of an alcohol (OH) group.

Stevia is derived from a South American shrub, with the leaves being the sweet part. The components responsible for this sweet taste are a group of compounds known as steviol glycosides. The structure of steviol is shown below.

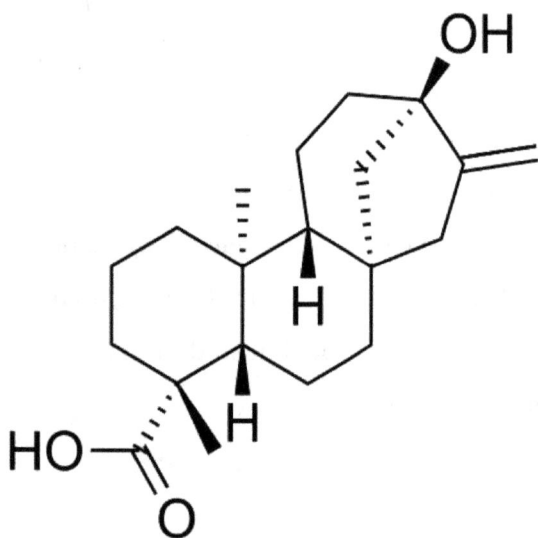

Figure 30. Structure of steviol

The term glycoside means that there are sugar molecules bonded to steviol. The two predominant steviol glycosides are stevioside and rebaudioside A. The structure of these two steviol glycosides are very similar. The structure of stevioside is shown below as an example.

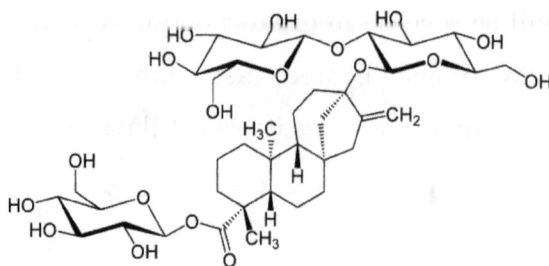

Figure 31. Structure of stevioside

Stevia in whole or extract form and sweeteners containing primarily rebaudioside A (known as 'rebiana'[13]) are becoming increasingly common "natural" sweeteners.

Thaumatin is a protein that functions as a low-calorie sweetener and flavour modifier. The protein is often used primarily for its flavour-modifying properties and not exclusively as a sweetener.

The thaumatins were first found as a mixture of proteins isolated from the katemfe fruit (Thaumatococcus daniellii Bennett) of West Africa. Some proteins in the thaumatin family of sweeteners are roughly 2000 times more potent than sugar. Although very sweet, thaumatin's taste is markedly different from sugar. The sweetness of thaumatin builds gradually and in high concentrations leaves a liquorice-like after-taste. It is highly heat- and acid-stable and water soluble.

2.6.1 The Effects of Alternative Sweeteners on Human Health

The effects of non-nutritive sweeteners on human health is poorly understood. While once thought of as a viable alternative to sugar for preventing obesity and cardio-metabolic challenges arising from excessive sugar and calories, the picture is not now so clear.

The current consensus at this stage appears to be that the non-nutritive sweeteners are generally considered safe and that they may help with reduction of calories, reduction of sugar and aid weight-loss, but there are significant question marks with respect to some studies showing adverse effects on glucose status, satiety and there may be further challenges as we begin to discover more about the role of these sweeteners on the human microbiome. A 2012 review by Raben and Richelsen concluded that despite some short-term studies indicating divergent results with respect to appetite regulation, overall artificial sweeteners cannot be claimed to affect hunger, and that artificial sweeteners may positively affect bodyweight, liver fat levels, fasting and post-prandial glycaemia, insulinaemia and lipidaemia when compared to sugar[20]. A more recent review in the Journal *Nutrition* cautions that "The clinical and epidemiologic data available at present are insufficient to make definitive conclusions regarding the benefits of NNS in displacing caloric sweeteners as related to energy balance, maintenance or decrease in body weight, and other cardiometabolic risk factors."[21]

It has been demonstrated that artificial sweeteners saccharin, acesulfame-K and aspartame are metabolised by various bacteria in the gut and the steviosides from the natural sweetener stevia are metabolised by Bacteroides[19] the effect of non-nutritive sweeteners on the human microbiome and health or performance is at this stage still unclear.

2.6.2 Starch

Starch is the storage form of glucose in plants. There are two forms of starch: amylose and amylopectin. Structurally they differ in that amylose is a linear polysaccharide, whereas amylopectin is branched. The linear portion of both amylose and amylopectin contains alpha 1-4 glycosidic bonds, while the branches of amylopectin are made up of alpha 1-6 glycosidic bonds.

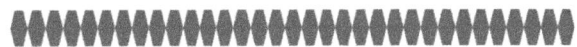

Figure 32. Structure of amylose

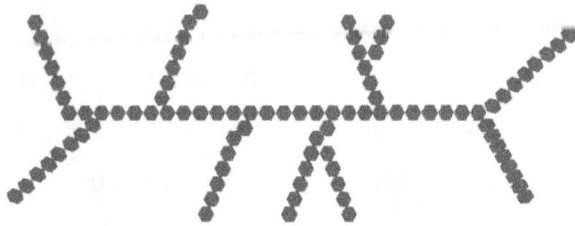

Figure 33. Structure of amylopectin

Amylopectin is more common than amylose (4:1 ratio on average) in starch.[15, 22] Starchy foods include grains, tubers and legumes.

Table 5. Amylose and amylopectin content of foods

High amylose and amylopectin foods

Source	Amylopectin %	Amylose %
Potato	79	21
Maize	72	28
Wheat	74	26
Tapioca	83	17
Waxy Maize	100	-

2.6.2.1 Glycogen

Glycogen is like starch in that it is a storage form of glucose. Glycogen, however, is the carbohydrate storage form in animals, rather than plants. It is even more highly branched than amylopectin, as shown below.

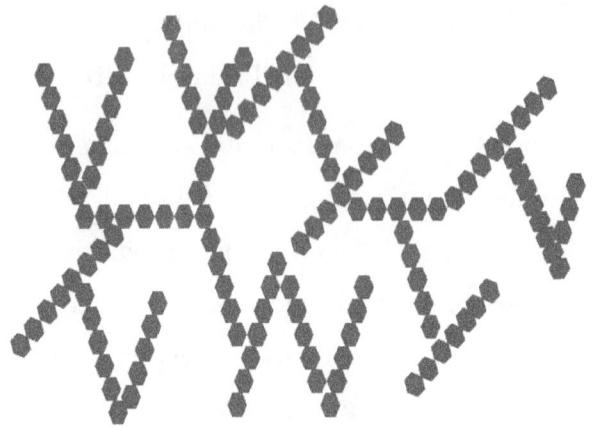

Figure 34. Structure of glycogen

Like amylopectin, the branch points of glycogen are alpha 1-6 glycosidic bonds, while the linear bonds are alpha 1-4 bonds, as shown below.

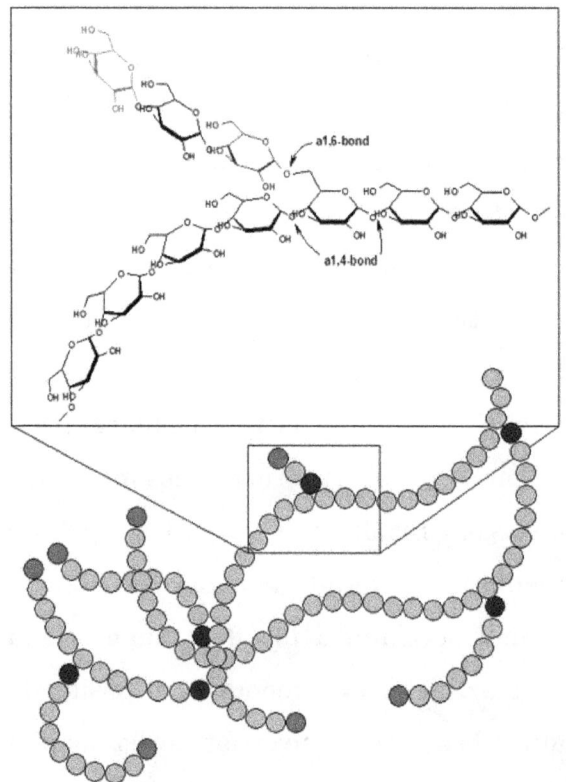

Figure 35. Additional structure of glycogen

The advantage of glycogen's highly branched structure is that the multiple ends (shown in red above) are where enzymes start to cleave off glucose molecules. As a result, with many ends available, it can provide glucose much more quickly to the body than it could if it was a linear molecule like amylose with only two ends. We consume almost no glycogen, because it is rapidly broken down by enzymes in animals after slaughter[18] and further degraded by cooking.[23]

2.6.3 Fibre

The simplest definition of fibre is indigestible matter. Indigestible means that it survives digestion in the small intestine and reaches the large intestine. There are three major fibre classifications[24]:

- Dietary fibre — non-digestible carbohydrates and lignin that are intrinsic and intact in plants
- Functional fibre — isolated, non-digestible carbohydrates that have beneficial physiological effects in humans
- Total fibre — dietary fibre + functional fibre

The differences between dietary and functional fibre are compared in the table below:

Table 6. Differences in fibre types

Dietary Fibre	Functional Fibre
Intact in plants	Isolated, extracted, or synthesized
Carbohydrates + lignans	Only carbohydrates
Only from plants	From plants or animals
No proven benefit	Must prove benefit

Dietary fibre is always intact in plants, whereas functional fibre can be isolated, extracted or synthesized. Functional fibre is only carbohydrates, while dietary fibre also includes lignans. Functional fibre can be from plants or animals, while dietary fibre is only from plants. Functional fibre must be proven to have a physiological benefit, while dietary fibre does not. Polysaccharide fibre differs from other polysaccharides in that it contains beta-glycosidic bonds (as opposed to alpha-glycosidic bonds). To illustrate these differences, consider the structural differences between amylose and cellulose (type of fibre). Both are linear chains of glucose, the only difference is that amylose has alpha-glycosidic bonds, while cellulose has beta-glycosidic bonds as shown below.

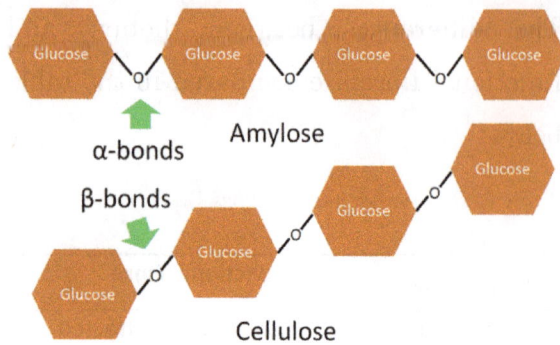

Figure 36. Structure of amylose vs cellulose

The beta-bonds in fibre cannot be broken down by the digestive enzymes in the small intestine so they continue into the large intestine.

Fibre can be classified by its physical properties. In the past, fibres were commonly referred to as soluble and insoluble. This classification distinguished whether the fibre was soluble in water. However, this classification is being phased out in the nutrition community. Instead most fibres that would have been classified as insoluble fibre are now referred to as non-fermentable and/or non-viscous and soluble fibre as fermentable, and/or viscous because these better describe the fibre's characteristics.[25] Fermentable refers to whether the bacteria in the colon can ferment or degrade the fibre into short chain fatty acids and gas. Viscous refers to the capacity of certain fibres to form a thick gel-like consistency. The following table lists some of the common types of fibre and provides a brief description about each.

Table 7. Description of celluloses and lignin

Fibre	Description
Cellulose	Main component of plant cell walls
Hemicellulose	Surround cellulose in plant cell walls
Lignan	Non-carbohydrate found within "woody" plant cell walls

Fibre	Description
Hemicellulose	Surround cellulose in plant cell walls
Pectin	Found in cell walls and intracellular tissues of fruits and berries
Beta-glucans	Found in cereal brans
Gums	Viscous, usually isolated from seeds

The following table gives the percentage of total dietary fibre in five foods.

Table 8. Fibre quantities in selected foods[26]

Food	Total Dietary Fibber
Cereal, all bran	30.1
Blueberries, fresh	2.7
Broccoli, fresh, cooked	3.5
Pork and beans, canned	4.4
Almonds, with skin	8.8

The table below shows the amount of non-fermentable, non-viscous fibre in these same five foods.

Foods that are useful sources of non-fermentable, non-viscous fibre include whole-grains, broccoli, and other vegetables. This type of fibre is believed to decrease the risk of constipation and colon cancer, because it increases stool bulk and reduces transit time.[15] This reduced transit time theoretically means shorter exposure to consumed carcinogens in the intestine, and thus lower cancer risk.

Fermentable, viscous fibre can be found in: oats, rice bran, psyllium seeds, soy, and some fruits. This type of fibre is believed to decrease blood cholesterol and sugar levels, thus also lowering the risk of heart disease and diabetes, respectively.[15]

2.6.3.1 Resistant Starch (RS)

Resistant starches are those that escape digestion in the small intestine. They deliver some of the benefits of both soluble and insoluble fibres, being fermentable (thus feeding intestinal bacteria) and being somewhat hydrophilic (attracting water) to aid stool consistency.

They are considered a dietary fibre, if naturally present in food, and as a functional fibre when added to a food or created through cooking or cooking-cooling processes. Sugars and most starches are rapidly broken down and absorbed as glucose in the small intestine, whereas RS resists digestion and passes through to the large intestine where it functions like fibre.

There are four categories of resistant starch:

RS1: Physically indigestible resistant starch, found in seeds or legumes and unprocessed whole grains

RS2: Resistant starch that occurs in its natural granular form in foods such as uncooked potato, green banana and high amylose corn

RS3: A 'retrograde' resistant starch that is formed when starch-containing foods such as legumes, potatoes, sushi rice or pasta are cooked and cooled, and found in some cooked (and cooled) processed foods such as breads and cornflakes.

RS4: Starches that have been chemically modified to resist digestion. This type of resistant starches can have a wide variety of structures and are not found in nature.

There is some discussion about resistant dextrins being described as 'resistant starch'. Resistant dextrins are not starches, and they can be soluble or insoluble. They might be described as "starch degradation products," a phrase which is included in the EURESTA definition, but their characteristics and performance are very different from those of insoluble resistant starches.

Resistant starches and fibres are found in many vegetables, tubers, fruits, berries and grains. It is assumed that a diet based around natural, whole and unprocessed foods provides a range and quantity of these fibres that is conducive to optimised gut-health. Some processed foods (such as cornflakes) also provide resistant starch (RS) in the form of a 'retrograde' starch. This results from structural changes induced by cooking and cooling. However, one must be aware that these foods, while containing some RS also contain substantial amounts of fast-digesting carbohydrate that may overload your tolerance and thus promote weight-gain. For all but the most carb-tolerant individuals, my advice is to get your RS from natural, whole-foods!

Table 9. Selected sources of resistant starch

Natural Resistant Starch

Food	Serving Size	Resistant starch (grams)	Carbohydrate content (grams)
Banana, raw, slightly green	1 medium peeled	4.7	27
Oats rolled	¼ cup uncooked	4.4	26
Green peas, frozen	1 cup cooked	4.0	18
White beans	½ cup, cooked	3.7	23
Lentils	½ cup, cooked	2.5	20
Cold Potato	½ medium	0.6-0.8	19

Residual amounts of fibres and resistant starches are to be found in the lower-carbohydrate vegetables too. For those needing to follow lower-carb diets, the above options may provide too much glycaemic load and are thus unsuitable. In these cases, the naturally occurring fibres and starches from vegetables and berries are likely to be sufficient to aid gut health.

2.6.3.1.1 Potential benefits of Resistant Starch

Resistant starches are prebiotic. For this reason they are considered health promoting.[27]

Public health authorities around the world see resistant starch as a beneficial carbohydrate. Research on resistant starch (in particular RS2) found that the high amylose content can be beneficial to intestinal/colonic health, as well as in glycaemic management, satiety and hunger. [27] It is however important to note that different types of resistant starch are metabolised and fermented differently and therefore you should consider them individually.[28]

2.7 Protein

Proteins are another major macronutrient that, like carbohydrates, are made up of small repeating units. But instead of sugars, proteins are made up of amino acids. In the following sections, you will learn more about how proteins are synthesized and why they are important in the body.

2.7.1 Amino Acids

Like carbohydrates, proteins contain carbon (C), hydrogen (H), and oxygen (O). However, unlike carbohydrates (and lipids) proteins also contain nitrogen (N). Proteins are made up of smaller units called amino acids. This name, amino acid, signifies that each contains an amino (NH_2) and carboxylic acid (COOH) group. The only structural difference in the 20 amino acids is the side group represented by the R below.

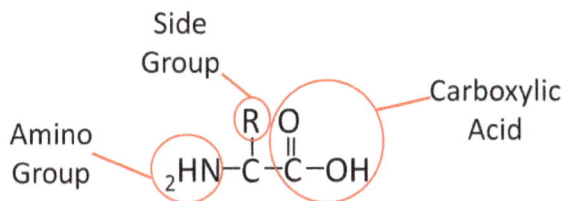

Figure 37. Structure of an amino acid

To illustrate the differences in the side group we will consider glycine and alanine, the two simplest amino acids. For glycine the R group is hydrogen (H), while in alanine the R group is a methyl (CH_3). The structures of these two amino acids are shown below.

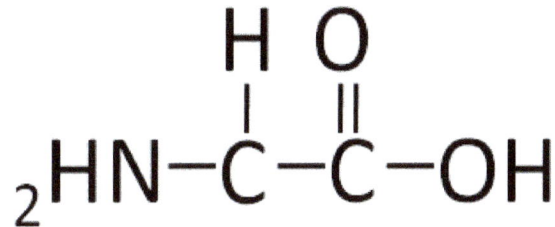

Figure 38. Structure of glycine

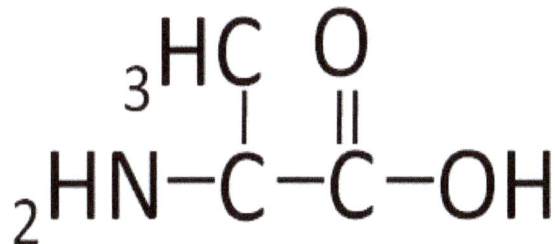

Figure 39. Structure of alanine

Individual amino acids are bonded together through a dehydration reaction (-H_2O) forming a dipeptide (2 amino acids). This bond between amino acids is known as a peptide bond.

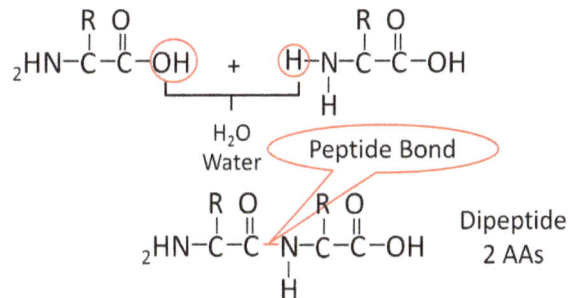

Figure 40. Peptide bond formation

Amino acids can also come together to form tripeptides (three amino acids), oligopeptides (3-10 amino acids), and polypeptides (10 or more amino acids). A polypeptide is a chain of amino acids as shown below.

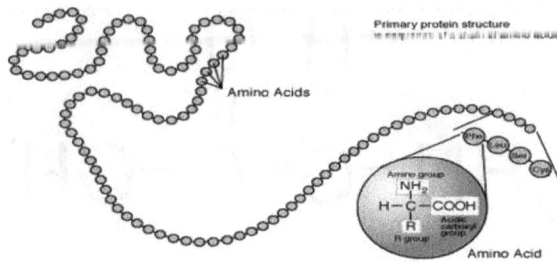

Figure 41. A polypeptide chain[v]

Proteins, known as ribosomes, assist with translation. After translation, the polypeptide can be folded, or gain structure as shown below and will be discussed in the next subsection (Protein Structure).

2.7.2 Protein Synthesis

Protein synthesis is a relatively complex process. DNA contains the genetic code that is used as a template to create mRNA in a process known as transcription. The mRNA then moves out of the nucleus into the cytoplasm where it serves as the template for translation, where tRNAs bring in individual amino acids that are bonded together to form a polypeptide.

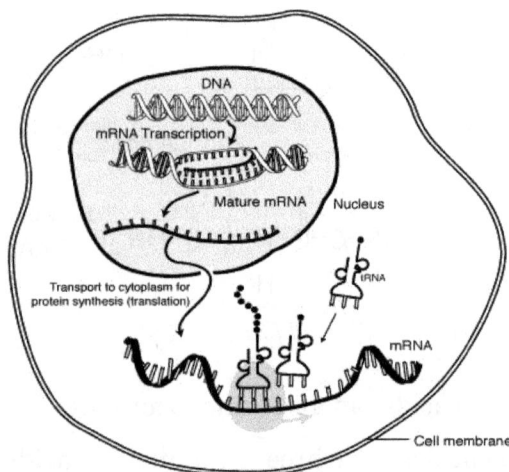

Figure 42. The process of creating a polypeptide (protein)[vi]

---

[v] http://www.genome.gov/Pages/Hyperion/DIR/VIP/Glossary/Illustration/amino_acid.cfm?key=amino%20acids

[vi] http://www.genome.gov/Pages/Hyperion/DIR/VIP/Glossary/Illustration/mrna.cfm?key=messenger%20RNA

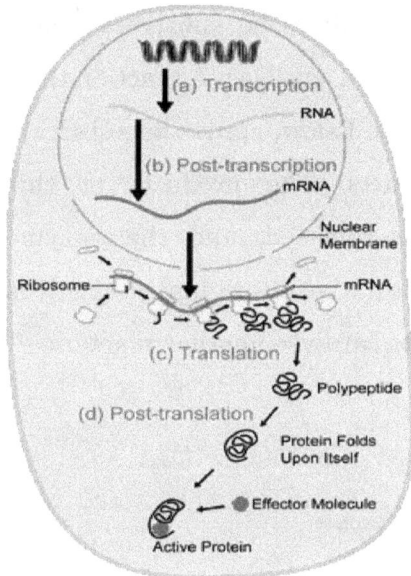

Figure 43. Protein synthesis and processing[vii]

2.7.3   Protein Structure

There are four levels of protein structure. Primary structure is the linear polypeptide chain. Secondary structure occurs when hydrogen bonding between amino acids in the same polypeptide chain causes the formation of structures such as beta-pleated sheets and alpha-helices. Tertiary structure occurs because of an attraction between different amino acids of the polypeptide chain and interactions between the different secondary structures. Finally, certain proteins contain quaternary structure where multiple polypeptide chains are bonded together to form a larger molecule. Haemoglobin is an example of a protein

with quaternary structure. The figure below illustrates the various levels of protein structure.

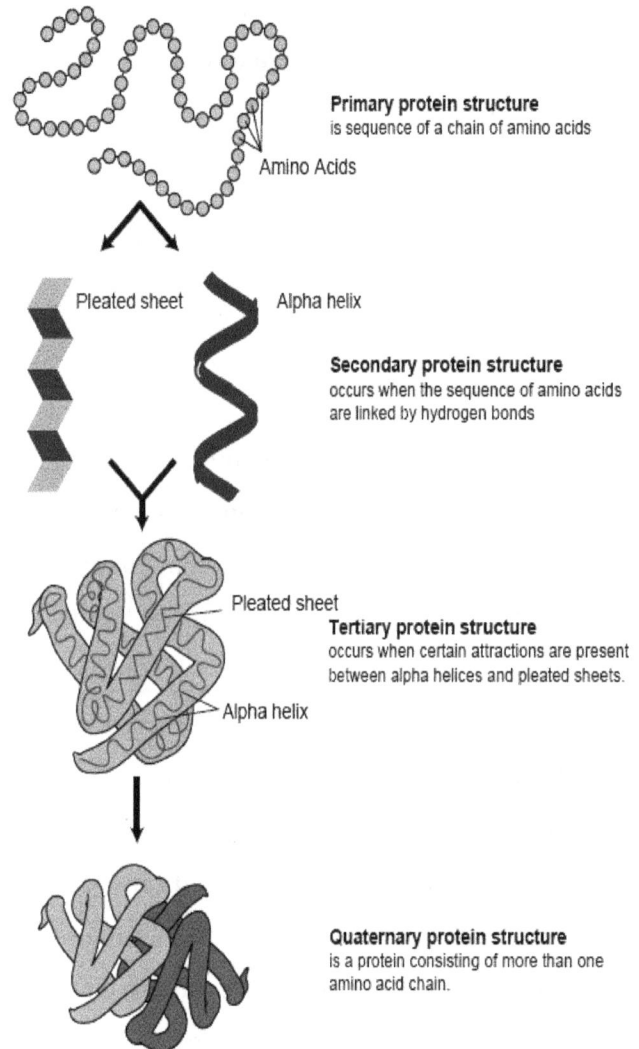

Figure 44. The four levels of protein structures[viii]

2.8   Protein Functions

Proteins, those chains of amino acids, provide the structure for practically every cell, tissue and organ in the human body –

[vii] http://en.wikipedia.org/wiki/File:Proteinsynthesis.png
[viii] In the public domain, from the National Human Genome Research Institute of the National Institutes of Health

so if we are to define the function of protein we could simply use the term 'structure'.

2.8.1.1 Connective Tissue

Proteins, such as collagen, serve as the scaffolding of the body, and thus are important for the structure of tissues.

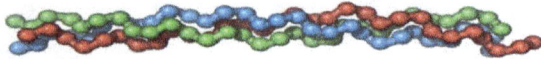

Figure 45. The triple helix structure of collagen[ix]

2.8.1.2 Enzymes

Most enzymes are proteins. Enzymes catalyse chemical reactions, this allows for reactions to occur at a much faster rate (thousands of times faster) and for those reactions to be 'directed'. Without this rapidity cellular functions would be unable to be performed and essential processes may not occur in a timely enough fashion to allow preservation of the organism. The key part of an enzyme is its "active site". The active site is where a compound that is to be acted upon (a substrate) attaches. Enzymes are specific for their substrates; they do not catalyse reactions for random compounds they may be in proximity to. You might have heard the "lock and key" analogy used for enzymes and substrates, respectively. After entering the active site, the enzyme slightly changes shape

(conformation) after the substrate binds. The enzyme then catalyses a reaction that, in the example below, splits the substrate into two parts. The products of this reaction are released, and the enzyme returns to its native or original shape. It is then ready to catalyse another reaction.

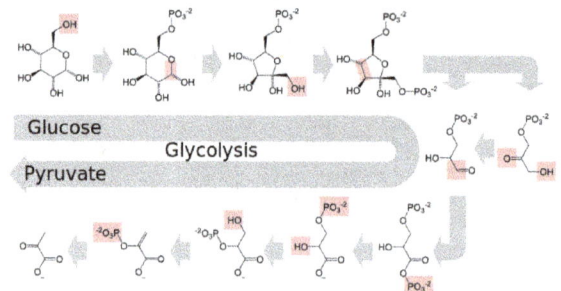

Figure 46. The function of enzymes demonstrated by glycolysis[x]

Enzymes' names commonly end in '-ase', and many are named for their substrate. For example, the enzyme amyl*ase* cleaves bonds found in amylose and amylopectin, and sucr*ase* cleaves sucrose (table sugar) into fructose and glucose.

2.8.1.3 Hormones and neurotransmitters

Many hormones and other chemical 'messengers' known as neurotransmitters, are proteins. An endocrine hormone is a compound that is produced in one tissue, released into circulation, then influences a different organ. Most hormones are

---

[ix] http://en.wikipedia.org/wiki/File:Collagentriplehelix.png

[x] https://commons.wikimedia.org/wiki/File:Glycolysis_metabolic_pathway.svg CC4.0 share alike, by Thomas Shafee

produced from several organs, collectively known as endocrine organs. Insulin is an example of a hormone that is a protein. Other protein hormones:

- Ghrelin
- Human Growth Hormone
- Bradykinin
- Oxytocin
- Glucagon

Hormones may also have autocrine, paracrine and juxtacrine roles.

Autocrine signalling occurs when a cell secretes a hormone or chemical messenger (an 'autocrine agent') that binds to autocrine receptors on the same cell. Paracrine signalling refers to when the target cell is near the signal-releasing cell and Juxtacrine signalling is a type of intercellular communication that is transmitted via oligosaccharide, lipid, or protein components of a cell membrane, and may affect either the emitting cell or the immediately adjacent cells.

2.8.1.4 Fluid Balance

Proteins help to maintain the balance between fluids in the plasma and the interstitial fluid. Interstitial fluid is the fluid that surrounds cells. Interstitial fluid and plasma (fluid part of blood) are the components of extracellular fluid, or the fluid outside of cells. Acid-Base Balance

Proteins also serve as buffers. This means that they help to prevent the pH of the body from getting too high or too low.

2.8.1.5 Transport

Transport proteins move molecules through circulation or across cell membranes. One example is haemoglobin that transports oxygen through the body.

2.8.1.6 Immune Function

Antibodies are proteins that recognize antigens (foreign substances that generate antibody or inflammatory response) and bind to and inactivate them. Antibodies are important in our ability to ward off disease.

2.8.1.7 Energy Provision

Direct oxidation of protein only provides insignificant amounts of energy (up to 15% of daily caloric demands) but can be important in times of stress and starvation. Most amino acids from protein can also be used to create energy substrates via the creation of glucose (gluconeogenesis) or ketone bodies (ketogenesis).

Table 10. Ketogenic and glucogenic amino acids

Glucogenic	Glucogenic and Ketogenic	Ketogenic
Glycine	Phenylalanine	Leucine

Serine   Isoleucine   lysine
Valine   Threonine
Histidine   Tyrosine
Arginine   Tryptophan
Cysteine
Proline
Alanine
Glutamate
Glutamine
Aspartate
Asparagine
Methionine

2.9 Types of Amino Acids

There are 20 'proteinogenic' (protein forming) amino acids our body uses to synthesize proteins. These amino acids can be classified as essential, non-essential, or conditionally essential. The table below shows how the 20 amino acids are classified.

Table 11. Essential and conditionally essential amino acids

Essential	Conditionally Essential	Non-essential
Histidine	Arginine	Alanine
Isoleucine	Cysteine	Asparagine
Leucine	Glutamine	Aspartic Acid or Aspartate
Lysine	Glycine	Glutamic Acid or Glutamate
Methionine	Proline	Serine
Phenylalanine	Tyrosine	
Threonine		
Tryptophan		
Valine		

The body cannot synthesize nine amino acids; therefore, they are 'essential' because they need to be consumed in the diet. These amino acids are known as essential, or indispensable, amino acids. Non-essential, or dispensable, amino acids can be made in our body, so we do not need to consume them, although emerging research is indicating the importance for optimal performance of consuming ample amounts of all the proteinogenic amino acids. 'Conditionally essential' amino acids become essential for individuals in certain situations. It must be noted that our knowledge of, and the benefits and thus 'conditionality' of amino acids continues to grow. An example of a condition when an amino acid becomes essential is the disease phenylketonuria (PKU). Individuals with PKU have a mutation in the enzyme phenylalanine hydroxylase, which normally adds an alcohol group (OH) to the amino acid phenylalanine to form tyrosine as shown below.

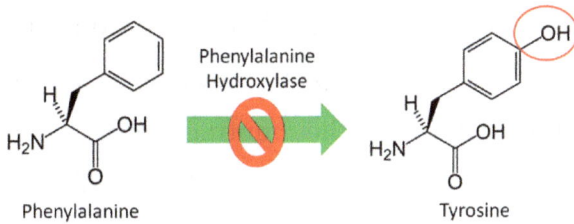

Figure 47. Phenylketonuria results from a mutation in the phenylalanine hydroxylase enzyme[xi]

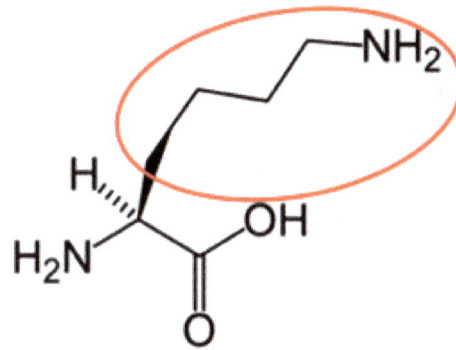

Figure 48. Lysine

Since tyrosine cannot be synthesized by people with PKU, it becomes essential for them. Thus, tyrosine is a conditionally essential amino acid. Individuals with PKU must eat a very low protein diet and avoid the alternative sweetener aspartame, because it can be broken down to phenylalanine. If individuals with PKU consume too much phenylalanine, a toxic phenylalanine metabolic product can build up that causes severe and irreversible damage to the brain.

2.9.1   Amino Acid Structures

It is helpful to have a general idea of the structure of different amino acids and to be able to recognise them as amino acids. Each amino acid differs only by its side group, which is circled in red in each figure of selected amino acids below.

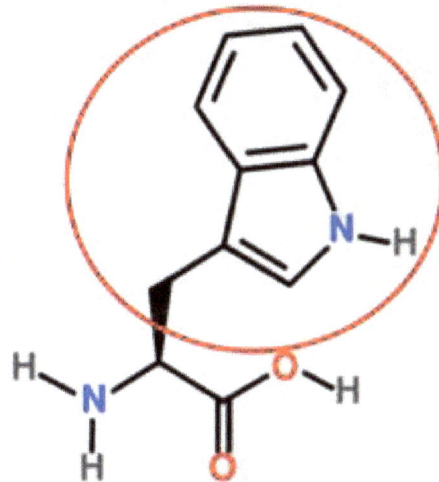

Figure 49. Tryptophan

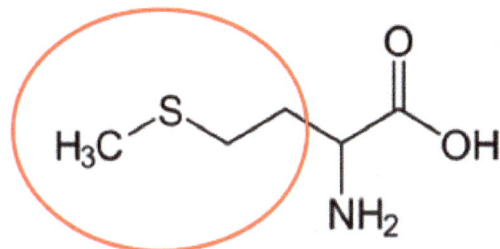

Figure 50. Methionine

The branch chain amino acids (BCAAs), which are all essential amino acids are illustrated below.

---

xi Brian Lindshield, Adapted from http://en.wikipedia.org/wiki/File:L-phenylalanine-skeletal.png and http://en.wikipedia.org/wiki/File:L-tyrosine-skeletal.png

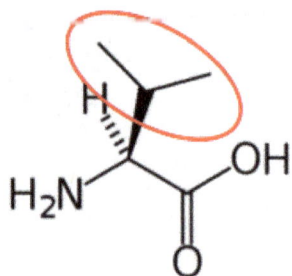

Figure 51. Valine

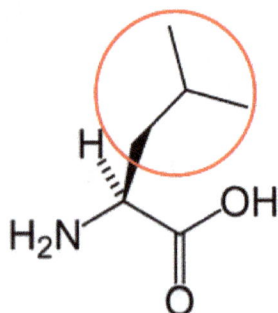

Figure 52. Leucine

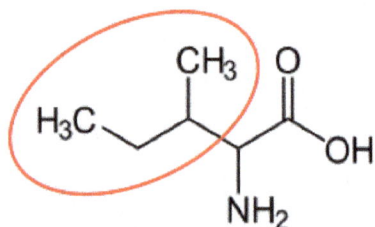

Figure 53. Isoleucine

2.9.2 Protein Quality

Proteins can be classified as either complete or incomplete. Complete proteins provide adequate amounts of all nine essential amino acids. Animal protein foods, such as meat, fish, milk, and eggs are good examples of complete proteins. Incomplete proteins do not contain adequate amounts of one or more of the essential amino acids. For example, if a protein doesn't provide enough of the essential amino acid leucine it would be considered incomplete. Leucine would be referred to as the limiting amino acid, because there is not enough of it for the protein to be complete. Most plant foods are incomplete proteins, with a few exceptions such as soy and newer iterations of pea proteins. Whilst some of these 'complete' plant foods contain lower levels of one or more amino acids they are considered complete because they contain all nine essential amino acids and when consumed at a recommended (per meal) dose, more than satisfy recommendations for amino acid intake. The table below shows the limiting amino acids in some plant foods.

Food	Limiting Amino Acid(s)
Beans and other legumes	Methionine, Tryptophan
Tree nuts and seeds	Methionine, Lysine
Grains	Lysine
Vegetables	Methionine, Lysine

Figure 54. Limiting amino acids in some common plant foods[17]

2.9.2.1 Complementary Proteins

Even though most plant foods do not contain complete proteins, this does not mean that they aren't useful protein sources. Differing foods with both adequate levels of amino acids and some inadequate can be paired to make complete proteins. It is possible to pair foods containing incomplete proteins with different limiting amino acids to provide adequate amounts of the essential amino acids. These proteins can be termed 'complementary proteins', because they supply the amino acid(s) missing in the other protein.

Two examples of complementary proteins are shown below.

Peanut Butter and Jelly Sandwich

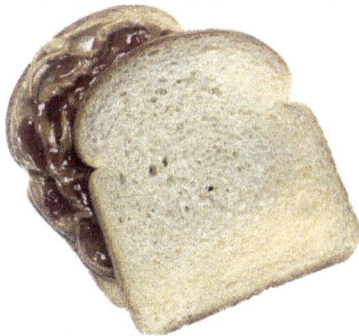

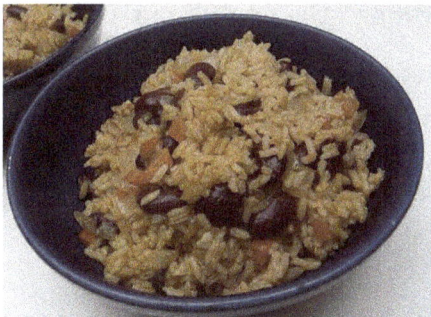

Red Beans and Rice

Figure 55. Examples of complementary protein combinations

It should be noted that complementary proteins do not need to be consumed at the same time or meal. It is current recommended that essential amino acids be met on a daily basis, meaning that if a grain is consumed at one meal a legume could be consumed at a later meal and the

proteins would still complement one another.[29] The concept of consuming protein with the recommended ratios of amino acids in every meal has been a concern for vegetarians and vegans in particular, however it is now considered unnecessary to combine protein types in order to provide all essential amino acids at all meals as a mixed diet (including one based solely on plant foods) can supply all necessary amino acids and encourage optimal protein status.

According to the World Health Organisation (WHO) complete proteins should contain the following amounts of amino acids per gram of protein and should be consumed in these amounts per day (minimum)

Table 12. WHO amino acid recommended amounts

	WHO recommended mg/g protein	Amino Acids Recommended per day (average) by the WHO
Leucine	59	2418
Isoleucine	30	1240
Valine	32	1612
Tryptophan	7	248
Methionine + cysteine	22	930
Methionine	*16*	
Cysteine	*6*	
Histidine	15	620
Lysine	45	1860
Threonine	27	930

45

Phenylalanine	47	1550
+ tyrosine		

Note: This amino acid profile also compares very favourably with the recommended amino acid pattern proposed by the Institute of Medicine of the United States National Institutes of Health*. [30, 31]

2.9.2.2 *Measures of Protein Quality*

How do you know the quality of the protein in the foods you consume?

The protein quality of most foods has been determined by one of the methods below.

- Biological Value (BV) - (grams of nitrogen retained / grams of nitrogen absorbed) x 100

- Protein Efficiency Ratio (PER) - (grams of weight gained / grams of protein consumed). This method is commonly performed in growing rats.

- Chemical or Amino Acid Score (AAS) - (Test food limiting essential amino acid (mg/g protein) / needs of same essential amino acid (mg/g protein))

- Protein Digestibility Corrected Amino Acid Score (PDCAAS) - (Amino Acid Score) x Digestibility

- This is the most widely used method and is preferred by the Food and Agriculture Organization and World Health Organization (WHO).[32]

The following table shows the protein quality measures for some common foods.

Table 13. Measures of protein quality

Protein	PER	Digestibility	AAS (%)	PDCAAS
Egg	3.8	98	121	100*
Milk	3.1	95	127	100*
Beef	2.9	98	94	92
Soy	2.1	95	96	91
Wheat	1.5	91	47	42

PDCAAS scores are truncated (cut off) at 100. These egg and milk scores are 118 and 121 respectively.

Protein efficiency ratios are typically no longer considered to be a valid indicator of protein quality in most cases, due to the differences between the needs of the growing rat and the adult human. Because of the lack of difference in most studies comparing protein types, PDCAAs are a valid 'real-world' measure of protein quality.

How do I find out the protein quality of what I'm eating and identify complementary proteins?

Nutrition Data is compiled from USDA food databases and is a useful resource for determining protein quality and identifying complementary proteins. To use the site, go to www.nutritiondata.com, type in the name of the food you would like to know about in the search bar and hit

Enter. When you have selected your food from the list of possibilities, you will be given information about this food. Included in this information is the Protein Quality section. This will give you an amino acid score and a figure that illustrates which amino acid(s) is limiting. If your food is an incomplete protein, you can click "Find foods with a complementary profile". This will take you to a list of dietary choices that will provide complementary proteins for your food. You can read more about this option in the link below.

2.9.3 Protein-Energy Malnutrition

Protein deficiency rarely occurs in isolation, but instead it is often coupled with insufficient energy intake. As a result, the condition is called protein-energy malnutrition (PEM). This condition is not common in the U.S. but is more prevalent in less developed countries. The two forms of protein energy malnutrition are *Kwashiorkor* and *Marasmus*. They differ in the severity of energy deficiency as shown in the figure below.

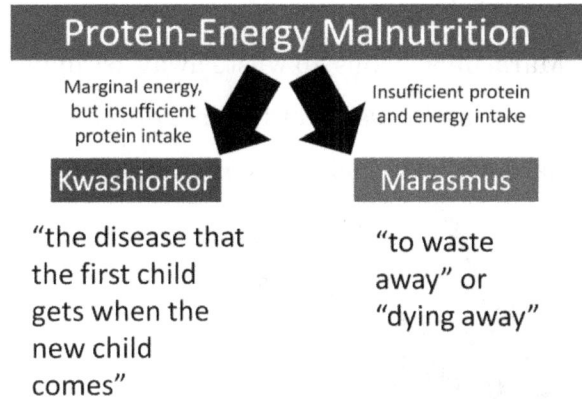

Figure 56. The two types of protein-energy malnutrition

Kwashiorkor is a Ghanaian word that means "the disease that the first child gets when the new child comes[15]." The characteristic symptom of kwashiorkor is a swollen abdomen. Energy intake could be adequate, but protein consumption is too low.

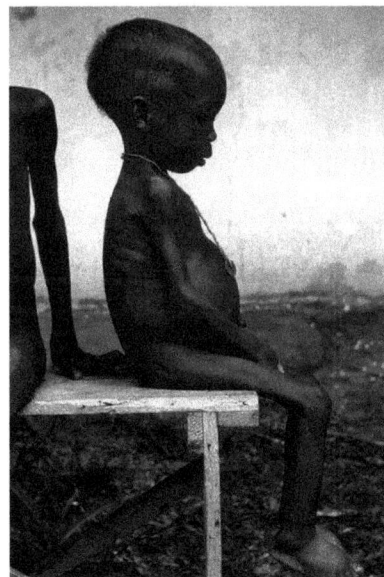

Figure 57. A child with Kwashiorkor[xii]

[xii] http://en.wikipedia.org/wiki/File:Starved_girl.jpg

Marasmus means 'to waste away' or 'dying away', and thus occurs in individuals who have severely limited energy intakes.

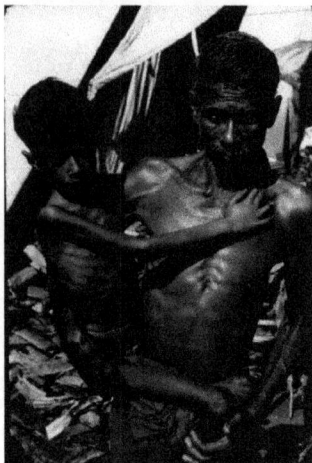

Figure 58. Two people with Marasmus[xiii]

2.10 Lipids

Lipids, commonly referred to as fats, have a garnered a poor reputation in nutrition due to the idea that ingested fat will cause body-fat accretion. We do however need to consume essential fats and we need to incorporate other fats into our diets for optimal health.

In this section we will dive deeper into fats and why they do not need to be feared.

2.10.1 How Does Fat Differ from Lipids?

The answer you receive from this question will depend on who you ask, so it is important to understand lipids and fats from a chemical and nutritional perspective.

To a chemist, lipids consist of:

- Triglycerides
- Fatty Acids
- Phospholipids
- Sterols

These compounds are grouped together because of their structural and physical property similarities. For instance, all lipids have hydrophobic (water-fearing) properties. Chemists further separate lipids into fats and oils based on their physical properties at room temperature:

Fats are solid at room temperature
Oils are liquid at room temperature

From a nutritional perspective, the definition of lipids is the same. The definition of a fat differs, however, because nutrition-oriented people define fats based on their caloric contribution rather than whether they are solid at room temperature. Thus, from a nutrition perspective:

Fats are triglycerides, fatty acids, and phospholipids that provide 9 kcal/g.

The other difference is that from a caloric perspective, an oil is a fat. For example, let's consider olive oil.

[xiii] http://en.wikipedia.org/wiki/File:Starved_child.jpg

Clearly, it is an oil according to a chemist definition, but from a caloric standpoint it is a fat because it provides 9 kcal/g.

2.10.2 Fatty Acids

Fatty acids are lipids themselves, and they are also components of triglycerides and phospholipids. Like carbohydrates, fatty acids are made up of carbon (C), hydrogen (H), and oxygen (O).

On one end of a fatty acid is a methyl group (CH_3) that is known as the methyl or omega end. On the opposite end of a fatty acid is a carboxylic acid (COOH). This end is known as the acid or alpha end. The figure below shows the structure of fatty acids.

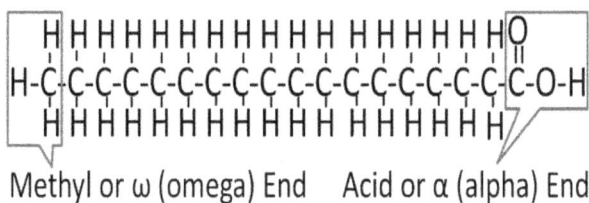

Methyl or ω (omega) End   Acid or α (alpha) End

Figure 59. Structure of a saturated fat

Fatty acids can be defined and described in several ways:

1. Carbon chain length (i.e. 6 carbons vs. 18 carbons)

2. Saturation/unsaturation

3. Double bond configuration (cis vs. trans)

2.10.2.1 Carbon Chain Length

Fatty acids differ in their carbon chain length (number of carbons in the fatty

acid). Most fatty acids contain somewhere between 2-24 carbons, with even numbers (i.e. 8, 18) of carbons occurring more frequently than odd numbers (i.e. 9, 19). Fatty acids are classified as short-chain fatty acids, medium-chain fatty acids, and long-chain fatty acids based on their carbon chain length using the criteria shown in the table below.

Table 14. Fatty acid classification by chain-length

Classification	# of carbons
Short-Chain Fatty Acid	< 6
Medium-Chain Fatty Acid	6-12
Long-Chain Fatty Acid	≥14

Carbon chain length also impacts the physical properties of the fatty acid. As the number of carbons in a fatty acid chain increases, so does the melting point as illustrated in the figure below.

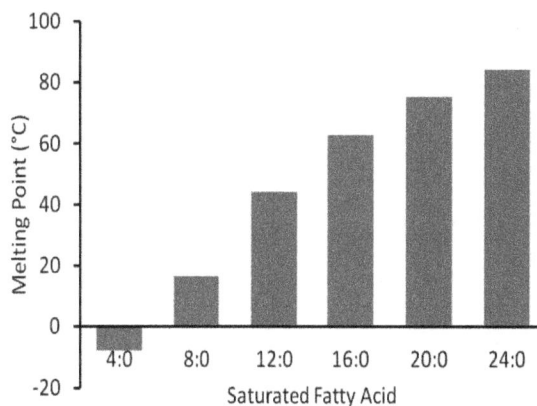

Figure 60. The melting point of saturated fatty acids of various lengths[1]

Thus, shorter chain fatty acids are more likely to be liquid, while longer chain fatty acids are more likely to be solid at room temperature (20-25°C, 68-77°F). It has also been demonstrated that the shorter the chain length, the greater the primary deposition into the bloodstream (the hepatic portal vein) and thus, the greater the effect on encouraging ketogenesis. There may also be an inverse correlation between chain length and effect on HDL-c levels.

2.10.3 2. Saturation/Unsaturation

A saturated fatty acid is one that contains the maximum number of hydrogens possible, and no carbon-carbon double bonds. Carbon normally has four bonds to it. Thus, a saturated fatty acid has hydrogens at every position except carbon-carbon single bonds and carbon-oxygen bonds on the acid end.

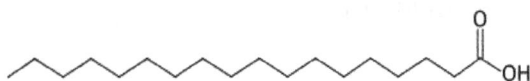

Figure 61. A simplified view of 18 carbon saturated fatty acid stearic acid2. Each corner of the zigzag pattern represents a carbon, and the hydrogens are not shown to allow quicker recognition of the carbon chain

Unsaturation means the fatty acid doesn't contain the maximum number of hydrogens on each of its carbons. Instead, unsaturated fatty acids contain a carbon-carbon double bond and only 1 hydrogen off each carbon. The simplest example of unsaturation is a monounsaturated fatty acid. Mono means one, so these are fatty acids with one degree of unsaturation, or one double bond (shown below).

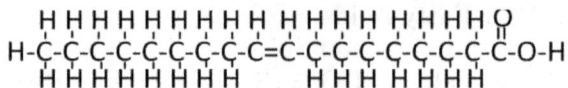

Figure 62. Structure of the monounsaturated fatty acid (oleic acid)

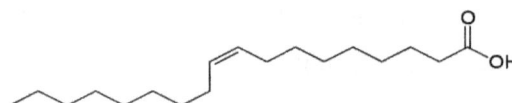

Figure 63. The simplified structure of the monounsaturated fatty acid (oleic acid)

Any fatty acid that has two or more double bonds is considered a polyunsaturated fatty acid. As you may remember from the polysaccharide section, poly means many. A simple example of a polyunsaturated fatty acid is linoleic acid (shown below).

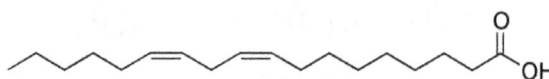

Figure 64. Structure of the polyunsaturated fatty acid linoleic acid, a polyunsaturated fatty acid with two carbon-carbon double bonds

2.10.3.1 Double Bond Configuration (Shape)

Double bonds in unsaturated fatty acids are in one of two structural orientations: cis or trans. In a trans orientation, the hydrogens on the carbons involved in the double bond are opposite of one another. In the cis orientation the hydrogens are on the same side of the bond. Steric hindrance in the cis orientation causes the chain to take on a more bent shape.

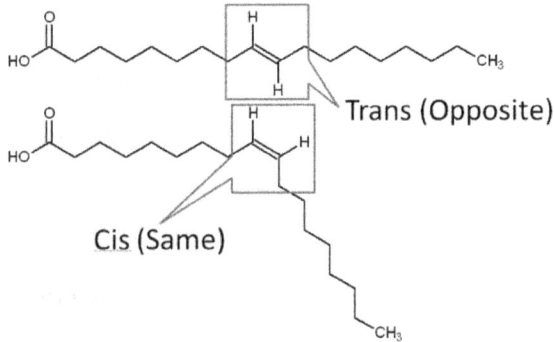

Figure 65. *Cis and trans structural conformations of a monounsaturated fatty acid.*

Most natural unsaturated fatty acids are in the cis conformation. As can be seen in Figure 2.327, the cis fatty acids have a more of kinked shape, which means they do not pack together as well as the saturated or trans fatty acids. As a result, the melting point is much lower for cis fatty acids compared to trans and saturated fatty acids. To illustrate this difference, the figure below shows the difference in the melting points of saturated, trans-, and cis-monounsaturated 18 carbon fatty acids.

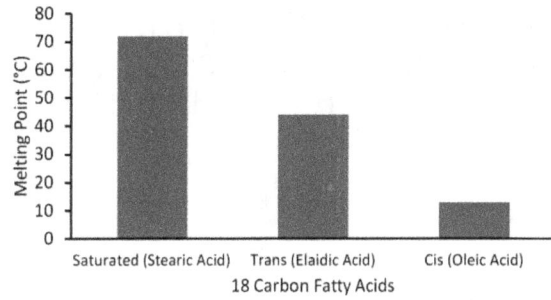

Figure 66. *The melting point of saturated, trans, and cis 18 carbon monounsaturated fatty acids[1]*

There are some naturally occurring trans fatty acids, such as conjugated linoleic acid (CLA) and vaccenic acids in dairy products. These would generally be healthy fats. However, for the most part, trans fatty acids in our diets are not natural; instead, they have been produced synthetically. The primary source of trans fatty acids in our food supply is partially hydrogenated vegetable oil. The 'hydrogenated' means that the oil has gone through the process of hydrogenation. Hydrogenation, like the name implies, is the addition of hydrogen. If an unsaturated fatty acid is completely hydrogenated it would be converted to a saturated fatty acid as shown below.

H H H H H H H HI I H HH H H H H H O
‖
H-C-C-C-C-C-C=C-C-C=C-C-C-C-C-C-C-C-C-C-O-H
H H H H H   H   H H H H H H H

↓

H H H H H H H H H H H H H H H H H H HO
‖
H-C-C-C-C-C-C-C-C-C-C-C-C-C-C-C-C-C-C-C-O-H
H H H H H H H H H H H H H H H H H H H

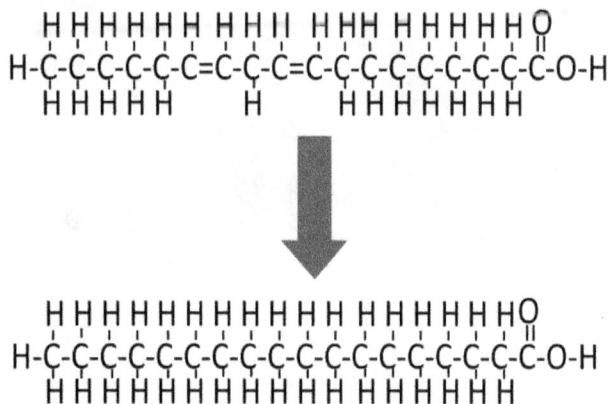

Figure 67. Fatty acid hydrogenation

However, this isn't/wasn't always desirable, thus partially hydrogenated vegetable oil became widely used. To visualize the difference in the amount of hydrogenation consider the difference between tub margarine and stick margarine.

Stick margarine is more fully hydrogenated leading it to have a much harder texture. This is one of the two reasons to hydrogenate, to get a more solid texture. The second reason is that it makes it more shelf stable, because the double bond(s) of unsaturated fatty acids are susceptible to oxidation, which causes them to become rancid.

Partial hydrogenation causes the conversion of cis to trans fatty acids along with the formation of some saturated fatty acids. Originally, it was thought that trans fatty acids would be a better alternative to saturated fat (think margarine vs. butter). However, it turns out that trans-fat is

worse than saturated fat in altering biomarkers associated with cardiovascular disease and saturated fats are not in actuality negatively affective for cardiovascular disease markers in most people. Trans-fats generally increase LDL and decrease HDL levels, while saturated fat may increase LDL whilst increasing HDL levels, or these may be unchanged, and there may be beneficial effects of saturated fats on lipid sub-fractions (i.e. small vs. large particle LDL).

2.10.4 Fatty Acid Naming & Food Sources

There are three naming systems used for fatty acids:

1. Delta nomenclature
2. Omega nomenclature
3. Common names

The omega nomenclature and common names are used more in the field of nutrition than the delta nomenclature when describing specific fatty acids.

2.10.5 Delta Nomenclature

For delta nomenclature you need to know 3 things:

1. Number of carbons in the fatty acid
2. Number of double bonds
3. Number of carbons from the carboxylic acid (alpha) end to the first carbon in the double bond(s)

Let's consider the example in the figure below.

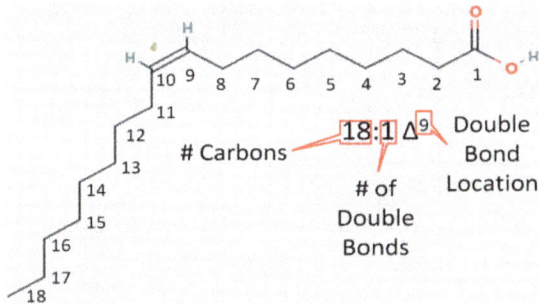

Figure 68. Delta Nomenclature

1. Number of carbons in the fatty acid = 18
2. Number of double bonds = 1
3. Number of carbons from the carboxylic acid end to the first carbon in the double bond = 9

2.10.6 Omega Nomenclature

The omega nomenclature is almost the same as the delta nomenclature, the only difference being that carbons are counted from the methyl (omega) end instead of the carboxylic acid end and the omega symbol is used instead of the delta symbol.

For omega nomenclature you need to know 3 things:

1. Number of carbons in the fatty acid
2. Number of double bonds
3. Number of carbons from the methyl end (aka Omega end) to the first carbon in the double bond closest to the methyl end

We will again consider the same fatty acid.

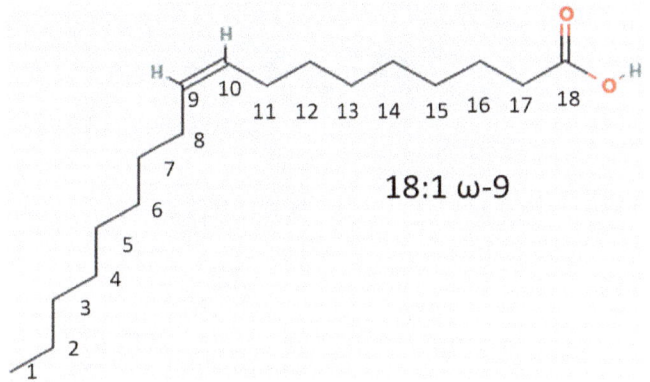

Figure 69. Omega Nomenclature

1. Number of carbons in the fatty acid = 18
2. Number of double bonds = 1
3. Number of carbons from the methyl (aka omega) end to the first carbon in the double bond closest to the methyl end = 9

If it is a saturated fatty acid, then the omega nomenclature is not added to the end of the name. If it is an 18-carbon saturated fatty acid, then it would be named 18:0.

This is written as shown in figure 2.332. Instead of an omega prefix, the prefix n- (i.e. n-3) is also commonly used.

2.10.7 Common Names

The common names of fatty acids are something that, for the most part, must be learned/memorized. The common name of the fatty acid we have been naming in this section is oleic acid.

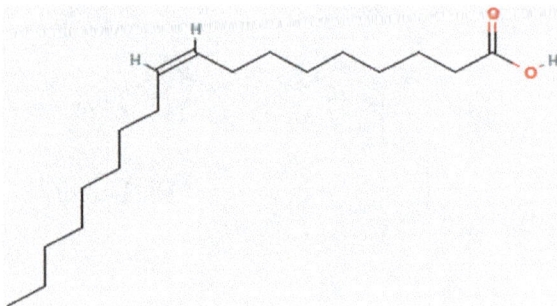

Figure 70. Oleic acid

However, it can also be called oleate. The only difference is that, instead of a carboxylic acid on the end of the fatty acid, it has been ionized to form a salt (shown below). This is what the -ate ending indicates and the two names are used interchangeably.

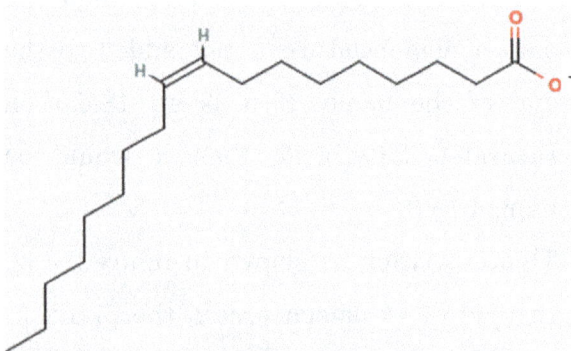

Figure 71. Oleate

The table below gives the common names and food sources of some common fatty acids.

Table 15. Common names of fatty acids

Omega Name	Common Name	Common Food Source
4:0	Butyric Acid	Butter and various milks (horse, goat)
6:0	Caproic	Goats milk

8:0	Caprylic	Goats milk
10:0	Capric	Goats milk, coconut oil
12:0	Lauric Acid	Coconut oil
14:0	Myristic Acid	Coconut oil, palm kernel oil, butter
16:0	Palmitic acid	Palm oil, palm kernel oil
18:0	Stearic Acid	Animal fats
20:0	Arachidic Acid	Corn oil, peanut oil, macadamias
24:0	Lignoceric Acid	Peanut oil
18:1 (n-9)	Oleic Acid	Olive oil
18:2 (n-6)	Linoleic Acid	Common seed oils
18:3 (n-3)	Alpha-linolenic Acid	Flaxseed oil
20:4 (n-6)	Arachidonic Acid	Meat and fish
20:5 (n-3)	Eicosapentanoic Acid	Oily fish
22:6 (n-3)	Docosahexanoic Acid	Oily fish

2.11 Food Sources of Fatty Acids

After going through this wide array of fatty acids, you may be wondering where they are found in nature. The figure below shows the fatty acid composition of certain oils and oil-based foods. As you can see, most foods contain a mixture of fatty acids. Stick margarine is the only product in the figure that contains an appreciable amount of trans fatty acids. Corn, walnut, and soybean are rich sources of n-6 polyunsaturated fatty acids, while flax seed is unique among plants in that it is a reliable source of n-3 polyunsaturated fatty acids. Canola and olive oil are rich sources of monounsaturated fatty acids. Lard, palm oil, butter and coconut oil all contain a significant amount of saturated fatty acids.

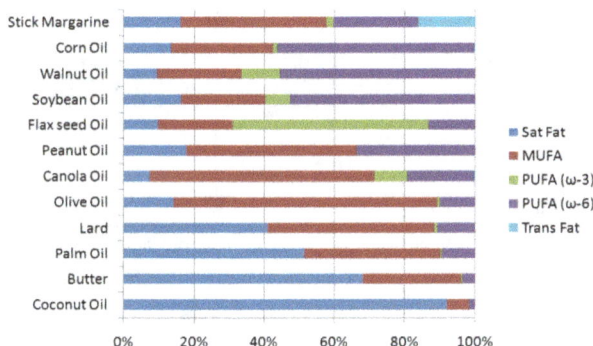

Figure 72. Fatty acid composition of foods and oils[xiv]

2.34 Essential Fatty Acids & Eicosanoids

The two essential fatty acids are:

1. linoleic acid (omega-6)

2. alpha-linolenic (omega-3)

These fatty acids are essential because we can't synthesize them. This is because we do not have an enzyme capable of adding a double bond (desaturating) beyond the omega-9 carbon counting from the alpha end (the omega-6 and 3 positions). The structures of the two essential fatty acids are shown below.

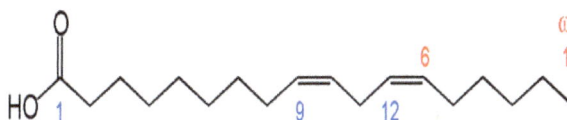

Figure 2.341 Linoleic acid[1]

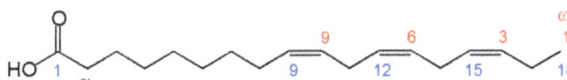

Figure 2.342 Alpha-linolenic acid[2]

However, we do possess enzymes that can take the essential fatty acids, elongate them (add two carbons to them), and then further desaturate them (add double bonds) to other omega-6 and omega-3 fatty acids. Thus, there are 2 families of fatty acids that most of the polyunsaturated fatty acids fit into as shown below.

_____

[xiv] Information derived from nutritiondata.com

Eicosanoids

Omega-3 family   pg = prostaglandin   tx = thromboxane   **Omega-6 family**
pgi = prostacyclin   lt = leukotriene

☐ = less inflammatory
☐ = more inflammatory

Omega-3 family		Omega-6 family
α-linolenic acid $18:3\ \omega\text{-}3$		linoleic acid $18:2\ \omega\text{-}6$

$\Delta6$ desaturase

| stearidonic acid $18:4\ \omega\text{-}3$ | | γ-linolenic acid GLA $18:3\ \omega\text{-}6$ |

elongase

| eicosatetraenoic acid $20:4\ \omega\text{-}3$ | $pge_1\ pgf_{1\alpha}$ txa_1 blocks lt_4 | dihomo γ-linolenic acid DGLA $20:3\ \omega\text{-}6$ |

$\Delta5$ desaturase

| eicosapentaenoic acid EPA $20:5\ \omega\text{-}3$ | $pgd_3\ pge_3\ pgf_{3\alpha}$ $pgi_3\ txa_3$ $lta_5\ ltb_5\ ltc_5\ ltd_5$ | $pgd_2\ pge_2\ pgf_{2\alpha}$ $pgi_2\ txa_2\ lta_4\ ltb_4$ $ltc_4\ ltd_4\ lte_4$ main | arachidonic acid AA $20:4\ \omega\text{-}6$ |

Sprecher's Shunt

elongase

| docosapentaenoic acid DPA $22:5\ \omega\text{-}3$ | | docosatetraenoic acid $22:4\ \omega\text{-}6$ |

$\Delta4$ desaturase

| docosahexaenoic acid DHA $22:6\ \omega\text{-}3$ | A/J-Ring Neuroprostane 17S Resolvins blocks prostanoids | docosapentaenoic acid $22:5\ \omega\text{-}6$ |

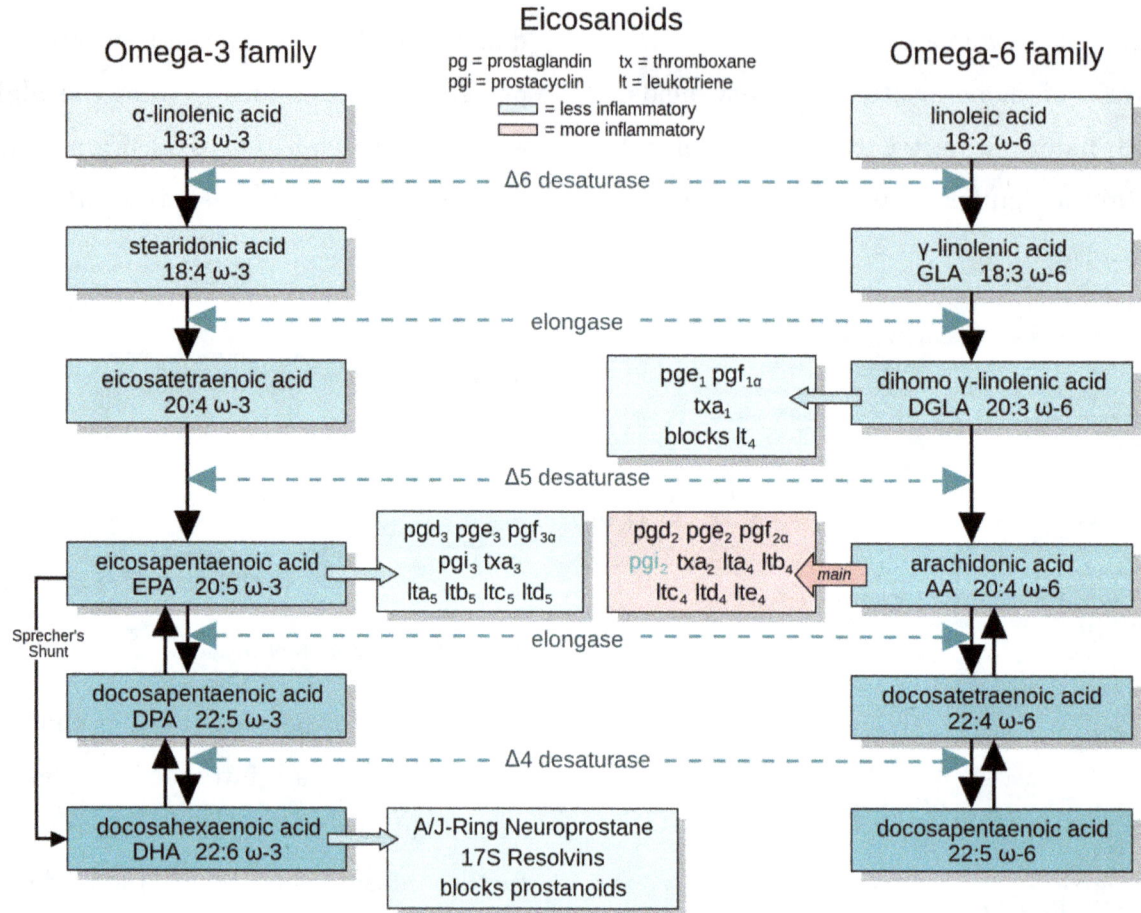

Figure 73. Omega-3 and omega-6 fatty acids and eicosanoid production

The same enzymes are used for both omega-6 and omega-3 fatty acids. However, we cannot convert omega-3 fatty acids to omega-6 fatty acids or omega-6 fatty acids to omega-3 fatty acids. Among these families, the omega-3 fatty acid, eicosapentaenoic acid (EPA), and the omega-6 fatty acids, dihomo gamma-linolenic acid and arachidonic acid (AA), are used to form compounds known as eicosanoids. These 20 carbon fatty acid derivatives are biologically active in the body (like hormones, but they act locally in the tissue they are produced). There are four classes of eicosanoids:

Prostaglandins (PG)

Prostacyclins (PC)

Thromboxanes (TX)

Leukotrienes (LT)

The difference in the effects and outcomes of omega-6 and omega-3 fatty acid intake is primarily a result of the eicosanoids produced from them. Omega-6 fatty acid derived eicosanoids are more inflammatory than omega-3 fatty acid derived eicosanoids. As a result, omega-3 fatty acids are considered anti-inflammatory because replacing the more inflammatory omega-6 fatty acid derived eicosanoids with omega-3 fatty acid derived eicosanoids will decrease inflammation. As an example of the action of eicosanoids, aspirin works by inhibiting the enzymes cyclooxygenase (Cox)-1 and Cox-2. These enzymes convert arachidonic acid into inflammatory prostaglandins.

You have probably heard that you should get more omega-3s in your diet, and in general polyunsaturated fatty acids are considered healthy. However, since omega-3 fatty acids are competing for the same enzymes as omega-6 fatty acids, and because the omega-6 fatty acids are more inflammatory, consuming too many omega-6s is probably more detrimental than helpful. As a result, many people talk about the omega-3: omega-6 fatty acid ratio in peoples' diets. For many on the western world, the ratio is believed to be too high, at almost 10-20 times more omega-6 fatty acids than omega-3 fatty acids.[33] The table below shows food sources of some selected omega-3 and omega-6 fatty acids.

Table 16. Food sources of selected omega-3 and omega-6 fatty acids

Fatty Acid	Food Sources
Linoleic Acid (LA, n-6)	Safflower Oil, Corn Oil, Sunflower Oil
Arachidonic Acid (AA, n-6)	Eggs, Meat
Alpha-Linolenic Acid (ALA, n-3)	Walnuts, Flaxseed (linseed), Canola (rapeseed), and Soybean Oils
Eicosapentaenoic Acid (EPA, n-3)	Fatty Fish & Fish Oils
Docosahexanoic Acid (DHA, n-3)	Fatty Fish & Fish Oils

Conversion of alpha-linolenic acid to EPA and DHA, this conversion is actually quite limited; 0.2-8% of ALA is converted to EPA and 0-4% of ALA is converted to DHA.[34] Thus, dietary consumption is the most effective way to get the longer chain fatty acids (EPA and DHA) in our bodies. It is less clear whether ALA consumption is as beneficial as EPA and DHA, but a recent study found it to be equally effective in decreasing blood triglyceride concentrations. In that study, DHA had the added positive benefit of increasing HDL. These are all positive outcomes that are expected to reduce the risk of developing cardiovascular disease.

2.11.1 Essential Fatty Acid Deficiency

Essential fatty acid deficiency is rare and unlikely to occur, but the symptoms are:

Growth retardation

Reproductive problems

Skin lesions

Neurological and visual problems

2.12 Triglycerides

Triglycerides are the most common lipid in our bodies and in food. Fatty acids are not typically found in a free form in nature, but instead are found in triglycerides. The name *triglyceride* tells a lot about its structure. "Tri" refers to the three fatty acids, and "glyceride" refers to the glycerol backbone that the 3 fatty acids are bonded to. Thus, a monoglyceride contains one fatty acid and a diglyceride contains two fatty acids.

Triglycerides perform the following functions in our bodies:

- Provide energy, especially at rest and at lower levels of movement intensity
- Primary form of energy storage in the body
- Insulate and protect the body and vital organ
- Aid in the absorption and transport of fat-soluble vitamins and some related compounds (like the pro-vitamin carotenoids).

A triglyceride is formed via a dehydration reaction between a glycerol and three fatty acids as shown below.

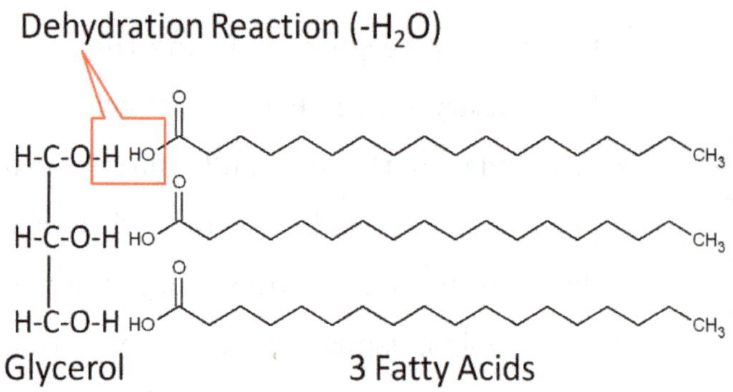

Figure 74. Triglyceride formation

When a fatty acid is added to the glycerol backbone, this process is called esterification. This process is so named, because it forms an ester bond between each fatty acid and glycerol. Three molecules of water are also formed during this process as shown below.

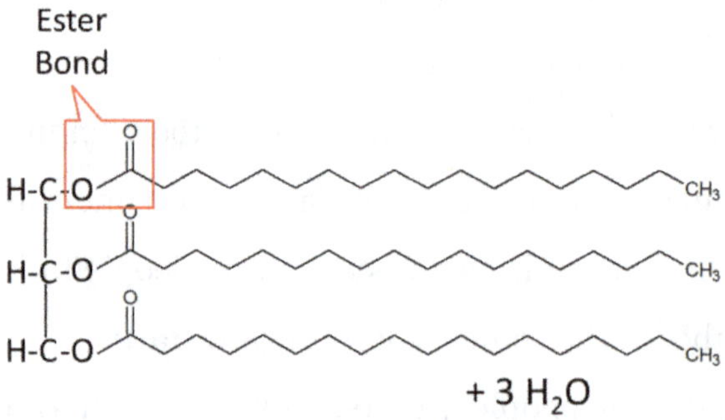

Figure 75. Esterification of three fatty acids to glycerol

A stereospecific numbering (sn) system is used to number the three fatty acids in a triglyceride sn-1, sn-2, and sn-3 respectively. A triglyceride can also be simply represented as a polar (hydrophilic) head, with 3 nonpolar (hydrophobic) tails as shown below.

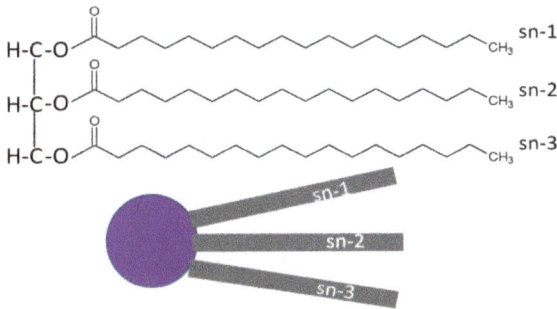

Figure 76. Stereospecific numbering (sn) of triglycerides

The three fatty acids in a triglyceride can be the same or can each be a different fatty acid. A triglyceride containing different fatty acids is known as a mixed triglyceride. An example of a mixed triglyceride is shown below.

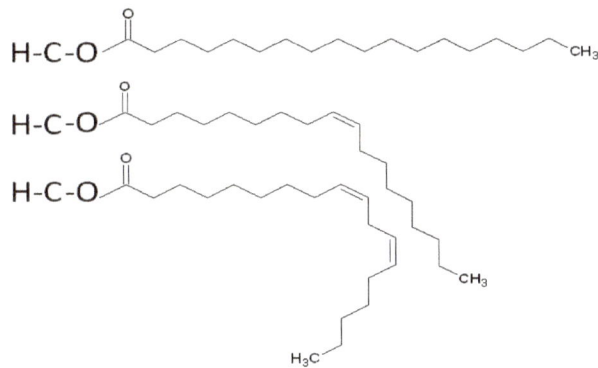

Figure 77. Structure of a mixed triglyceride

2.13 Phospholipids

Phospholipids are similar in structure to triglycerides, with the only difference being a phosphate group and nitrogen-containing compound in the place of a fatty acid.

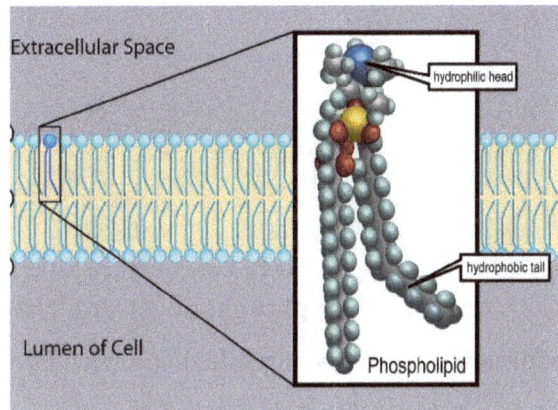

Figure 78. A phospholipid[xv]

The best-known phospholipid is phosphatidylcholine (aka lecithin). As you can see in the structure below, it contains a choline off the phosphate group.

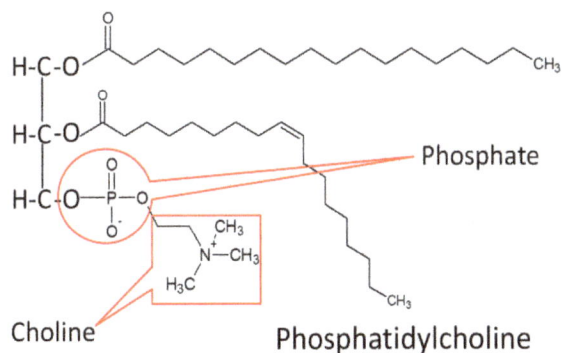

Figure 79. Structure of phosphatidylcholine (lecithin)

[xv] Creative Commons Attribution-Share Alike 4.0 International license. By SuperScience71421 https://commons.wikimedia.org/wiki/File:Phospholipid_TvanBrussel.edit.jpg

However, you will not normally find phospholipids arranged like a triglyceride, with the 3 tails opposite the glycerol head. This is because the phosphate/nitrogen tail of the phospholipid is polar. Thus, the structure will look like the 2 figures below.

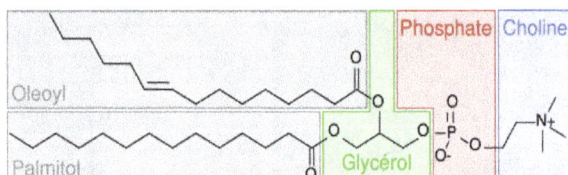

Figure 80. Structure of phosphatidylcholine[xvi]

Like triglycerides, phospholipids are also represented as a hydrophilic head with two hydrophobic tails as shown below.

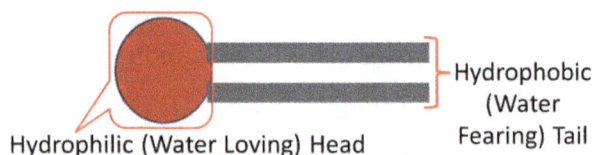

Figure 81. Schematic of a phospholipid

2.13.1 Phospholipid Functions

Because its structure allows it to be at the interface of water-lipid environments, there are two main functions of phospholipids:

1. Key Component of the Cell's Lipid Bilayer

2. Emulsification

Number 1 in the figure below is a cell's lipid bilayer, while 2 is a micelle that is formed by phospholipids to assist in emulsification.

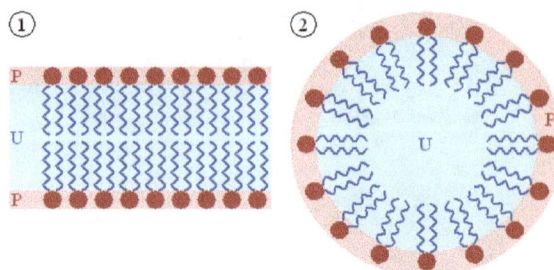

Figure 82. Lipid bilayer (1) and micelle (2)[xvii]

2.13.2 Key Component of Cells' Lipid Bilayers

Phospholipids are a vital component of the lipid bilayers of cells. A cross section of a lipid bilayer is shown below. The hydrophilic heads are on the outside and inside of the cell; the hydrophobic tails are on the interior.

---

xvi http://commons.wikimedia.org/wiki/File:Popc_details.svg

xvii http://en.wikipedia.org/wiki/File:Lipid_bilayer_and_micelle.png

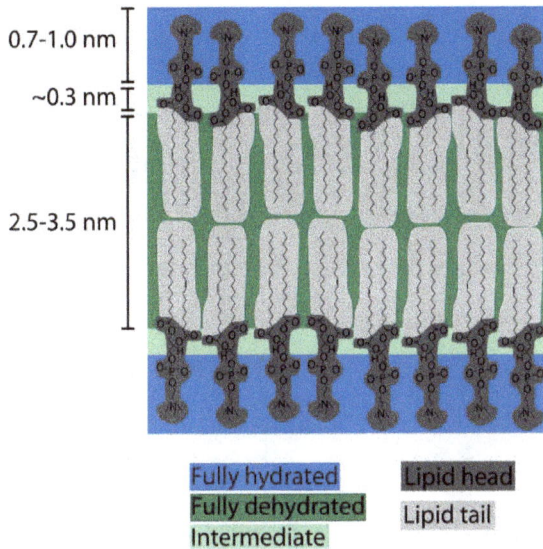

0.7-1.0 nm
~0.3 nm
2.5-3.5 nm

Fully hydrated   Lipid head
Fully dehydrated   Lipid tail
Intermediate

Figure 83. Phospholipids in a bilayer[xviii]

2.13.3 Emulsification

As emulsifiers, phospholipids help hydrophobic substances mix in a watery environment. It does this by forming a micelle as shown below. The hydrophobic substance is trapped on the interior of the micelle away from the aqueous environment.

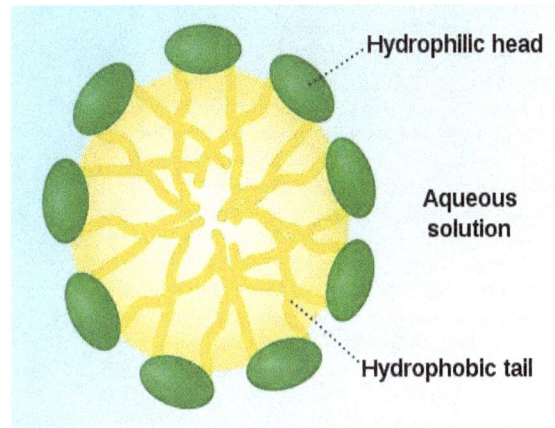

Hydrophilic head

Aqueous solution

Hydrophobic tail

Figure 84. Structure of a micelle[xix]

As a result, it can take a hydrophobic liquid (oil) and allow it to mix with hydrophilic liquid (water).

[xviii] http://en.wikipedia.org/wiki/File:Bilayer_hydration_profile.svg

[xix] http://en.wikipedia.org/wiki/File:Micelle_scheme-en.svg

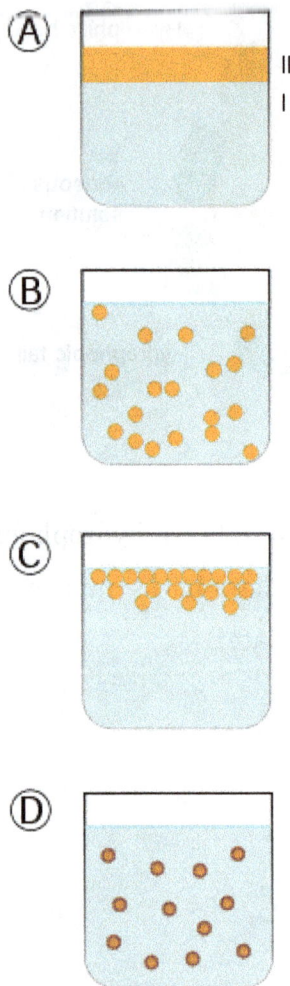

Figure 85. How emulsions allow the dispersion of a hydrophobic substance into a hydrophilic environment[xx]

Foods rich in phosphatidylcholine include: egg yolks, liver, soybeans, wheat germ, and peanuts[16]. Egg yolks serve as an emulsifier in a variety of recipes. Your body makes all the phospholipids that it needs, so they do not need to be consumed (not essential).

2.142.37 Sterols

The last category of lipids are the sterols. Their structure is quite different from the other lipids because sterols are made up of several carbon rings. The generic structure of a sterol is shown below.

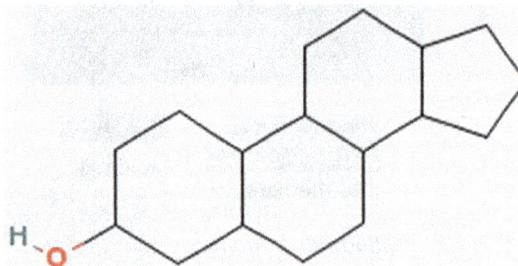

Figure 86. Generic structure of a sterol

The primary sterol that we consume is cholesterol. The structure of cholesterol is shown below.

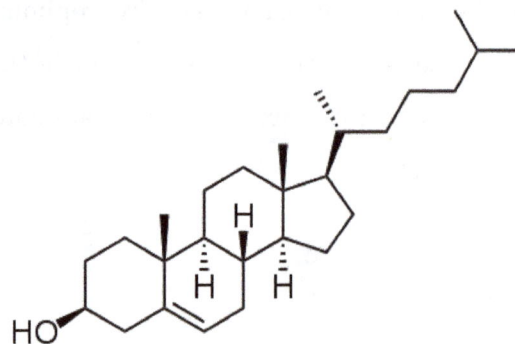

Figure 87. The structure of cholesterol

Cholesterol is frequently found in foods as a cholesterol ester, meaning that there is a fatty acid attached to cholesterol. The structure of a cholesterol ester is shown below.

---

xx http://en.wikipedia.org/wiki/File:Emulsions.svg

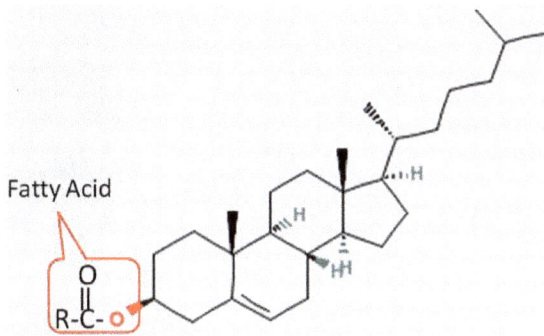

Fatty Acid

Figure 88. Structure of a cholesterol ester

All sterols have a similar structure to cholesterol. Cholesterol is only found in foods of animal origin.

2.14.1 Function

Although cholesterol has acquired the status of a nutritional "villain", it is a vital component of cell membranes and is used to produce vitamin D, hormones, and bile acids. You can see the similarity between the structures of vitamin D and oestradiol, one of the forms of oestrogen shown below.

We do not need to consume any cholesterol from our diets (not essential) because our bodies can synthesize the required amounts. In fact, the regulation of cholesterol is so finely balanced that if one eats more cholesterol they will produce less and if they eat less they will produce more internally to preserve required levels within the body.

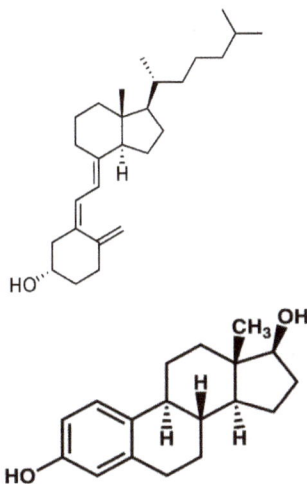

Figure 89. Structures of vitamin D3 and oestradiol (a form of oestrogen)

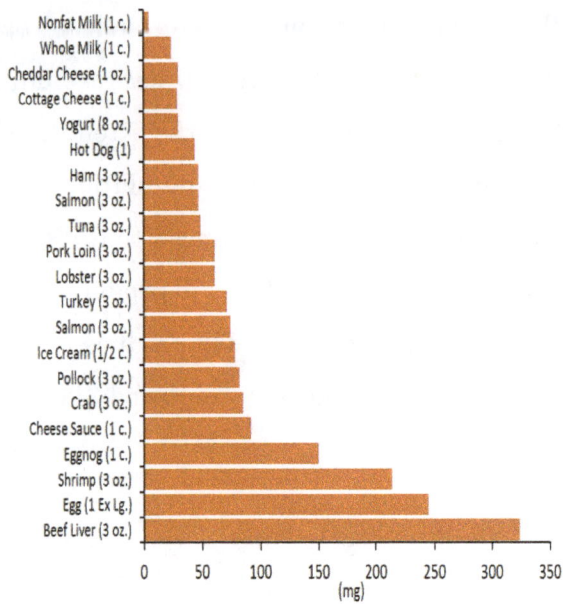

Figure 90. Cholesterol content of various foods[xxi]

There is neither bad nor good cholesterol, despite these descriptions being commonly used for LDL and HDL, respectively. Cholesterol is cholesterol. HDL and LDL contain cholesterol but are lipoproteins that will be described in a later chapter.

[xxi] http://www.nal.usda.gov/fnic/foodcomp/Data/SR21/nutrlist/sr21w601.pdf

3 Macronutrient Digestion

3.1 Digestion at a Glance

Digestion is the process of breaking down food to be absorbed or excreted. Food travels through the gastrointestinal (GI) tract (or 'digestive tract') to be digested.

In simple terms it can be described as a "tube within a tube" As illustrated below. The trunk of our body is the outer tube and the GI tract is the interior tube. Therefore, even though the GI tract is contained within the body, the interior of the tract is technically an exterior surface (like your skin or the mucous membranes of our various body cavities). This is because the contents must be absorbed into the body. If it's not absorbed, it will be excreted and never enter the body itself.

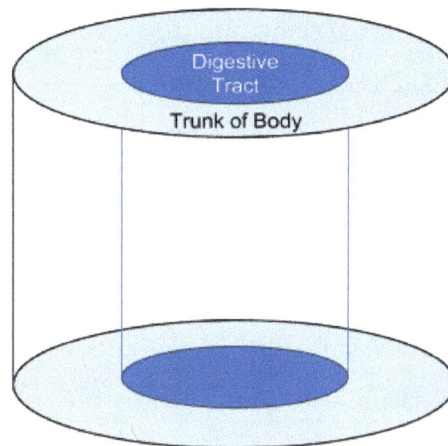

Figure 91. The digestive tract, also known as the gastrointestinal tract, is a "tube within a tube"

Several organs are involved in digestion, which collectively are referred to as the digestive system.

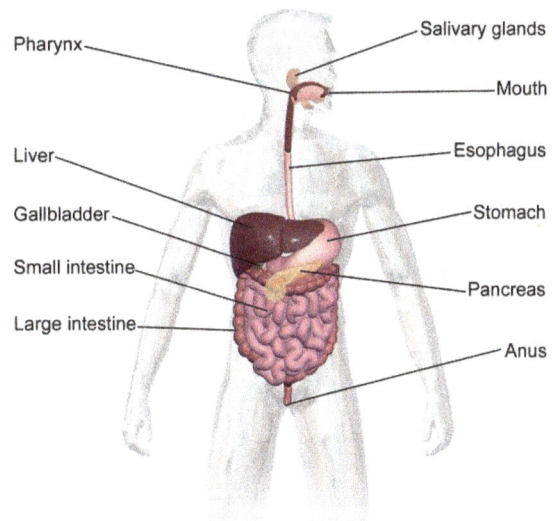

The Components of the Digestive System

Figure 92. The human digestive system[xxii]

---

xxii Blausen.com staff (2014). "Medical gallery of Blausen Medical 2014". *WikiJournal of Medicine* 1 (2). DOI:10.15347/wjm/2014.010. ISSN 2002-4436.

The organs that form the gastrointestinal tract (mouth, oesophagus, stomach, small intestine, large intestine (aka colon), rectum, and anus) come into direct contact with the food or digestive content.

The journey through the gastrointestinal tract starts in the mouth and ends in the anus as shown below:

Mouth → Oesophagus → Stomach → Small Intestine → Large Intestine → Rectum → Anus

In addition to the GI tract, there are digestion accessory organs (salivary glands, pancreas, gallbladder, and liver) that play an integral role in digestion. The accessory organs do not come directly in contact with food or digestive content.

There are several enzymes that are involved in digestion. We will go through each one in detail, but this table should help give an overview of which enzymes are active at each location of the GI tract.

Table 17. Digestive enzymes

Location	Enzyme/Coenzyme
Mouth	Salivary amylase Lingual lipase Lysozyme
Stomach	Pepsin Gastric lipase
	Pancreatic alpha-amylase Brush border disaccharidases Pancreatic lipase
Small Intestine	Colipase Phospholipase-A2 Cholesterol esterase Proteases Brush border peptidases

3.2 Mouth to the Stomach

Digestion begins in the mouth, both mechanically and chemically. Mechanical digestion is called mastication, or the chewing and grinding of food into smaller pieces. The salivary glands release saliva, mucus, and the enzymes, salivary amylase and lysozyme.

Salivary amylase cleaves the alpha 1-4 glycosidic bonds in the starch molecules, amylose and amylopectin. However, salivary amylase cannot cleave the branch points in amylopectin where there are alpha 1-6 glycosidic bonds, as shown in the figure below. Overall this enzyme accounts for a small, albeit important amount of carbohydrate digestion. The amounts of salivary amylase are determined by the copy number of the gene that codes for salivary amylase (AMY 1 CNV) and this is an interesting area of research for determining overall carbohydrate tolerance.

α 1-4 glycosidic bonds

Glycoside = sugar

Amylose – All α 1-4 glycosidic bonds

α 1-4 glycosidic bonds

Branch points are α 1-6 glycosidic bonds, amylase can't cleave

Amylopectin

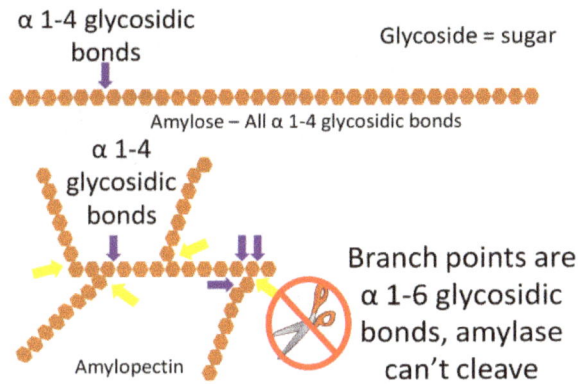

Figure 93. Enzymatic action of salivary amylase. Purple arrows point to alpha 1-4 glycosidic bonds that can be cleaved. The yellow arrows point to the alpha 1-6 glycosidic bonds that cannot be cleaved

Lysozyme helps break down bacteria cell walls to prevent a possible infection. Another enzyme, lingual lipase, is also released in the mouth. Although it is released in the mouth, it is most active in the stomach where it preferentially cleaves short-chain fatty acids in the sn-3 position. Lingual lipase has a small role in digestion in adults, but may be important for infants to help break down triglycerides in breast milk.[35]

3.2.1 Swallowing

After food has been thoroughly chewed and formed into a bolus, it can proceed down the throat to the next stage of digestion. The bolus moves down the pharynx where it reaches a "fork in the road", with the larynx as one road and the oesophagus as the other. The oesophagus leads to the stomach; this is the direction that food

should go. The other road, through the larynx, leads to the trachea and ultimately the lungs. This is not where you want your food or drink going, as this is the pathway for the air you breathe.

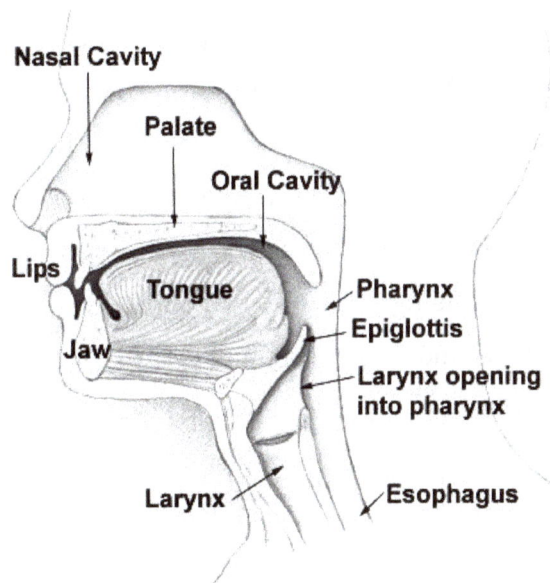

Nasal Cavity
Palate
Oral Cavity
Lips
Tongue
Jaw
Pharynx
Epiglottis
Larynx opening into pharynx
Larynx
Esophagus

Figure 94. Cross section of the human head

Fortunately, our body was designed in such a way that a small mass of tissue, the epiglottis, covers the opening to the trachea. It directs the food down the correct 'road'.

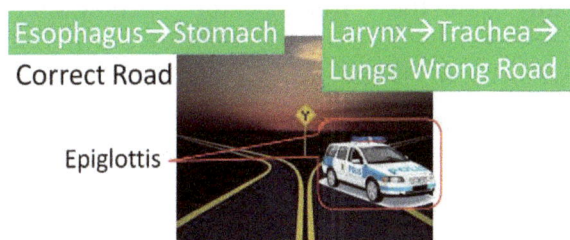

Esophagus→Stomach Correct Road
Larynx→Trachea→Lungs Wrong Road
Epiglottis

Figure 95. Epiglottis is like a traffic cop guiding food down the correct digestion road

3.2.2 Oesophagus

Before being correctly guided into the oesophagus, the bolus of food will travel through the upper oesophageal sphincter. Sphincters are circular muscles that are found throughout the gastrointestinal tract that essentially serve as gates between the different sections. Once in the oesophagus, wavelike muscular movements, known as peristalsis, occur, to guide the food down the GI tract.

At the end of the oesophagus the bolus will encounter the lower oesophageal sphincter. This sphincter keeps the harmful acids of the stomach out of the oesophagus. However, in many people this sphincter is leaky, which allows stomach acid to reflux, or creep up, the oesophagus. Stomach acid is very acidic (has a low pH). The diagram below gives you an idea of just how acidic the stomach is. Notice that the pH of gastric (term used to describe the stomach) fluid is lower (more acidic) than any of the listed items besides battery acid.

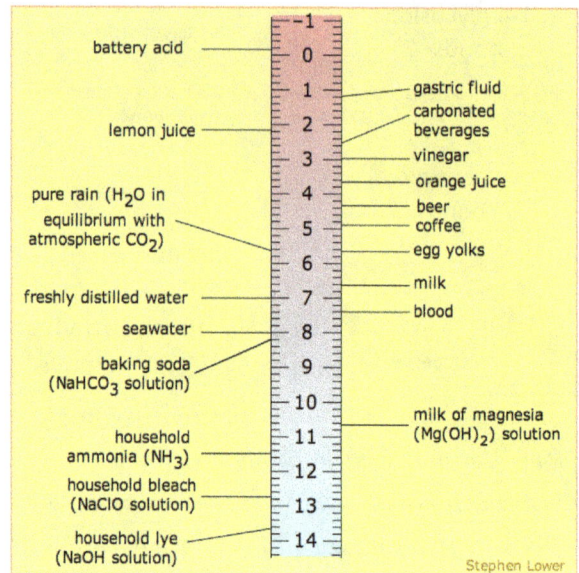

Figure 96. pH of common items[xxiii]

The leaking of the very acidic gastric contents results in a burning sensation, commonly referred to as "heartburn." If this occurs more than twice per week and is severe, the person may have gastroesophageal/gastro-oesophageal reflux disease (GERD or GORD).

Table 18. Chemical digestion in the mouth

Macronutrient	Action
Carbohydrates	Salivary amylase cleaves 1,4-glycosidic bonds
Lipids	Release of lingual lipase
Protein	None

3.2.3 Stomach

After going through the lower oesophageal sphincter, food enters the stomach. Our stomach is involved in both chemical and

---

mechanical digestion. Mechanical digestion occurs as the stomach churns and grinds food into a semisolid substance called chime, consisting of partially digested food.

The lining of the stomach is made up of different layers of tissue. The mucosa is the outermost layer.

The mucosa is not a flat surface. Instead, its surface is lined by gastric 'pits'. Gastric pits are indentations in the stomach's surface that are lined by four distinct types of cells.

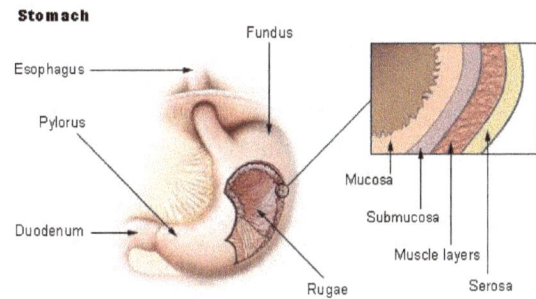

Figure 97. Anatomy of the stomach

At the bottom of the gastric pit are the G cells that secrete the hormone gastrin. Gastrin stimulates the parietal and chief cells that are found above the G cells. The chief cells secrete the zymogen pepsinogen and the enzyme gastric lipase. A zymogen is an inactive precursor of an enzyme that must be altered to form the active enzyme. The parietal cells secrete hydrochloric acid (HCl), which lowers the pH of the gastric juice (water + enzymes + acid). The HCl inactivates salivary amylase and catalyses

the conversion of pepsinogen to pepsin. Finally, the top of the pits are the neck cells that secrete mucus to prevent the gastric juice from digesting or damaging the stomach mucosa.[36] The table below summarizes the actions of the different cells in the gastric pits.

Table 19. Cells involved in the digestive processes in the stomach

Type of Cell	Secrete
Neck	Mucus
Chief	Pepsinogen and gastric lipase
Parietal	HCl
G	Gastrin

The figure below shows the action of all these different secretions in the stomach.

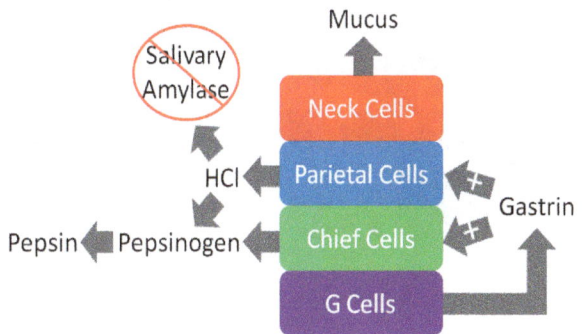

Figure 98. The action of gastric secretions in the stomach

To reiterate, the figure above illustrates that the neck cells of the gastric pits secrete mucus to protect the mucosa of the stomach from essentially digesting itself. Gastrin from the G cells stimulates the parietal and chief cells to secrete HCl and enzymes, respectively.

69

The HCl in the stomach denatures salivary amylase and other proteins by breaking down their structure and, thus, function. HCl also converts pepsinogen to the active enzyme pepsin. Pepsin is a protease, meaning that it cleaves bonds in proteins. It breaks down the proteins in food into individual peptides (shorter segments of amino acids). The other enzyme that is active in the stomach is gastric lipase. This enzyme preferentially cleaves the sn-3 position of triglycerides to produce 1,2-diglyceride and a free fatty acid, as shown below.[22] It is responsible for up to 20% of triglyceride digestion.[36]

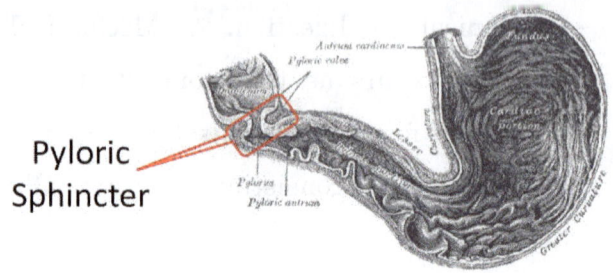

Figure 100. Cross section of the stomach showing the pyloric sphincter[xxiv]

Table 20. Summary of chemical digestion in the stomach

Chemical or Enzyme	Action
Gastrin	Stimulates chief cells to release pepsinogen Stimulates parietal cells to release HCl
HCl	Denatures salivary amylase Denatures proteins Activates pepsinogen to pepsin
Pepsin	Cleaves proteins to peptides
Gastric lipase	Cleaves sn-3 FA of triglycerides

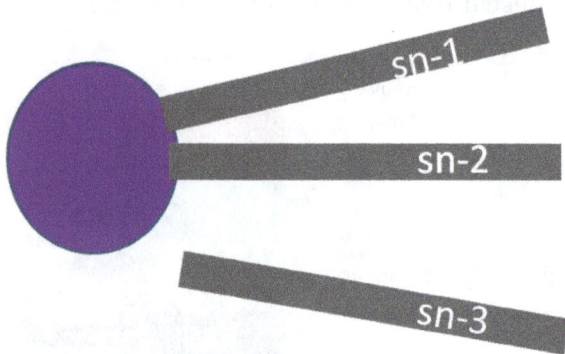

Figure 99. Gastric Lipase action results in production of 1,2-diglyceride and a free fatty acid

The chyme will then leave the stomach and enter the small intestine via the pyloric sphincter (shown below).

3.3 Small Intestine

The small intestine is the primary site of digestion. It is divided into three sections: the duodenum, jejunum, and ileum (shown below). Chyme leaves the stomach and first encounters the duodenum.

[xxiv] Public Domain. From Anatomy of the Human Body. Henry Gray, 1918

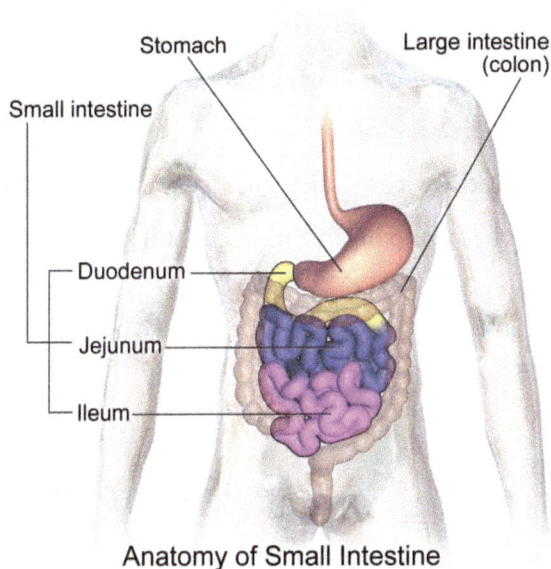

Anatomy of Small Intestine

Figure 101. Anatomy of the small intestine[xxv]

The small intestine consists of many layers. We are going to focus on the external layer—the epithelium, which meets the chyme and is responsible for absorption. The 'channel' or the space within the intestinal cavity is known as the 'lumen'.

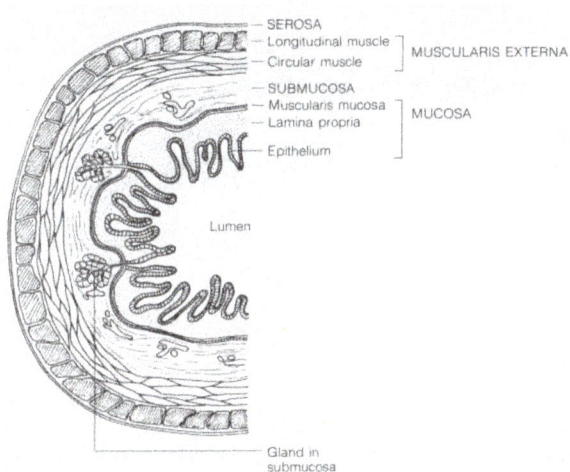

Figure 102. Cross-section of the intestinal lumen[xxvi]

The organization of the small intestine is in such a way that it contains circular folds and finger-like projections known as villi.

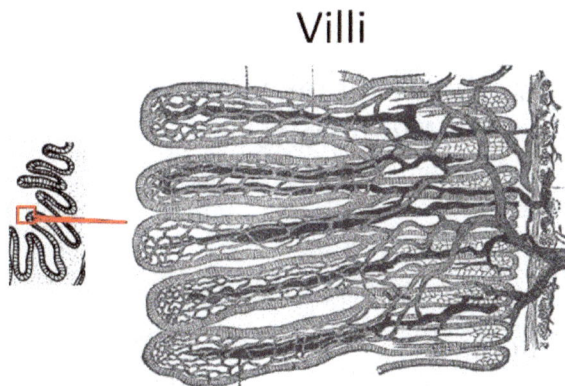

Figure 103. Villi line the surface of the small intestine[xxvii]

If we were to zoom in even closer, we would be able to see that enterocytes (small intestine absorptive cells) line villi as shown below.

xxv Blausen.com staff (2014). "Medical gallery of Blausen Medical 2014". *WikiJournal of Medicine* **1** (2). DOI:10.15347/wjm/2014.010. ISSN 2002-4436

xxvi Author unknown, NCI, http://visualsonline.cancer.gov/details.cfm?imageid=1781

xxvii Public Domain. Anatomy of the Human Body by Henry Gray, 1918. http://commons.wikimedia.org/wiki/Image:Gray1061.png

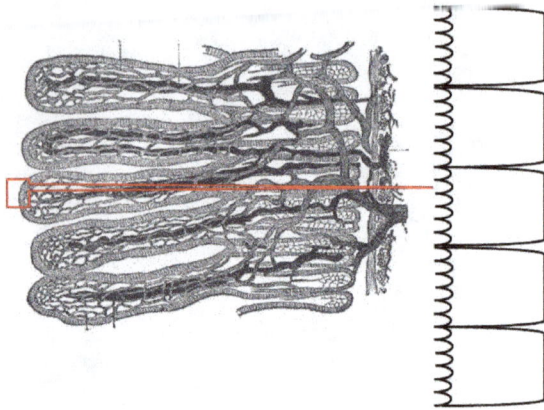

Figure 104. Enterocytes lining the villi

The side, or membrane, of the enterocyte that faces the lumen is not smooth either. It is lined with microvilli and is known as the brush border (or *apical*) membrane, as shown below.

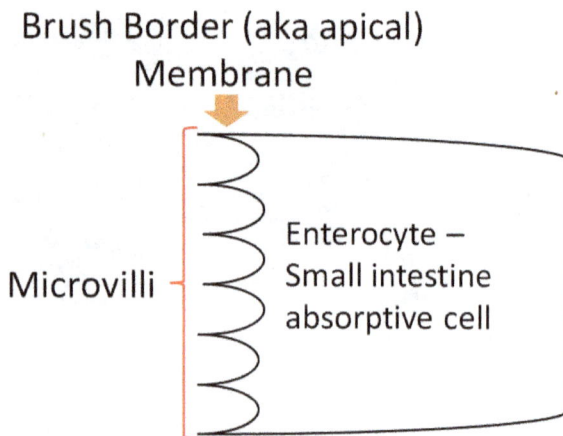

Figure 105. Enterocyte, or small intestinal absorptive cell is lined with microvilli. This lined surface is referred to as the brush border membrane

Together these features (folds + villi + microvilli) increase the surface area some 600-fold over a smooth surface. This greater surface area provides for more contact surface between food particles and their constituents and the enterocytes and thus, increases absorption.[15]

The surface of the microvilli is further covered by the hair-like glycocalyx, made up of glycoproteins and carbohydrates as shown below.

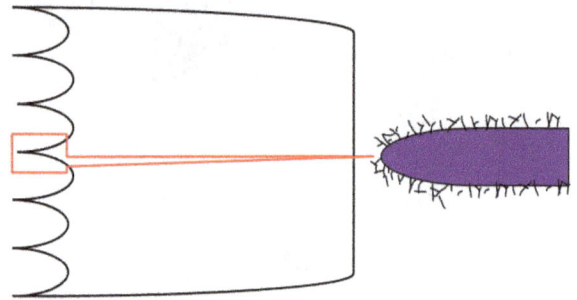

Figure 106. Glycocalyx lines the microvilli

3.4 Digestive Hormones, Accessory Organs & Secretions

Before we go into the digestive details of the small intestine, it is important that you have a basic understanding of the anatomy and physiology of the following digestion accessory organs: pancreas, liver, and gallbladder. Digestion accessory organs assist in digestion but are not part of the gastrointestinal tract.

How are these organs involved?

Upon entering the duodenum, chyme causes the release of two hormones from the small intestine: secretin and cholecystokinin (CCK, previously known as pancreozymin) in response to acid and fat, respectively. These hormones have multiple effects on different tissues. In the pancreas, secretin stimulates the secretion of bicarbonate (HCO_3), while CCK stimulates the secretion of digestive enzymes. The bicarbonate and digestive enzymes released together are collectively known as pancreatic juice, which travels to the small intestine, as shown below.

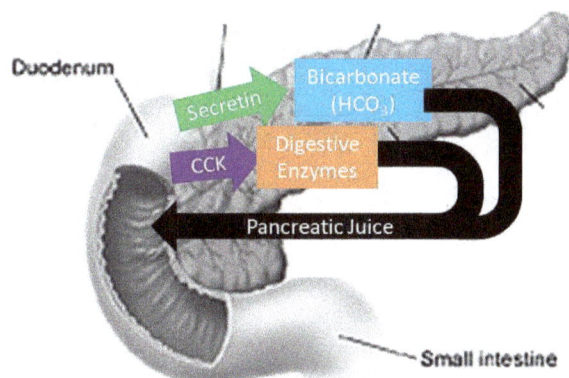

Figure 107. The hormones secretin and CCK stimulate the pancreas to secrete pancreatic juice[xxviii]

In addition, CCK also stimulates the contraction of the gallbladder causing the secretion of bile into the duodenum.

3.4.1 Pancreas

The pancreas is found behind the stomach and has two different portions. It has an endocrine (hormone-producing) portion that contains alpha and beta cells that secrete the hormones glucagon and insulin, respectively. However, most of the pancreas is made up of acini, or acinar

cells, that are responsible for producing pancreatic juice.

Bicarbonate is a base (high pH) meaning that it can help neutralize acid. You can find sodium bicarbonate ($NaHCO_3$, baking soda) on the ruler below to get an idea of its pH.

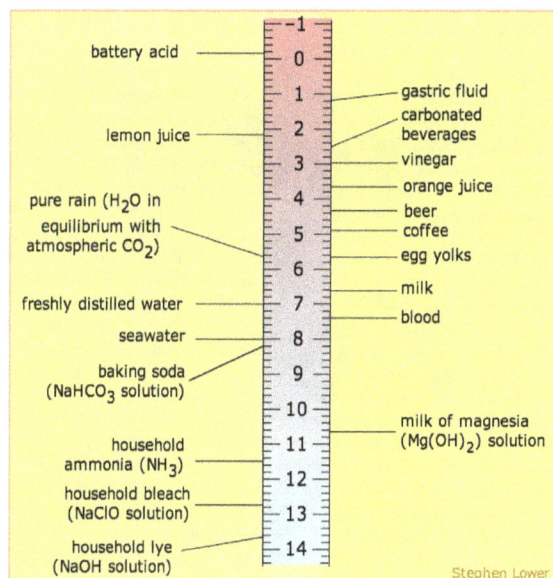

The main digestive enzymes in pancreatic juice are listed in the table below. Their function will be discussed further in later subsections.

Table 21. Enzymes in pancreatic juice

Enzyme
Pancreatic alpha-amylase
Proteases
Pancreatic lipase & procolipase*
Phospholipase A_2
Cholesterol Esterase

*Not an enzyme

---

xxviii Adapted from Don Bliss, NCI, http://visualsonline.cancer.gov

3.4.2   Liver

The liver is the largest internal and most metabolically active organ in the body. The figure below shows the liver and the accessory organs position relative to the stomach.

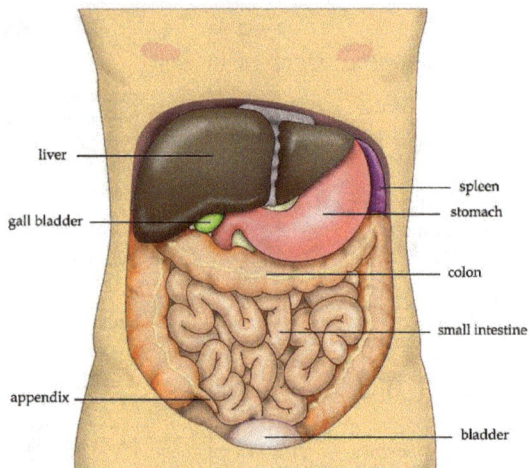

Figure 108. *Location of the digestive organs*

The liver is made up two major types of cells. The primary liver cells are hepatocytes, which carry out most of the liver's functions. Hepatic is another term for liver. For example, if you are going to refer to liver concentrations of a certain nutrient, these are often reported as hepatic concentrations. The other major cell type is the hepatic stellate ('Ito') cells. These are fat storing cells in the liver.

The liver's key role in digestion is to produce bile. This is a greenish-yellow fluid that is composed primarily of bile acids, but also contains cholesterol,

phospholipids, and the pigments bilirubin and biliverdin. Bile acids are synthesized from cholesterol. The two primary bile acids are chenodeoxycholic acid and cholic acid. In the same way that fatty acids are found in the form of salts, these bile acids can also be found as salts. These salts have an (-ate) ending, as shown below.

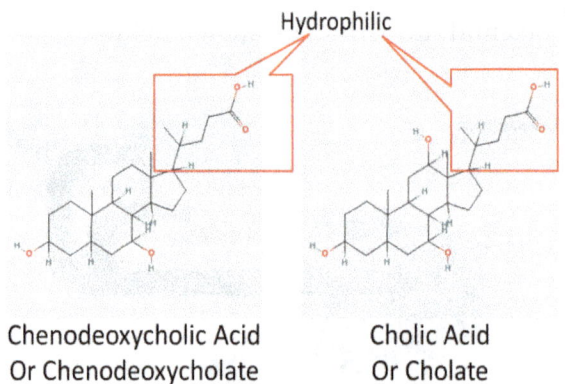

| Chenodeoxycholic Acid | Cholic Acid |
| Or Chenodeoxycholate | Or Cholate |

Figure 109. *Structures of the two primary bile acids*

Bile acids, like phospholipids, have a hydrophobic and hydrophilic end. This makes them excellent emulsifiers that are instrumental in fat digestion. Bile is then transported to the gallbladder.

3.4.3   Gallbladder

The gallbladder is a small, sac-like organ found just off the liver (see figures above). Its primary function is to store and concentrate bile made by the liver. The bile is then transported to the duodenum through the common bile duct.

3.4.3.1 Why do we need bile?

Bile is important because fat is hydrophobic and the environment in the lumen of the small intestine is watery. In addition, there is an unstirred water layer that fat must cross to reach the enterocytes to be absorbed.

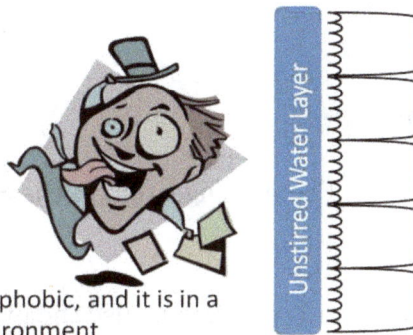

Fat is hydrophobic, and it is in a watery environment

Figure 110. Fat is not happy alone in the watery environment of the small intestine

Here triglycerides form large triglyceride droplets to keep the interaction with the watery environment to a minimum. This is inefficient for digestion, because enzymes cannot access the interior of the droplet. Bile acts as an emulsifier, or detergent. It, along with phospholipids, forms smaller triglyceride droplets that increase access for triglyceride digesting enzymes, as indicated below.

• Emulsifier or Detergent

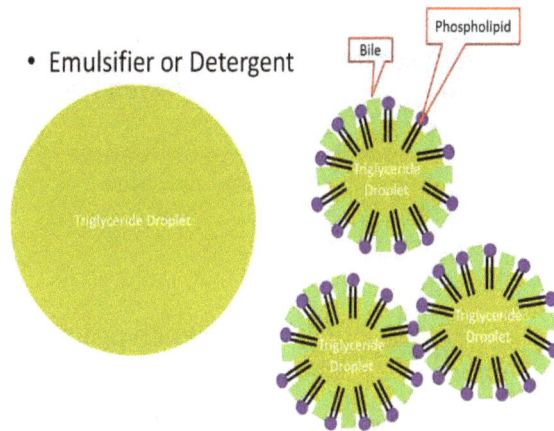

Figure 111. Bile acids and phospholipids facilitate the production of smaller triglyceride droplets

Secretin and CCK also control the production and secretion of bile. Secretin stimulates the flow of bile from the liver to the gallbladder. CCK stimulates the gallbladder to contract, causing bile to be secreted into the duodenum.

3.4.4 Carbohydrate Digestion in the Small Intestine

The small intestine is the primary site of carbohydrate digestion. Pancreatic alpha-amylase is the primary carbohydrate digesting enzyme. Pancreatic alpha-amylase, like salivary amylase, cleaves the alpha 1-4 glycosidic bonds of carbohydrates, reducing them to simpler carbohydrates, such as glucose, maltose, maltotriose, and dextrins (oligosaccharides containing 1 or more alpha 1-6 glycosidic bonds). Pancreatic amylase is also unable to cleave the branch point alpha 1-6 bonds.[36]

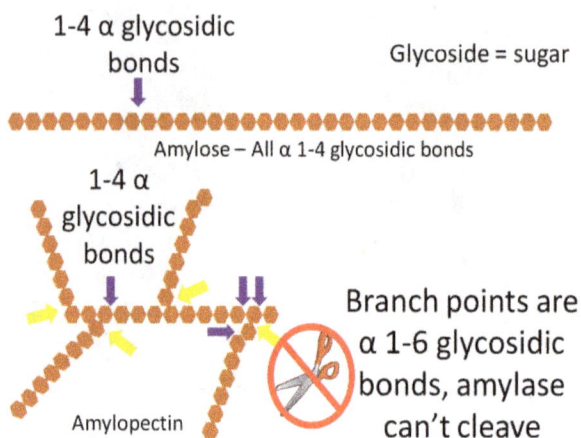

Figure 112. The function of pancreatic amylase

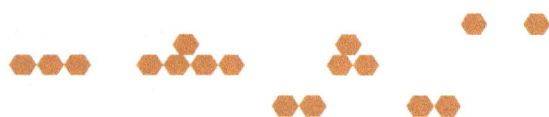

Figure 113. Products of pancreatic amylase

The pancreatic amylase products, along with the disaccharides sucrose and lactose, then move to the surface of the enterocyte. Here, there are disaccharidase enzymes (lactase, sucrase, maltase) on the outside of the enterocyte. Enzymes, like these, that are on the outside of cell walls are referred to as ectoenzymes. Individual monosaccharides are formed when lactase cleaves lactose, sucrase cleaves sucrose, and maltase cleaves maltose. There is also another brush border enzyme, alpha-dextrinase. This enzyme cleaves alpha 1-6 glycosidic bonds in dextrins, primarily the branch point bonds in amylopectin. The products from these brush border enzymes are the single monosaccharides glucose, fructose, and galactose that are ready for absorption into the enterocyte.[36]

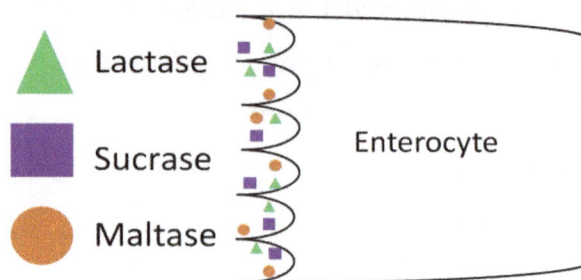

Figure 114. Disaccharidases on the outside of the enterocyte

3.4.5 Protein Digestion in the Small Intestine

The small intestine is also the major site of protein digestion by proteases (enzymes that cleave proteins). The pancreas secretes several proteases as zymogens into the duodenum where they must be activated before they can cleave peptide bonds.[1] This activation occurs through an activation cascade. A cascade is a series of reactions in which one step activates the next in a sequence that results in an amplification of the response. A cascade using trypsinogen → trypsin as an example, is shown below.

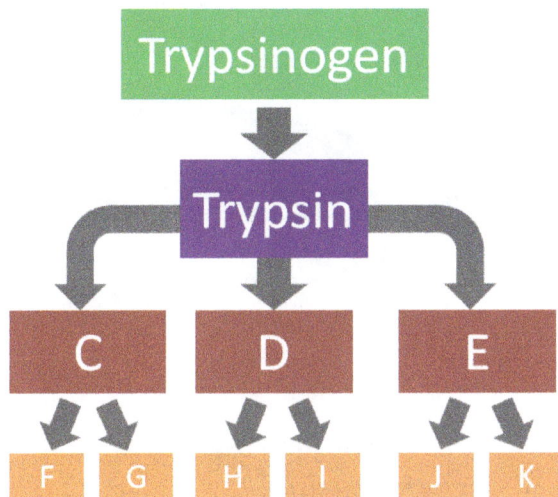

Figure 115. Example of a cascade

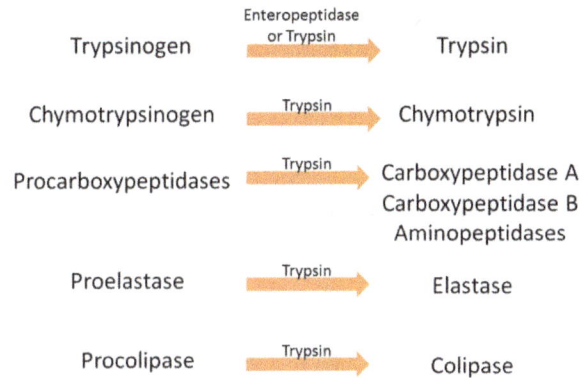

Figure 116. The protease/colipase activation cascade

In this example, A activates B, B activates C, D, and E, C activates F and G, D activates H and I, and E activates K and L. Cascades also help to serve as control points for certain process. In the protease cascade, the activation of B is important because it starts the cascade.

The protease/colipase activation scheme starts with the enzyme enteropeptidase (secreted from the intestinal brush border) that converts trypsinogen to trypsin. Trypsin can activate all the proteases (including itself) and colipase (involved in fat digestion)[1] as shown in the 2 figures below.

The products of the action of the proteases on proteins are dipeptides, tripeptides, and individual amino acids, as shown below.

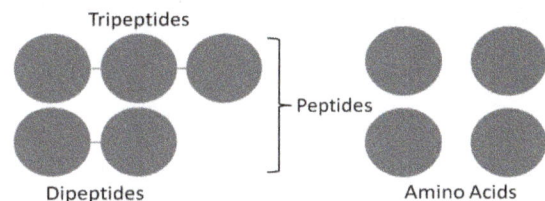

Figure 117. Products of pancreatic proteases

At the brush border, much like disaccharidases, there are peptidases that cleave some peptides down to amino acids. Not all peptides are cleaved to individual amino acids, because small peptides can be taken up into the enterocyte, thus, the peptides do not need to be completely broken down to individual amino acids. Thus the end products of protein digestion are primarily dipeptides and tripeptides, along with individual amino acids.[36]

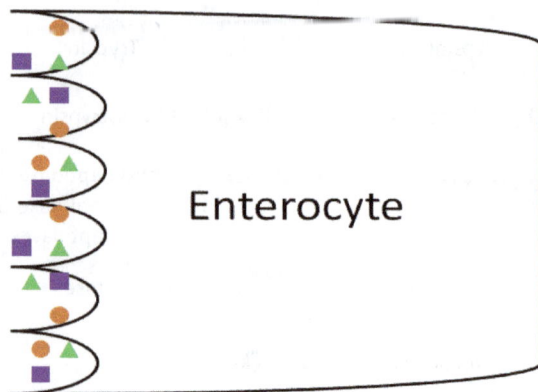

Figure 118. Peptidases are produced by the brush border to cleave some peptides

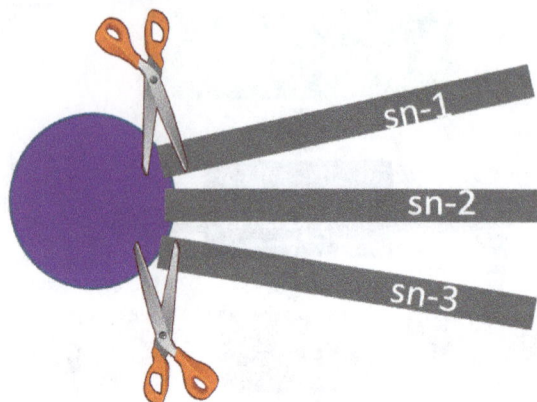

Figure 119. Pancreatic lipase cleaves the sn-1 and sn-3 fatty acids of triglycerides

3.4.6 Lipid Digestion in the Small Intestine

The small intestine is the major site for lipid digestion. There are specific enzymes for the digestion of triglycerides, phospholipids, and cleavage of esters from cholesterol. We will look at each in this section.

3.4.6.1 Triglycerides

The pancreas secretes pancreatic lipase into the duodenum as part of pancreatic juice. This major triglyceride digestion enzyme preferentially cleaves the sn-1 and sn-3 fatty acids from triglycerides. This cleavage results in the formation of a 2-monoglyceride and two free fatty acids as shown below.

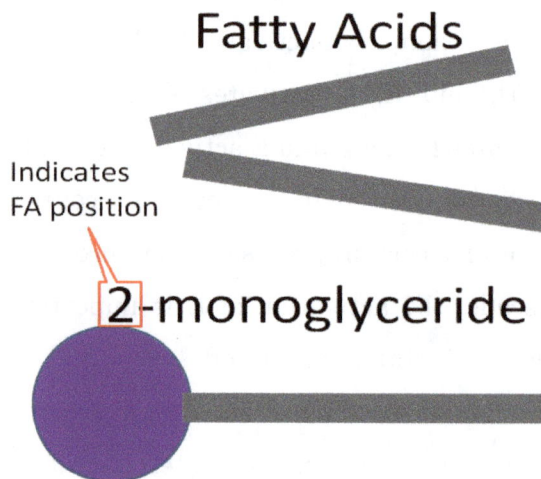

Figure 120. The products of pancreatic lipase are a 2-monoglyceride and two free fatty acids

To assist lipase, colipase serves as an anchor point to help lipase attach to the triglyceride droplet.

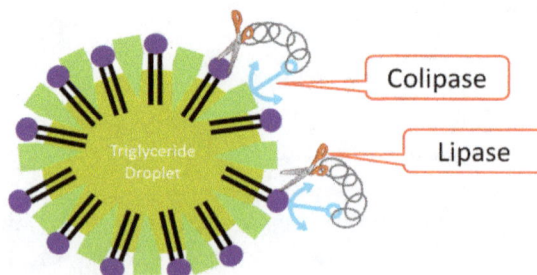

Figure 121. Colipase helps anchor lipase to the triglyceride droplet

3.4.6.2 Short and Medium Chain Fatty Acid Digestion

Not all triglycerides and their fatty acids are digested and absorbed via micellar and chylomicron mediated pathways. As a rule of thumb 'the shorter the fatty acid chain length, the more will be deposited (passively) directly into the hepatic portal vein.

This is important for the clinician to know as this has application for encouraging ketosis and ketogenesis and for use with those whose bile salt production of release is inhibited (for example those who have had their gall bladder removed.)

Table 22. Hepatic portal vein deposition of various fatty acids

Fatty Acid		Portal Vein Deposition (%)	Study Type
C8:0	Caprylic Acid	65	Pig[37]
C10:0	Capric Acid	54	Pig
C12:0	Lauric Acid	72	Rat[38]
C14:0	Myristic Acid	58	Rat
C16:0	Palmitic Acid	41	Rat
C18:0	Stearic Acid	28	Rat
C18:2	Linoleic Acid	58	Rat
C18:3	Linolenic Acid	68	Rat

3.4.6.3 Phospholipids

The enzyme phospholipase A_2 cleaves the C-2 fatty acid of lecithin, producing lysolecithin and a free fatty acid.

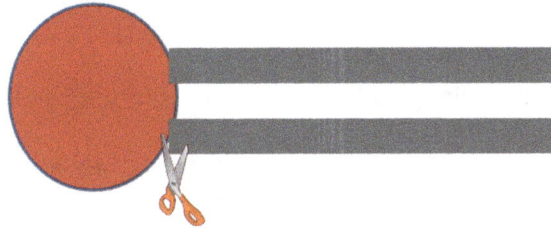

Figure 122. Phospholipase A2 cleaves the C-2 fatty acid of lecithin

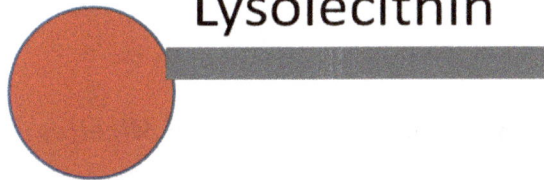

Figure 123. Products of phospholipase A2 cleavage

3.4.6.4 Cholesterol Esters

The fatty acid in cholesterol esters is cleaved by the enzyme, cholesterol esterase, producing cholesterol and a free fatty acid.

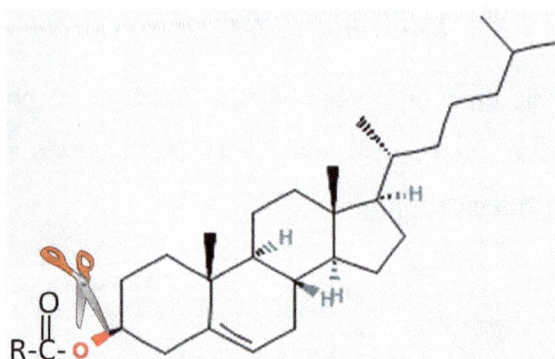

Figure 124. Cholesterol esterase cleaves fatty acids off cholesterol

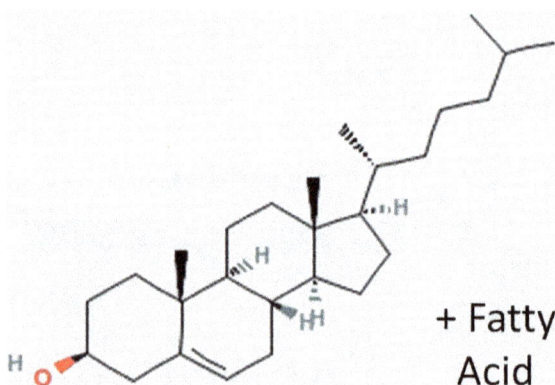

Figure 125. Products of cholesterol esterase

3.4.6.5 *Formation of Mixed Micelles*

If nothing else happened at this point, the 2-monoglycerides and fatty acids produced by pancreatic lipase would form micelles. The hydrophilic heads would be outward, and the fatty acids would be buried on the interior. These micelles are not sufficiently water-soluble to cross the unstirred water layer to get to the brush border of enterocytes. Thus, mixed micelles are formed containing cholesterol, bile acids, and lysolecithin in addition to the 2-monoglycerides and fatty acids, as illustrated below.[36]

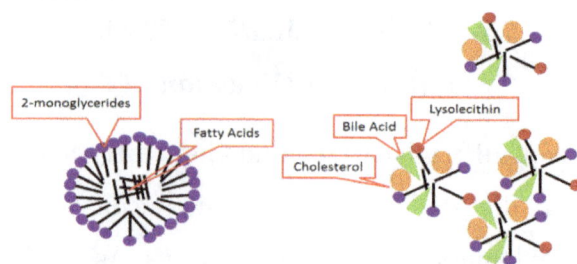

Figure 126. Normal (left) and mixed (right) micelles

Mixed micelles are more water-soluble, allowing them to cross the unstirred water layer to the brush border of enterocytes for absorption.

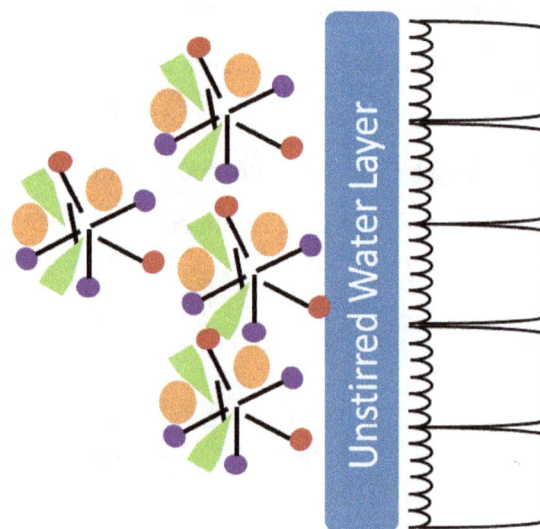

Figure 127. Mixed micelles can cross the unstirred water layer for absorption into the enterocytes

3.5 The Large Intestine

Anything that escapes digestion in the small intestine reaches the large intestine. The ileocaecal valve is the sphincter between the ileum and the large intestine. This name should make more sense as we go through the anatomy of the large intestine.

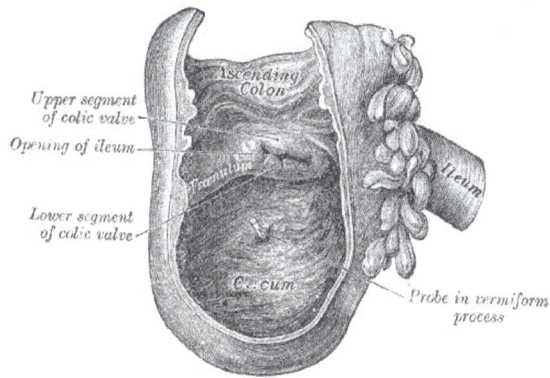

Figure 128. The ileocaecal valve[xxix]

The large intestine consists of the colon, the rectum, and the anus. The colon can be further divided into the caecum (hence the -caecal in ileocaecal valve, ileo- refers to ileum), ascending colon, transverse colon, descending colon, and sigmoid colon as shown below.

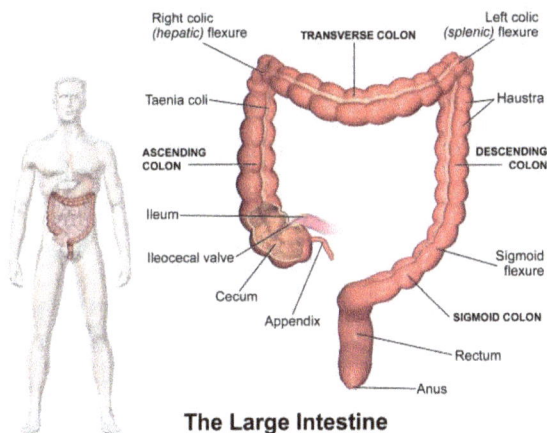

The Large Intestine

Figure 129. Anatomy of the large intestine and rectum[xxx]

The large intestine is responsible for absorbing remaining water and electrolytes (sodium, potassium, and chloride). It also forms and excretes faeces. The large intestine also contains copious amounts of microorganisms (microbiota) and forms a large part of our internal 'microbiome'. The large intestine can also be referred to as the gut. There are many microorganisms found throughout the gastrointestinal tract that collectively are referred to as the flora, microflora, biota, microbiome or microbiota. The terms microbiome and microbiota are generally used synonymously, although technically the microbiome refers to the collective genomes of the organisms, whereas the microbiota refers to the organisms themselves. For simplicity, we will use the terms interchangeably.

The human body contains well over ten times more microbial cells than human cells accounting for up to 3% of our total body-mass. These 'non-human' cells include over 10,000 varieties of bacteria, viruses, protozoa, prions and bacteriophages with over eight million unique, protein-coding genes (in comparison to our 22,000).[39] These various organisms that we house have co-evolved with since the beginning of time and we have reached a level of symbiosis, which by

---

[xxix] Public Domain. From Henry Gray (1918) *Anatomy of the Human Body*, Plate 1075

[xxx] Blausen.com staff (2014). "Medical gallery of Blausen Medical 2014". *WikiJournal of Medicine* 1 (2). DOI:10.15347/wjm/2014.010. ISSN 2002-4436. -

dofinition means that we need them, and they us. Suffice it to say that having a healthy balance of gut flora is essential to optimal health, body-composition and performance. As can be seen in the figure below, the density of microorganisms' increases as you move down the digestive tract.

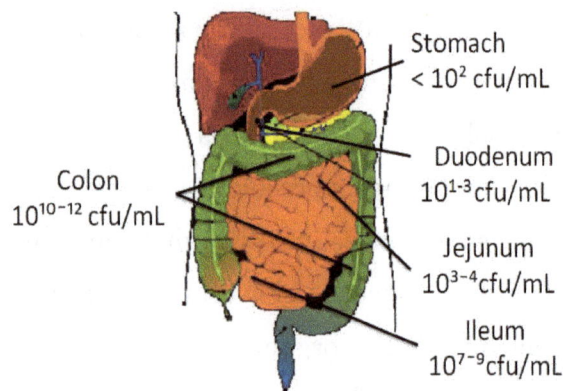

Figure 130. Relative number of bacteria in selected locations of the GI tract. cfu/ml = colony forming unit, a measure of the number of live microorganisms in 1 mL of digestive sample

As described in the fibre sections, there are two different fates for fibre once it reaches the large intestine. Fermentable, viscous fibre is fermented by bacteria. Fermentation is the metabolism of compounds by the microorganisms in the gut. An example of fermentation is the utilization of the oligosaccharides raffinose and stachyose by microorganisms that results in the production of gas, which can lead to flatulence. Also, some bile acids are fermented by microorganisms to form secondary bile acids that can be reabsorbed. These secondary bile acids represent approximately 20% of the total bile acids in our body. Fermentable fibres can be used to form short-chain fatty acids, such as butyrate (C:4:0), that can then be absorbed and used by the body. The nonfermentable, non-viscous fibre is not really altered and will be a component of faeces, which is then excreted through the rectum and anus. This process involves both an internal and external sphincter that are shown in figure 3.63 above.

3.5.1 Probiotics & Prebiotics

Increasing attention is being paid to the microbiome and its effect on health. Within the gastrointestinal system there are a variety of bacteria, some of which are considered health promoting and others health degrading, although it may simply be that we need a particular 'balance' of various microbes to ensure optimal health of the gut and the entire bodily system. In addition to bacteria there are yeasts, fungus, protozoa, viruses and bacteriophages that inhabit the gut and that have a role to play in local and general health, although much of this role is yet to be fully elucidated.

Probiotics and prebiotic compounds have garnered attention for improving various health outcomes.

A probiotic is a live microorganism that is consumed and colonizes in the body as shown in the figures below.

A prebiotic is a non-digestible food component that selectively stimulates the growth of beneficial intestinal bacteria. An example of a prebiotic is inulin.

The net result is the same for both prebiotics and probiotics, an increase in the ratio of beneficial to non-beneficial microorganisms.

Some examples of prebiotics other than inulin include, other fructose-containing oligosaccharides and polysaccharides, and resistant starch. Inulin is a polysaccharide that contains mainly fructoses that are joined by beta-bonds, which allows them to survive digestion. The structure of inulin is shown below.

about fibres and resistant starches can be found in the section on fibres in this text.

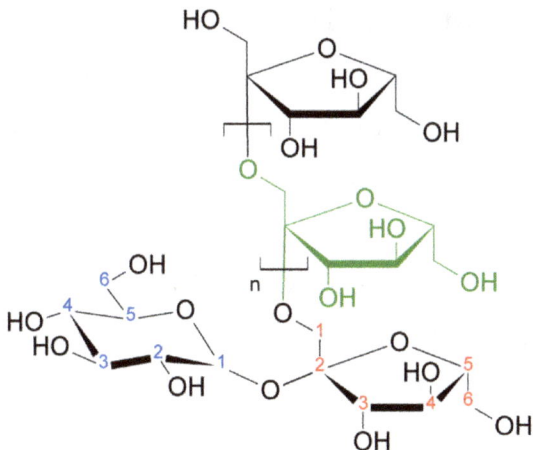

Figure 131. Structure of insulin

Resistant starch is so named because it is a starch that is resistant to digestion. More

4 Macronutrient Uptake, Absorption & Transport

The term absorption can have several different meanings. For clarity, when we refer to absorption, this is the uptake of a compound into the body's circulation. Thus, if something is taken up into the enterocyte, it is not necessarily absorbed. Hopefully after this chapter, the reasoning for this distinction will be clear.

4.1 Crypts of Lieberkuhn & Enterocyte Maturation

There are some additional anatomical and physiological features of the small intestine that are important to understand before we start talking about uptake and absorption. Crypts of Lieberkuhn are pits between villi.

The crypts of Lieberkuhn (often referred to simply as crypts) are like the gastric pits in the stomach. The crypts contain stem cells that can produce a number of different cell types, including enterocytes.[22] Immature enterocyte cells form and migrate up the villi as they mature. Thus, the tips at the top of villi are where the mature, fully functioning enterocytes are located.

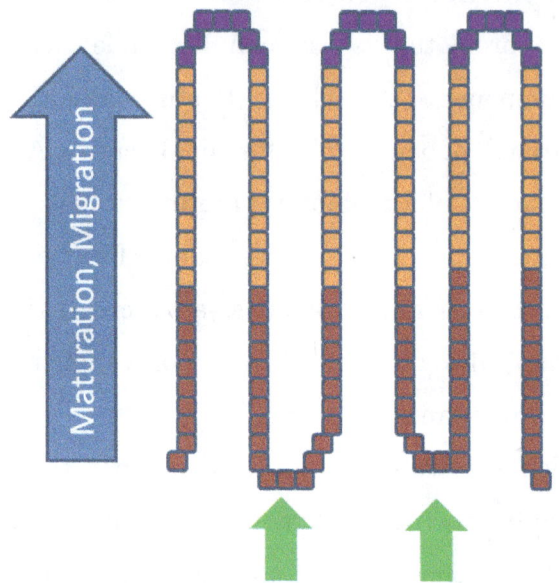

Figure 132. Crypts are represented by green arrows; fully mature enterocytes are represented by the purple cells at the top of the villi

This maturation and migration is a continuous process. The life cycle of an enterocyte is 72 hours once it enters the villus from the crypt.[36] At the top, enterocytes are sloughed off, and, unless they are digested (they predominantly contain proteins and lipid) and components are taken up by enterocytes still on villi, they will be excreted in faeces as depicted in Figure 133.

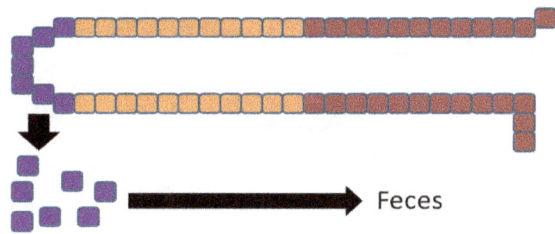

Figure 133. Enterocytes sloughed off the villus. Unless these cells are digested, and their components are taken up by other enterocytes on the villus, they will be excreted in faeces

Figure 4.13

So, we define absorption as reaching circulation within the body, because compounds taken up into enterocytes might not make it into body-circulation, and thus are not necessarily absorbed.

4.2 Uptake Line-up & Cell Membranes

Having completed digestion in the small intestine, a few compounds are ready for uptake into the enterocyte. The figure below shows the macronutrient uptake line-up, or what is ready to be taken up into the enterocyte.

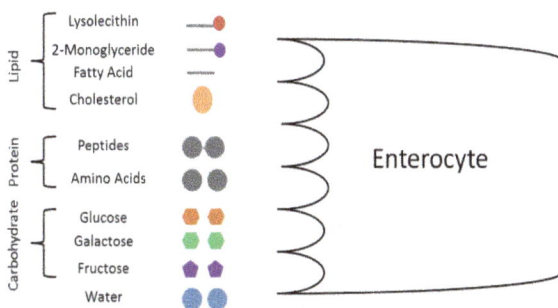

Figure 134. The macronutrient uptake line-up

From lipids, we have the lysolecithin (from phospholipid), 2-monoglyceride (from triglycerides), fatty acids, and cholesterol. From protein, there are small peptides (di- and tripeptides) and amino acids. From carbohydrates, only the monosaccharides glucose, galactose, and fructose will be taken up. The other macronutrient, water, has not been discussed so far because it does not undergo digestion.

However, these compounds must now cross the plasma (cell) membrane, which is a phospholipid bilayer. In the cell membrane, the hydrophilic heads of the phospholipids point into the lumen as well as towards the interior of the cell, while the tails are on the interior of the plasma membrane as shown below.

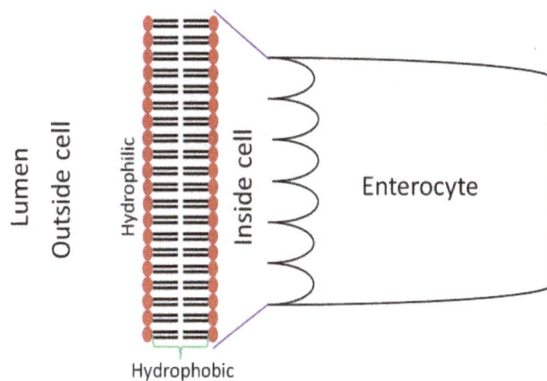

Figure 135. Plasma membrane of a cell

The plasma membrane contains proteins, cholesterol, and carbohydrates in addition to the phospholipids. Membrane proteins, such as channels and pumps, are important for the transport of some compounds across the cell membrane.

4.3 Carbohydrate Uptake, Absorption, Transport & Liver Uptake

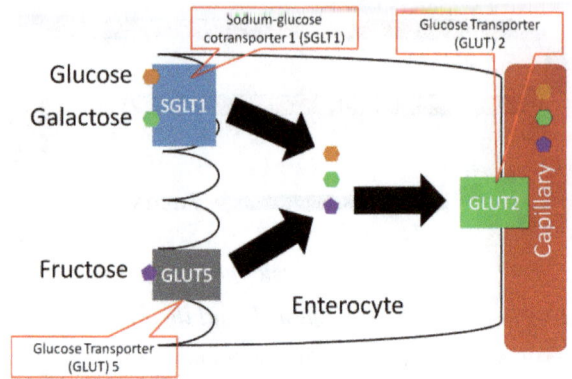

Figure 136. Carbohydrate uptake and absorption

Monosaccharides are taken up into the enterocyte. Glucose and galactose are taken up by the sodium-glucose cotransporter 1 (SGLT1, active carrier transport). The cotransporter part of the name of this transporter means that it also transports sodium along with glucose or galactose. Fructose is taken up by facilitated diffusion through glucose transporter (GLUT) 5. There are 12 glucose transporters that are named GLUT 1-12, and all use facilitated diffusion to transport monosaccharides. The different GLUTs have distinct functions and are expressed in different tissues. Thus, the intestine might be high in GLUT5, but not in GLUT12. Moving back to monosaccharides, inside the enterocyte, all three are then transported out of the enterocyte into the capillary (absorbed) through GLUT2 (figure 4.41.)

Inside of each villus there are capillaries and lacteal as shown below. Capillaries are the smallest blood vessels in the body, lacteal are also small vessels but are part of the lymphatic system, as will be described further in a later subsection.

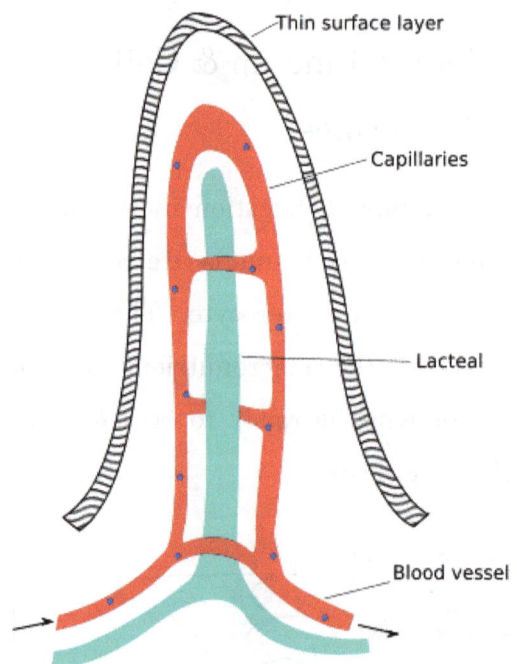

Figure 137. Anatomy of a villus

The capillaries in the small intestine join to the portal vein, which transports monosaccharides directly to the liver. The figure below shows the portal vein and all the smaller vessels from the stomach, small intestine, and large intestine that feed into it.

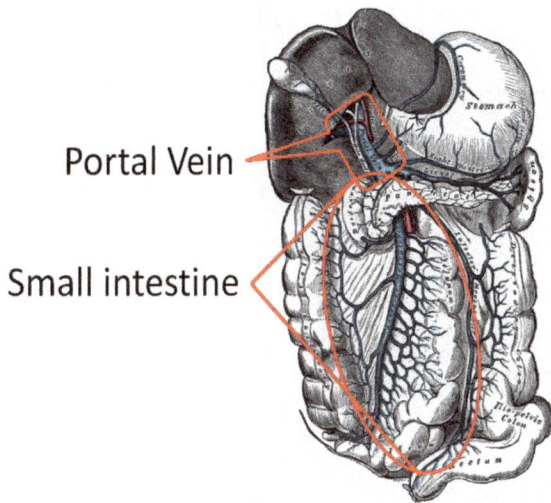

Figure 138. The portal vein transports monosaccharides, amino acids and some fatty acids to the liver

At the liver, galactose and fructose are completely taken up through GLUT5, while only 30-40% of glucose is taken up through GLUT2. After the monosaccharides are taken up, they are phosphorylated by their respective kinase enzymes forming galactose-1-phosphate, fructose-1-phosphate, and glucose-6-phosphate as shown below.

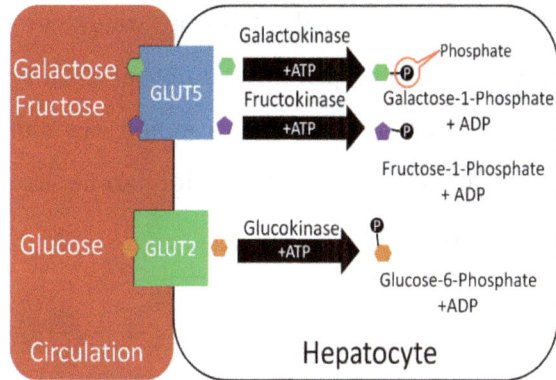

Figure 139. Hepatic monosaccharide uptake

Kinase enzymes normally phosphorylate substrates. Phosphorylation of the monosaccharides is important for maintaining the gradient (by keeping free monosaccharide levels within hepatocytes low) needed for facilitated diffusion through the GLUT transporters.[3]

4.4 Protein Uptake, Absorption, Transport & Liver Uptake

There are several similarities between carbohydrate and protein uptake, absorption, transport, and uptake by the liver. Hopefully after this section you'll understand these similarities.

Over 60% of all amino acids are taken up into the enterocyte as di- and tripeptides through the PepT1 transporter. Individual amino acids are taken up through a variety of amino acid transporters. Once inside the enterocyte, peptidases cleave the peptides to individual amino acids. These cleaved amino acids, along with those that were taken up as individual amino acids, are moved into the capillary by another variety of amino acid transporters (some are the same as on the brush border, some are different).

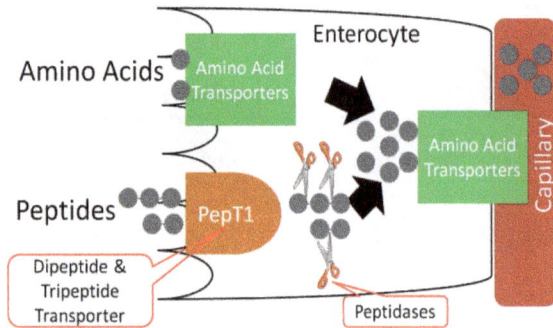

Figure 140. Protein uptake and absorption

The capillary inside a villus is shown below.

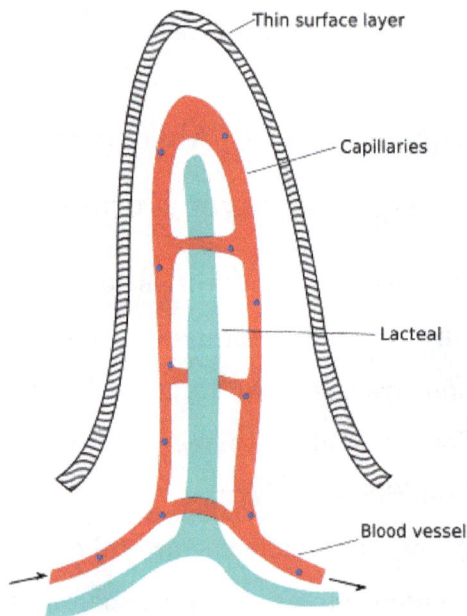

Figure 141. Anatomy of a villus

Like monosaccharides, amino acids are transported directly to the liver through the portal vein.

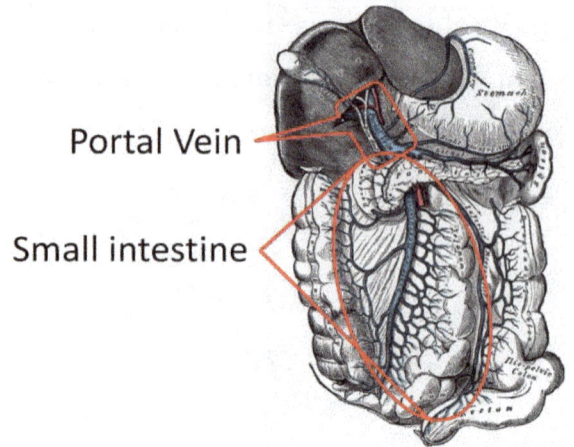

Figure 142. The portal vein transports monosaccharides amino acids and some fatty acids to the liver

Amino acids are taken up into the hepatocyte through a variety of amino acid transporters. The amino acids can then be used to either make proteins or broken down to produce glucose, as will be described in chapter 5.

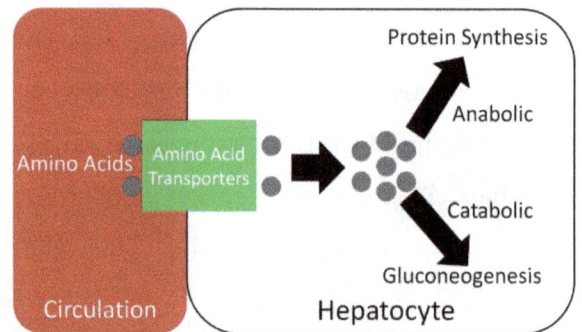

Figure 143. Hepatic amino acid uptake

4.5 Types of Cell Uptake/Transport

There are several different forms of uptake/transport utilized by your body. These can be classified as passive or active.

The difference between the two is whether energy is required and whether they move with or against a concentration gradient. Passive transport does not require energy and moves with a concentration gradient. Active transport requires energy to move against the concentration gradient.

The energy for active uptake/transport is provided by adenosine triphosphate (ATP), which is the energy currency in the body. ATP stores energy in its high-energy phosphate bonds. The structures of adenosine and phosphate are shown below.

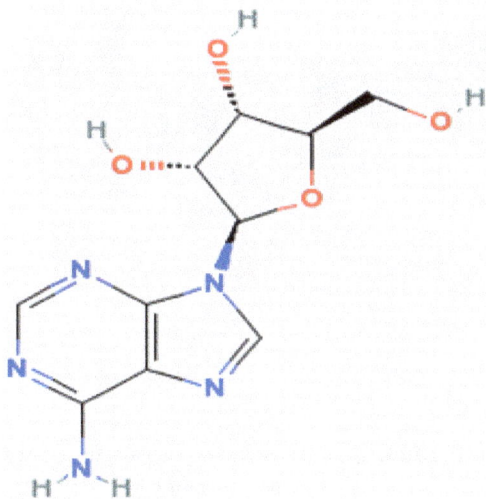

Figure 144. Structures of adenosine (left) and phosphate (right)

Tri- means three, thus ATP is adenosine with three phosphate groups bonded to it, as shown below.

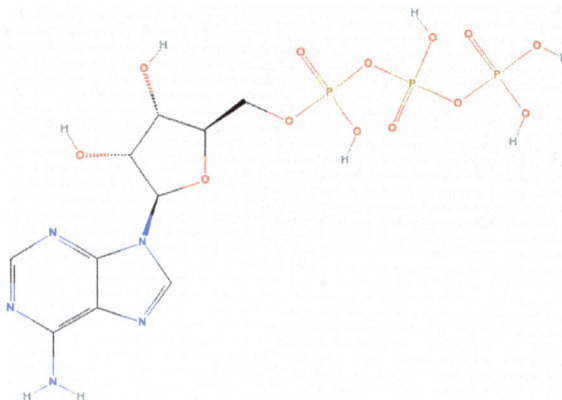

Figure 145. Structure of adenosine triphosphate

Phosphorylation is the formation of a phosphate bond. Dephosphorylation is removal of a phosphate bond. Phosphorylation requires energy to create the bond. Thus, when this bond is broken, energy is released.

The concentration gradient is a way to describe the difference between the concentration of the solute outside of a cell versus the concentration inside of a cell. A solute is what is dissolved in a solvent in a solution; the more solute the higher the concentration. Moving with the gradient is moving from a region of higher concentration to an area of lower concentration. Moving against the gradient is moving from an area of lower concentration to an area of higher concentration.

4.5.1 Passive Uptake/Transport

There are three forms of passive uptake/transport:

1. Simple Diffusion

2. Osmosis

3. Facilitated Diffusion

Below is more information of each type of uptake/transport.

1. Simple Diffusion

Simple diffusion is the movement of solutes from an area of higher concentration (with the concentration gradient) to an area of lower concentration without the help of a protein, as shown below.

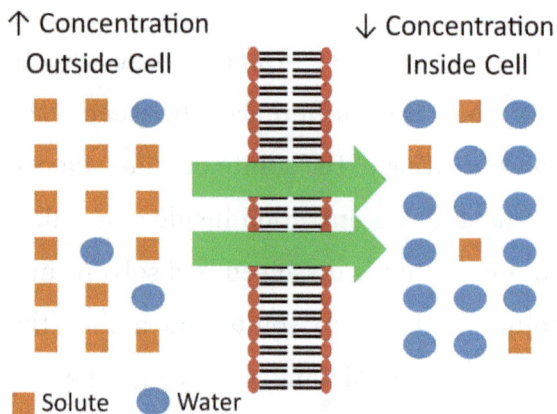

Figure 146. Simple diffusion

2. Osmosis

Osmosis is like simple diffusion, but water moves instead of solutes. In osmosis water molecules move from an area of lower concentration to an area of higher concentration of solute as shown below. The effect of this movement is to dilute the area of higher concentration.

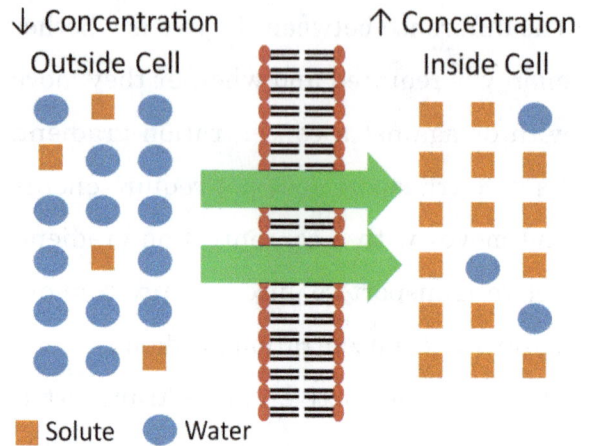

Figure 147. Osmosis

Another example illustrating osmosis is the red blood cells in different solutions shown below.

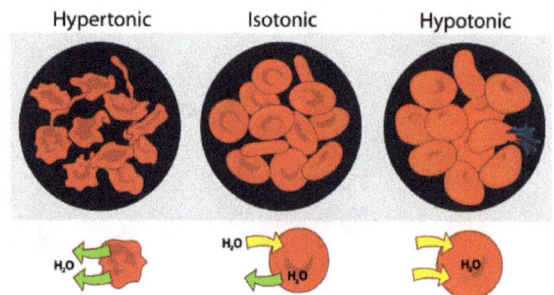

Figure 148. Effect of salt solution concentration on red blood cells

We will consider the simple example of salt as the solute. If the solution is hypertonic, that means that there is a greater concentration of salt outside (extracellular) the red blood cells than within them (intracellular). Water will then move out of the red blood cells to the area of higher salt concentration, resulting in the crenation (shrivelling) of the red blood cells depicted. Isotonic means that there is no difference between concentrations. There is an equal exchange of water between intracellular and extracellular fluids. Thus, the cells are normal, functioning red blood cells. A hypotonic solution contains a lower extracellular concentration of salt than the red blood cell intracellular fluid. As a result, water enters the red blood cells, possibly causing them to burst (lysis).

3. Facilitated Diffusion

The last form of passive absorption is like diffusion in that it follows the concentration gradient (higher concentration to lower concentration). However, it requires a carrier protein to transport the solute across the membrane (figure x.)

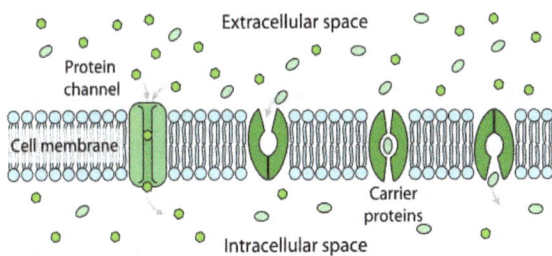

Figure 149. Facilitated diffusion examples

4.5.2   Active Uptake/Transport

There are two forms of active uptake/transport:

1. Active Carrier Transport

2. Endocytosis

1. Active Carrier Transport

Active carrier transport is like facilitated diffusion in that it utilises a protein carrier. Energy is used to move compounds against their concentration gradient (figure 4.321.)

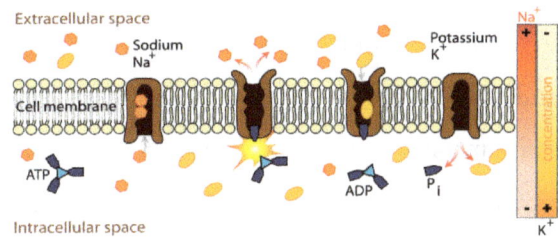

Figure 150. Sodium-potassium ATPase (aka sodium-potassium pump) an example of active carrier transport

2. Endocytosis

Endocytosis is the engulfing of particles or fluid to be taken up into the cell. If a particle is endocytosed, this process referred to as phagocytosis. If a fluid is endocytosed, this process is referred to as pinocytosis.

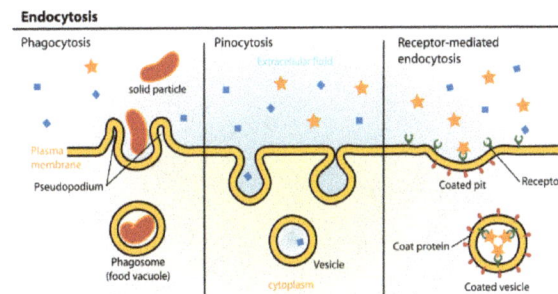

Figure 151. Different types of endocytosis[xxxi]

[xxxi] Public Domain. By Mariana Ruiz Villarreal

4.6 Glycaemic Response, Insulin, & Glucagon

Only 30-40% of glucose is taken up by the liver. The rest enters the blood stream and needs to be handled by the body. A large and consistent rise in blood glucose would be detrimental to health (because of the sugar-related damage known as 'glycation' and effects on blood volume) and so, the body must clear excess glucose from the blood. These processes are referred to as the glycaemic response. The pancreas senses changes in blood glucose levels and responds accordingly. After a meal, the pancreatic beta-cells sense that glucose levels are higher and secrete the hormone insulin (figure 4.51.)

Thus, as can be seen in the following figure, blood insulin levels rise and fall with blood glucose levels over the course of a day.

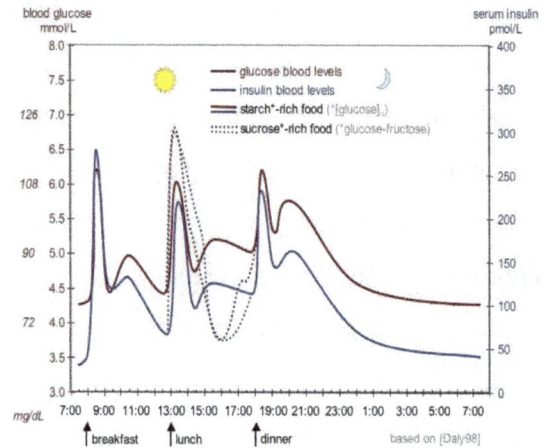

Figure 152. Representative figure of blood glucose and insulin levels during a 24-hour period[xxxii]

Figure 4.52

Blood glucose and insulin levels rise following carbohydrate consumption, and they drop after tissues have taken up the glucose from the blood (described below). Higher than normal blood sugar levels are referred to as hyperglycaemia, while lower than normal blood sugar levels are known as hypoglycaemia.

Insulin travels through the bloodstream to muscle and adipose cells. There, insulin binds to the insulin receptor. This causes GLUT4 transporters that are in vesicles inside the cell to move to the cell surface as shown below.

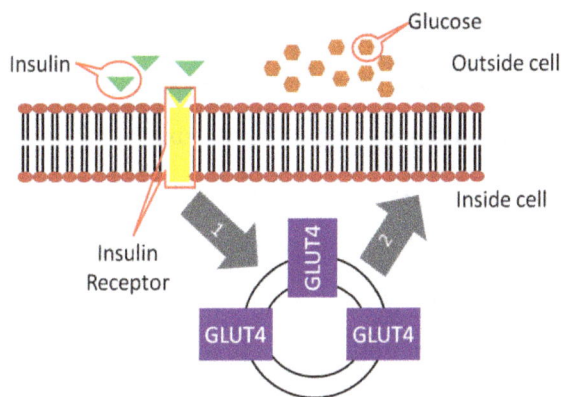

Figure 153. Response of muscle and adipose cells to insulin; 1) binding of insulin to its receptor, 2) movement of GLUT4 vesicles to the cell surface

The movement of the GLUT4 to the cell surface allows glucose to enter the muscle and adipose cells. The glucose is phosphorylated to glucose-6-phosphate by hexokinase (different enzyme but same function as glucokinase in liver).

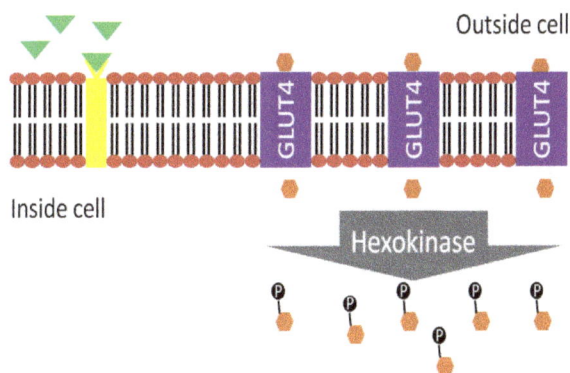

Figure 154. Response of muscle and adipose cells to insulin part 2; hexokinase phosphorylates glucose to glucose-6-phosphate

The hormone Glucagon has a roughly opposite action to that of insulin. Glucagon is secreted from the alpha-cells of the pancreas when they sense that blood glucose levels are low.

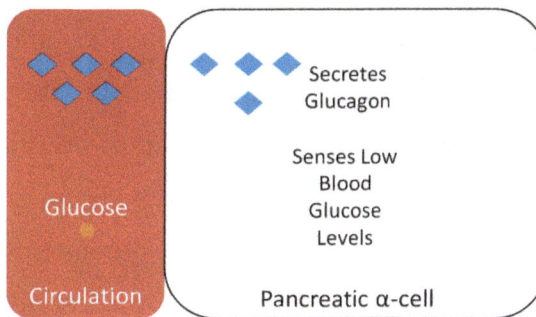

Figure 155. Glucagon secretion from pancreatic alpha-cells in response to low blood glucose levels

Glucagon binds to the glucagon receptor in the liver, which causes the breakdown of glycogen to glucose.

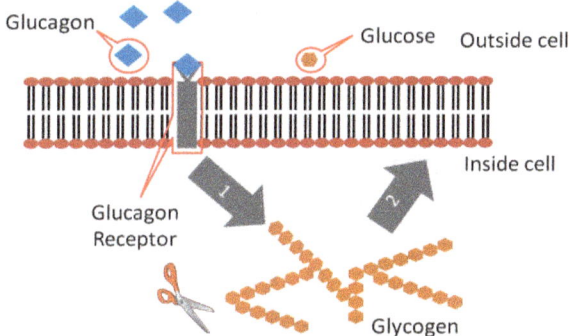

Figure 156. Glucagon binding to its receptor leads to the breakdown of glycogen to glucose

This glucose is then released into circulation to raise blood glucose levels as shown below.

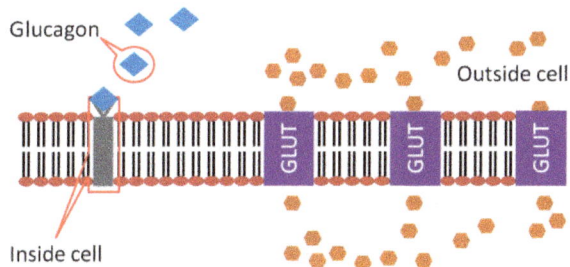

Figure 157. Glucagon leads to the release of glucose from the liver

93

Note. We have focussed on the basic, glucose modulating role of insulin and glucagon. It is important to remember that insulin is released in response to amino acids and certain chemicals in addition to carbohydrate. Insulin also has other roles in nutrient partitioning, including: increasing uptake of triglycerides (fat) into tissue, especially adipose tissue, and reducing the amount of fat released from adipocytes (fat cells). It is therefore a part of the system of interrelated processes involved with long-term weight gain and weight management.

Perhaps the most important and underappreciated role of insulin is inhibiting hepatic glucose output. This is the primary way it modulates blood glucose levels when non-insulin mediated glucose disposal (i.e. during exercise and in those very active) is at play.

4.7 Diabetes Mellitus

Diabetes mellitus is a condition characterised by chronically high blood sugar levels. The prevalence of diabetes in western nations, including New Zealand has been rapidly increasing. 2012-2013 data from New Zealand's Ministry of Health (MOH) suggests a prevalence of diagnosed diabetes of just under 6% of the adult population, with higher rates observed amongst the elderly, Pacific Island and Maori populations and those from poorer socio-economic areas.[40] However this rate is increasing and estimates suggest that metabolic disorder is rising rapidly.

There are two forms of diabetes, type 1 and type 2.

In type 1 diabetes, not enough insulin is produced.

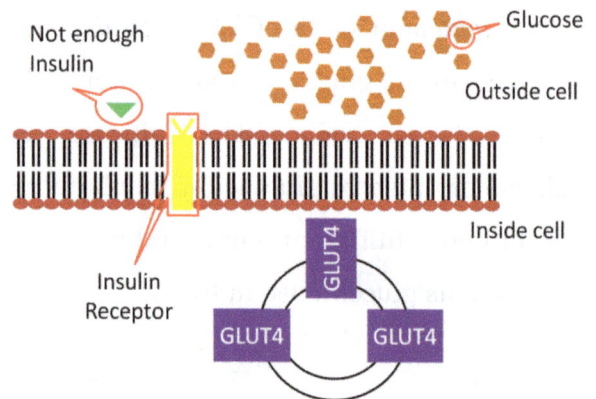

Figure 158. Type 1 diabetes

As a result, GLUT4 does not make it to the surface of muscle and adipose cells, meaning glucose is not taken up into these cells. Type 1 diabetes was previously known as juvenile-onset, or insulin-dependent diabetes and is estimated to account for 5-10% of diabetes cases.[1] Type 1 diabetics receive insulin through injections or pumps to manage their blood sugar.

In type 2 diabetes, the body (at least initially) produces insulin, but the person's body is resistant to it. In type 2 diabetics the binding of insulin to its receptor does not cause GLUT4 to move to the surface of the muscle and adipose cells, thus little glucose is taken up. Thus, a cascade of events can occur in which more insulin is required to be produced and the receptivity of tissue to insulin can continue to fall, encouraging greater and greater levels of insulin resistance.

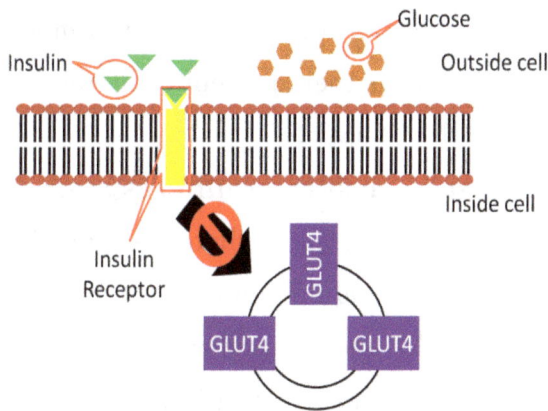

Figure 159. Type 2 diabetes

Type 2 diabetes accounts for 90-95% of diabetes cases and was once known as non-insulin-dependent diabetes or adult-onset diabetes.[1] However, concurrent with the increasing rates of obesity, many younger people are being diagnosed with type 2, making the latter definition no longer appropriate. Many people with type 2 diabetes can control their condition with a diet and exercise regimen. This regimen reduces their need for glucose as a primary fuel (for example by improving fat adaptation), increases insulin sensitivity, or their response to the body's own insulin.[2] Some with type 2 diabetes will also benefit from receiving insulin though. These individuals are producing enough insulin but are so resistant to it that more is needed for glucose to be taken up by their muscle and adipose cells or they have begun to exhaust the capacity of the beta-cells of the pancreas to produce insulin adequately. In this instance a type 2 → type 1 diabetes may be occurring.

4.7.1   Glycaemic Index

Research has indicated that hyperglycaemia is associated with chronic diseases and obesity. As a result, measures of the glycaemic response to food consumption have been developed so that people can choose foods with a smaller glycaemic response. The first measure developed for this purpose was the glycaemic index. The glycaemic index is the relative change in blood glucose after consumption of 50 g of carbohydrate in a test food compared to 50 g of carbohydrates of a reference food (white bread or glucose). Thus, a high glycaemic index food will produce a greater rise in blood glucose concentrations compared to a low glycaemic index food, as shown below.

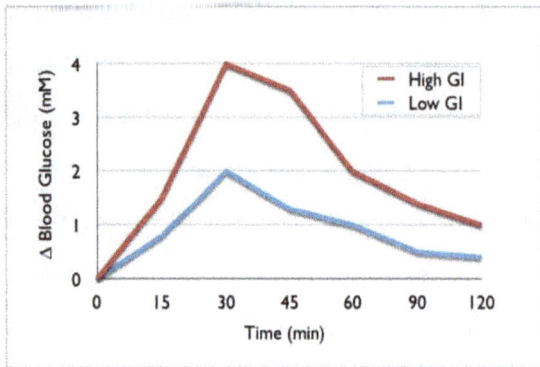

Figure 160. Blood glucose response to a high glycaemic index (GI) food compared to a low glycaemic index food

As a general guideline, a glycaemic index that is 70 or greater is high, 56-69 is medium, and 55 and below is low. A stop light graphical presentation has been designed to emphasize the consumption of the low glycaemic index foods while cautioning against the consumption of too many high glycaemic index foods[2].

There are however several problems with the glycaemic index however.

It does not consider serving sizes.

Let's take popcorn (glycaemic index 89-127) as an example. A serving size of popcorn is 20 g, 11 g of which is carbohydrate.[41] This is equal to approximately 2.5 cups of popcorn[4]. Thus, a person would have to consume over 11 cups of popcorn to consume 50 g of carbohydrate needed for the glycaemic index measurement. Another example is watermelon, which has a glycaemic index of 103, with a 120 g serving containing only

6 g of carbohydrates.[41] To consume the 50 g needed for glycaemic index measurement, a person would need to consume over 1000 g (1 kg) of watermelon. Assuming this is all watermelon flesh (no rind), this would be over 6.5 cups of watermelon.[4] These are obviously unlikely to be consumed and so the actual glycaemic response (and insulinergic effects) of these foods in a real-world situation are much different than their perception if related only to the GI scale.

It doesn't consider insulin response.

Several factors contribute to insulin response, including amino acid content and profile and non-calorific chemicals such as the various xanthines (such as caffeine.) The insulin response to foods may be somewhat different to their glycaemic index rating, and thus may affect the viability of a food for people with metabolic disorders.

The value of the glycaemic index has been brought into question and more recently other factors such as nutrient density of a food (i.e. relative calorie to micronutrient content), total glycaemic load, and fibre and resistant starch content, have gained greater prominence as indicators of food quality.

4.7.2 Glycaemic Load

To incorporate serving size into the calculation, another measure known as the glycaemic load has been developed. It is calculated as shown below:

Glycaemic Load = (Glycaemic Index X (g) Carbs/serving)/100

Thus, for most people, the glycaemic load is a more meaningful measure of the glycaemic impact of different foods. Considering the two examples from the glycaemic index section, their glycaemic loads would be:

Popcorn

(89-127 X 11 g Carbs/ Serving)/100= 10-14

Watermelon

(103 X 6 g Carbs/Serving)/100 = 6.18

A general guideline for glycaemic loads of foods is, 20 or above is high, 11-19 is medium, and 10 or below is low.

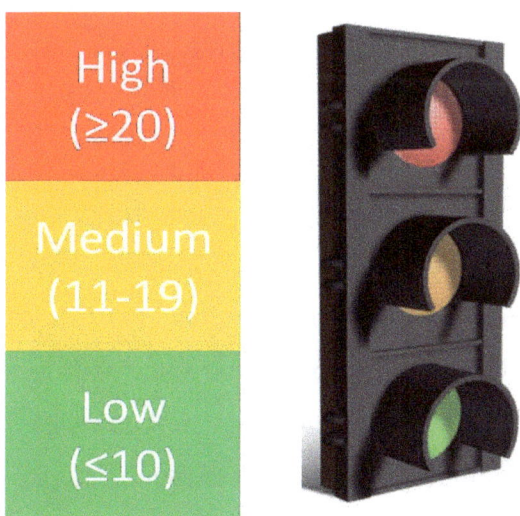

Figure 161. Food glycaemic load classifications1

Putting it all together, popcorn and watermelon have high glycaemic indexes, but medium and low glycaemic loads, respectively.

4.7.3 Lipoproteins

Lipoproteins, as the name suggests, are complexes of lipids and protein. The proteins within a lipoprotein are called apolipoproteins (aka apoproteins). There are several different apolipoproteins that are abbreviated apo-, then an identifying letter (i.e. Apo A) as shown in the chylomicron below.

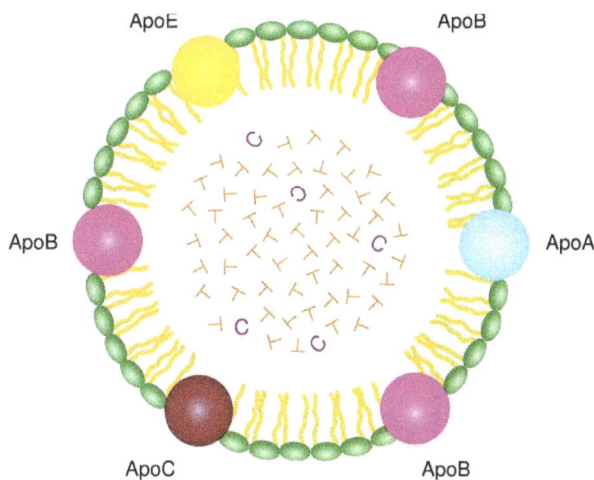

Figure 162. Structure of a chylomicron

There are several lipoproteins in the body. They differ by the apolipoproteins they contain, size (diameter), density, and composition. The table below shows the difference in density and diameter of different lipoproteins. Notice that as diameter decreases, density increases.

97

Table 23. The density and diameter of different lipoproteins

Lipoprotein	Density (g/dL)	Diameter (nm)
Chylomicrons	0.95	75-1200
VLDL (very low-density lipoproteins)	0.95-1.006	30-80
IDL (intermediate-density lipoproteins)	1.006-1.019	25-35
LDL (low-density lipoproteins)	1.019-1.063	18-25
HDL (high-density lipoproteins)	1.063-1.21	5-12

This inverse relationship is a result of the larger lipoproteins being composed of a higher percentage of triglyceride and a lower percentage of protein as shown below.

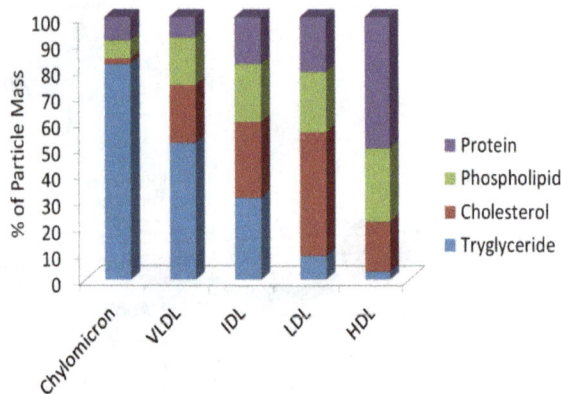

Figure 163. Composition of lipoproteins[36]

Protein is denser than triglyceride, thus the higher protein/lower triglyceride composition, the higher the density of the lipoprotein. Many of the lipoproteins are named based on their densities (i.e. very low-density lipoproteins).

As described in the last subsection, the lipoproteins released from the small intestine are chylomicrons.

The endothelial cells that line blood vessels, especially in the muscle and adipose tissue, contain the enzyme lipoprotein lipase (LPL). LPL cleaves the fatty acids from lipoprotein triglycerides so that the fatty acids can be taken up into tissues. The figure below illustrates how endothelial cells are in contact with the blood that flows through the lumen of blood vessels.

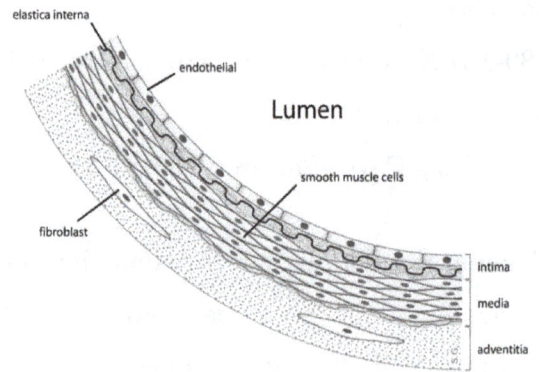

Figure 164. Lining of a blood vessel. The lumen is where the blood would be flowing, thus endothelial cells are those that are in contact with blood

LPL cleaves fatty acids from the triglycerides in the chylomicron, decreasing the amount of triglyceride in the lipoprotein. This lipoprotein with less triglycerides becomes what is known as a chylomicron remnant, as shown below.

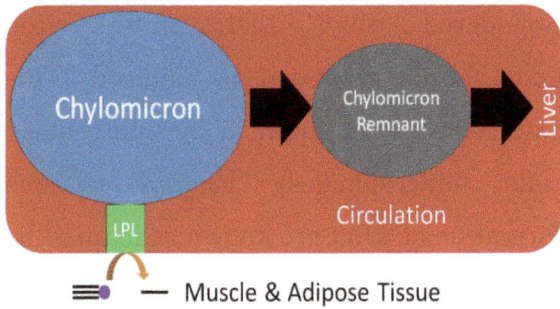

Figure 165. The cleavage of triglycerides by LPL from a chylomicron leads to the formation of a chylomicron remnant

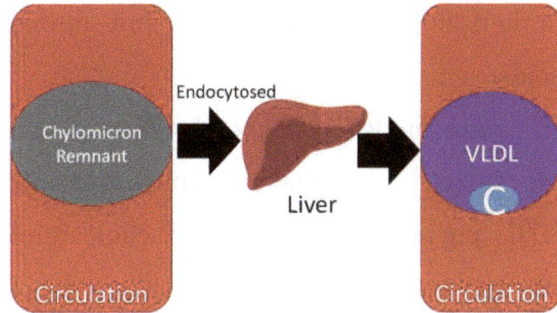

Figure 166. Chylomicron remnants are taken up by the liver. The liver secretes VLDL that contain cholesterol (C)

Now in the form of a chylomicron remnant, the digested lipid components originally packaged into the chylomicron are directed to the liver where the chylomicron remnant is endocytosed. This process of clearing chylomicrons from the blood takes 2-10 hours after a meal.[15] This is why people must fast 12 hours before having their blood lipids (triglycerides, HDL, LDL etc.) measured. This fast allows all the chylomicrons and chylomicron remnants to be cleared before blood is taken. After the chylomicron remnant is endocytosed, it is broken down to its individual components (triglycerides, cholesterol, protein etc.). In the liver, VLDL are produced, like how chylomicrons are produced in the small intestine. The individual components are packaged into VLDL and secreted into circulation as shown below.

Like it does to chylomicrons, LPL cleaves fatty acids from triglycerides in VLDL, forming the smaller IDL (aka VLDL remnant). Further action of LPL on IDL results in the formation of LDL. The C in Figures 4.715 and 4.716 represents cholesterol, which is not increasing; rather, since triglyceride is being removed, it constitutes a greater percentage of particle mass of lipoproteins. As a result, LDL is composed mostly of cholesterol, as depicted in the figure below.

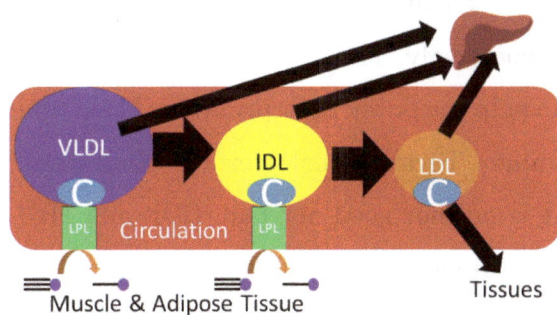

Figure 167. Formation of IDL and LDL from VLDL

LDL contains a specific apolipoprotein (Apo B100) that binds to LDL receptors on the surface of target tissues. The LDL are then endocytosed into the target tissue and broken down to cholesterol and amino acids.

HDL are made up of mostly protein and are derived from the liver and intestine. HDL participates in reverse cholesterol transport, which is the transport of cholesterol back to the liver. HDL picks up cholesterol from tissues/blood vessels and returns it to the liver itself or transfers it to other lipoproteins returning to the liver.

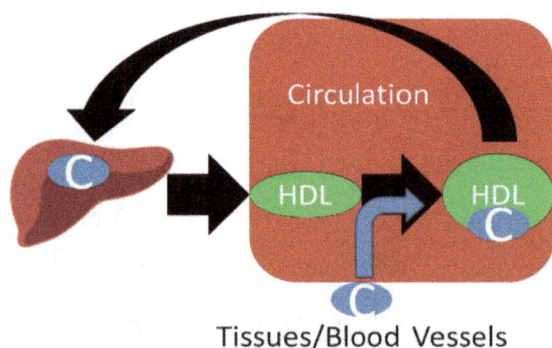

Figure 168. HDL is involved in reverse cholesterol transport

HDL and LDL are commonly referred to as "good cholesterol" and "bad cholesterol," respectively. This is an oversimplification to help the public interpret their blood lipid values, because cholesterol is cholesterol; it is neither good nor bad. LDL and HDL are lipoproteins (protein carriers for cholesterol), and as a result you can't consume good or bad cholesterol, nor produce 'good or 'bad' cholesterol.

LDL is labelled as 'bad' cholesterol because it has been linked to the formation of atherosclerosis. In this process it is considered that LDL enters the endothelium where it is oxidized. This oxidized LDL is engulfed by white blood cells (macrophages), leading to the formation of what are known as foam cells. The foam cells eventually accumulate so much LDL that they die and accumulate forming a fatty streak. From there the fatty streak, which is the beginning stages of a lesion, can continue to grow until it blocks the artery. This can result in a myocardial infarction (heart attack) or a stroke.

HDL is considered 'good' in that it scavenges cholesterol from other lipoproteins or cells and returns it to the liver.

These definitions and processes are oversimplified too, and there is a wealth of emerging evidence suggesting many factors, including, but not limited to: lipoprotein particle size, inflammatory status, glycation and others play a role in the development of atherosclerotic plaques and the further development of cardiovascular disease.

5 Macronutrient & Alcohol Metabolism

Now that we have digested, taken up, absorbed, and transported the macronutrients, the next step is to learn how these macronutrients are metabolised. Alcohol is also included, even though it is technically not a macronutrient, as it provides calories to the diet.

5.1 Metabolism Basics

Metabolism consists of all the chemical processes that occur in living cells. These processes/reactions can generally be classified as either anabolic or catabolic. Anabolic means to build up, whereas catabolic means to breakdown. If you have trouble remembering the difference between the two, remember that anabolic steroids are what some athletes use to build large amount of muscle mass.

An anabolic reaction/pathway requires energy to build something. A catabolic reaction/pathway generates energy by breaking down something. This is shown in the example below of glucose and glycogen. The same is true for other macronutrients. It is important to remember these functional aspects. People often think of anabolic (or building up) as

being 'good' whereas the breakdown of tissue (catabolism) is 'bad'. This is incorrect as both functions are essential for life as we build up and breakdown tissue constantly and we require the breakdown of molecules and chemicals to provide for the energy necessary to sustain life, and performance.

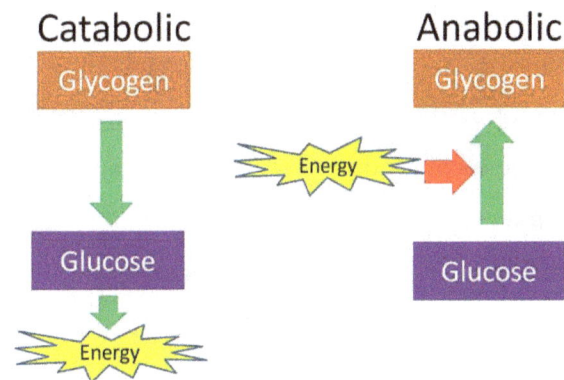

Figure 169. The breakdown of glycogen to glucose is catabolic. The glucose can then be used to produce energy. The synthesis of glycogen from glucose is anabolic and requires energy

Anabolic and catabolic can also be used to describe conditions in the body. For instance, after a meal there is often a positive energy balance, or there is more energy and macronutrients than the body needs at that time. Thus, some energy needs to be stored and the macronutrients will be used for synthesis, such as amino acids being used for protein synthesis. However, after a fast, or a prolonged period

101

without energy intake, the body is in negative energy balance and is considered catabolic. In this condition, macronutrients will be mobilized from their stores to be used to generate energy. For example, if a fast is prolonged enough, protein can be broken down and the released amino acids can be broken down to be directly used as an energy source, or more commonly converted to glucose for use as fuel.

Several the metabolic reactions oxidize or reduce compounds. A compound that is being oxidized loses at least one electron, while a compound that is reduced gains at least 1 electron. To remember the difference, a mnemonic device such as OIL (oxidation is lost), RIG (reduction is gained) is helpful. Oxidation-reduction reactions are illustrated in the figure below.

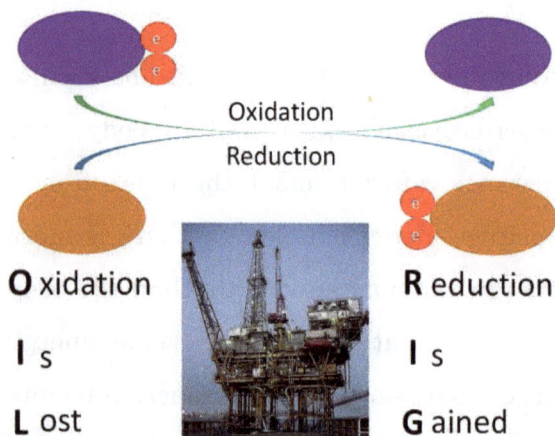

Figure 170. The purple compound is being oxidized, the orange compound is being reduced

Another way to remember oxidation versus reduction is **LEO goes GER** (like a lion)

Lose **E**lections = **O**xidize
Gain **E**lections = **R**educe

Iron is a good example we can use to illustrate oxidation-reduction reactions. Iron commonly exists in two oxidation states (Fe^{3+} or Fe^{2+}). It is constantly oxidized/reduced back and forth between the two states. The oxidation/reduction of iron is shown below.

$$Fe^{3+} + e^- \rightarrow Fe^{2+} \text{ Reduced}$$
$$Fe^{2+} + e^- \rightarrow Fe^{3+} \text{ Oxidized}$$

However, some oxidation reduction reactions are not as easy to recognize. There are some simple rules to help you recognize less obvious oxidation/reduction reactions that are based upon the gain or loss of oxygen or hydrogen. These are as follows:

Oxidation: gains oxygen or loses hydrogen
Reduction: loses oxygen or gains hydrogen

5.1.1 Cofactors

Several enzymes require cofactors to function. Some of these co-factors may be referred to as coenzymes. But for simplicity we are going to include these coenzymes in our definition of cofactors.

Thus, cofactors can be either organic or inorganic molecules that are required by enzymes to function. Many organic cofactors are vitamins or molecules derived from vitamins. Most inorganic cofactors are minerals. Cofactors can be oxidized or reduced for the enzymes to catalyse the reactions.

Two common cofactors that are derived from the B vitamins, niacin and riboflavin, are nicotinamide adenine dinucleotide (NAD) and flavin adenine dinucleotide (FAD), respectively. The structure of NAD and FAD are shown below.

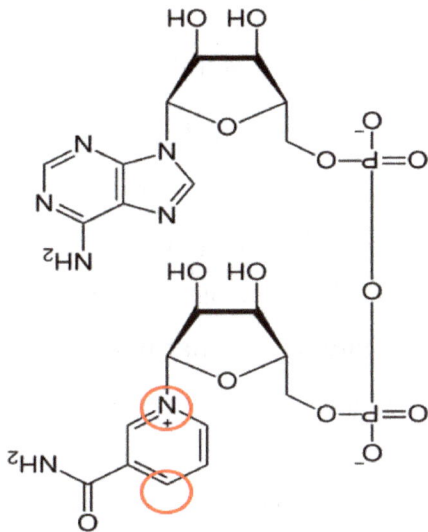

Figure 172. Structure of FAD[2]

Both cofactors can be reduced; NAD is reduced to form NADH, while FAD is reduced to form FADH$_2$ as shown in the 2 figures below.

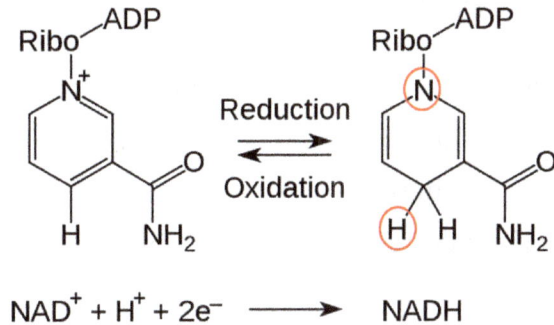

$$NAD^+ + H^+ + 2e^- \longrightarrow NADH$$

Figure 173. The reduction of NAD to form NADH[3]

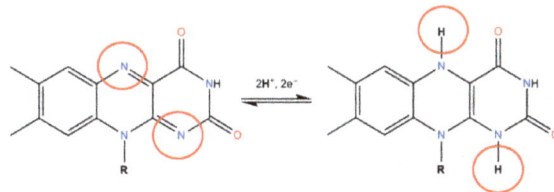

Figure 171. Structure of NAD[1] upside down

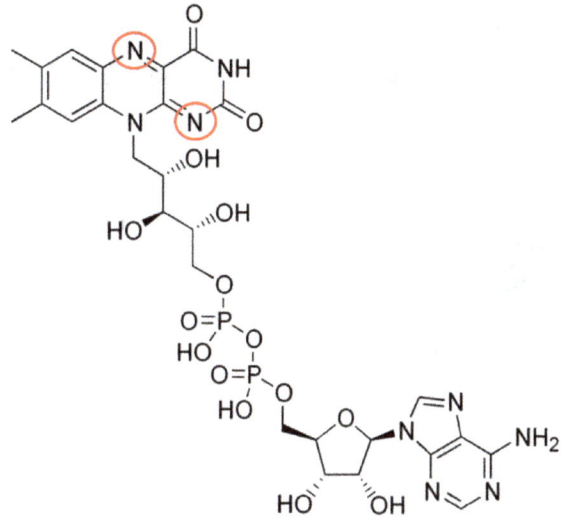

Figure 174. The reduction of FAD[4] to FADH$_2$

An example of a mineral that serves as a cofactor is Fe^{2+} for proline and lysyl hydroxylases. We will discuss later in detail why vitamin C (ascorbic acid) is needed to reduce iron to Fe^{2+} so that it can serve as a cofactor for proline and lysyl hydroxylases.

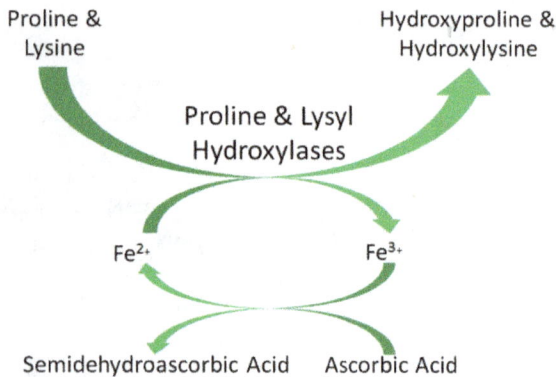

Proline & Lysine

Hydroxyproline & Hydroxylysine

Proline & Lysyl Hydroxylases

Fe^{2+} Fe^{3+}

Semidehydroascorbic Acid   Ascorbic Acid

Figure 175. Iron (Fe²+) is a cofactor for proline and lysyl hydroxylases

5.2 Carbohydrate Metabolism Pathways

There are many metabolic pathways (cycles, processes, or reactions) that are involved in the synthesis or degradation of carbohydrates and compounds formed from them. Please note that most of these pathways aren't specific to carbohydrates only. Gluconeogenesis will be covered in the protein section, because amino acids are a common substrate used for synthesizing glucose.

Carbohydrate Pathways/Cycles/Processes/Reactions

Glycogenesis

-glycogen synthesis

Glycogenolysis

-glycogen breakdown

Gluconeogenesis

-synthesis of glucose from a non-carbohydrate source

Glycolysis

-breakdown of glucose to pyruvate

Transition Reaction

-conversion of pyruvate to acetyl-CoA

Citric Acid (Tricarboxylic acid (TCA), Kreb's) Cycle

-acetyl-CoA combines with oxaloacetate to form citrate; ATP, NADH, and $FADH_2$ are produced in the cycle

Electron Transport Chain

-oxidative phosphorylation, producing ATP from NADH and $FADH_2$

5.2.1 Monosaccharide Metabolism

Since glucose is the body's preferred monosaccharide, galactose and fructose metabolism is a logical place to begin looking at carbohydrate metabolism. The figure below reminds you that in the liver, galactose (a monosaccharide derived from the breakdown of the disaccharide milk sugar lactose) and fructose (fruit sugar) have been phosphorylated.

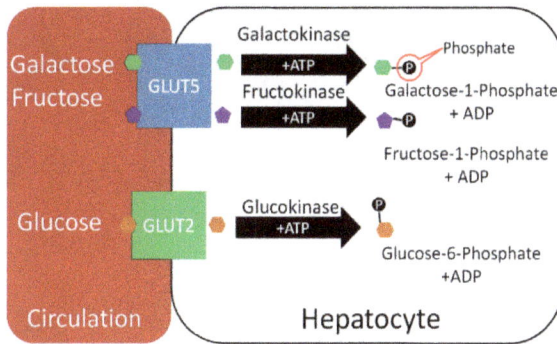

Figure 176. Uptake of monosaccharides into the hepatocyte

5.2.1.1 Galactose

In the liver, galactose-1-phosphate is converted to glucose-1-phosphate, before finally being converted to glucose-6-phosphate[36]. As shown below, glucose 6-phosphate can then be used in either glycolysis or glycogenesis, depending on the person's current energy state.

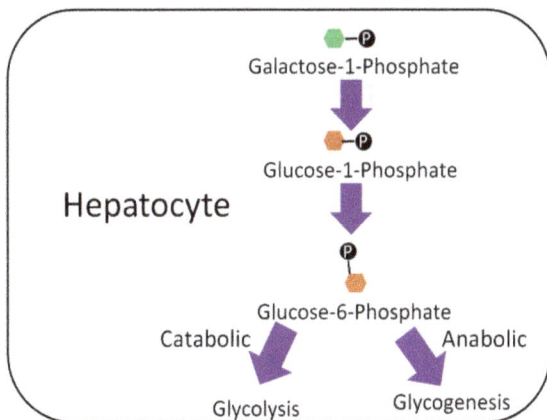

Figure 177. Conversion of galactose-1-phosphate to glucose-6-phosphate

5.2.1.2 Fructose

Unlike galactose, fructose cannot be used to form phosphorylated glucose. Instead, fructose-1-phosphate is cleaved in the liver

to form glyceraldehyde 3-phosphate, a glycolysis (pathway that breaks down glucose) intermediate. This occurs through multiple steps, as depicted below.

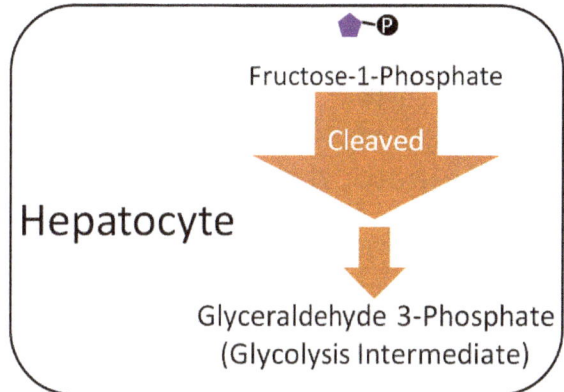

Figure 178. Conversion of fructose-1-phosphate to glyceraldehyde 3-phosphate

5.2.1.3 Glucose-6-Phosphate

Within hepatocytes or myocytes (muscle cells), glucose-6-phosphate can be used either for glycogenesis (glycogen synthesis) or glycolysis (breakdown of glucose for energy production). If the person is in an anabolic state, they will use glucose-6-phosphate for storage. If they are in a catabolic state, they will use it for energy production.

105

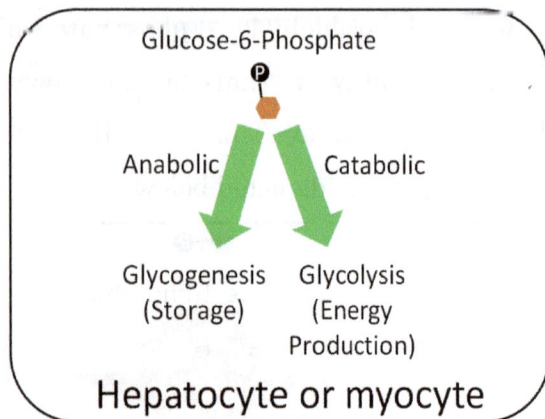

Figure 179. The "fork in the road" for glucose-6-phosphate

5.2.2   Glycogenesis & Glycogenolysis

As discussed earlier, glycogen is the animal storage form of glucose, like the polysaccharide starches found in plants. If a person is in an anabolic state, such as after consuming a meal, most glucose-6-phosphate within the myocytes (muscle cells) or hepatocytes (liver cells) is going to be stored as glycogen. The structure is shown below as a reminder.

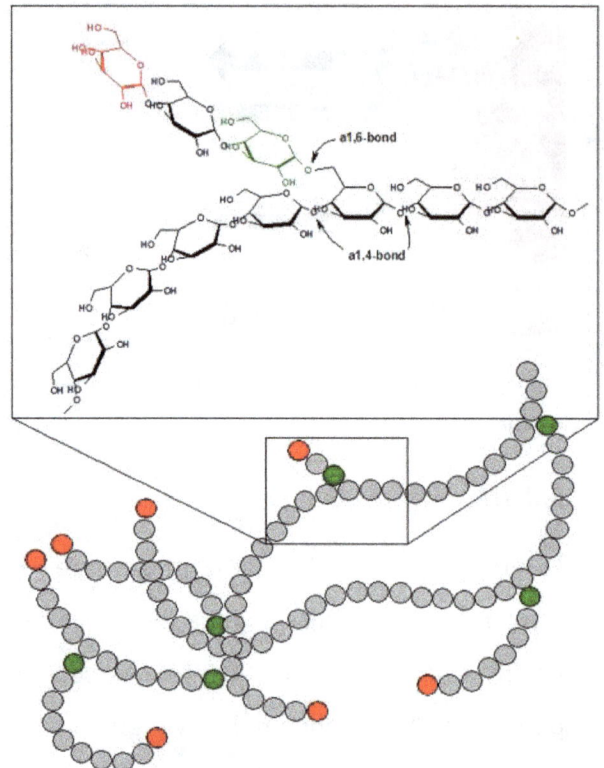

Figure 180. Structure of glycogen

Glycogen is mainly stored in the liver and the muscle. It makes up ~ 6% of the wet weight of the liver and only 1% of muscle wet weight. However, since we have far more muscle mass in our body, there is 3-4 times more glycogen stored in muscle than in the liver.[35] We have limited glycogen storage capacity. Thus, after a high-carbohydrate meal, our glycogen stores may reach capacity, although the ability of the body to store more glycogen (to 'supercompensate') may occur with 'carb-deloading and -loading' strategies.[42] After glycogen stores are filled, glucose will have to be metabolized in different ways for it to be stored in a different form—such as in the form of triglycerides in tissue, especially in stored fat-tissue (adipose), where it provides the backbone of triglycerides (along with three fatty-acid molecules) as glycerol.

5.2.2.1 Glycogenesis

The synthesis of glycogen from glucose is a process known as glycogenesis. Glucose-6-phosphate is not inserted directly into glycogen in this process. There are a couple of steps before it is incorporated. First, glucose-6-phosphate is converted to glucose-1-phosphate and then converted to uridine diphosphate (UDP)-glucose. UDP-glucose is inserted into glycogen by either the enzyme, glycogen synthase (alpha-1,4 bonds), or the branching enzyme (alpha-1,6 bonds) at the branch points[36].

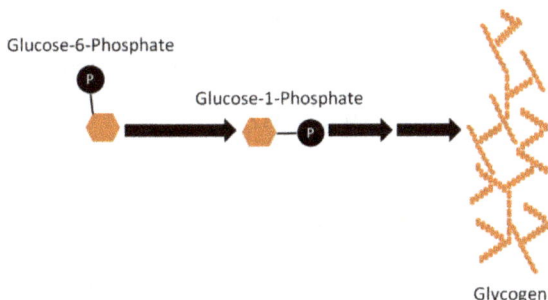

Figure 181. Glycogenesis

5.2.2.2 Glycogenolysis

The process of liberating glucose from glycogen is known as glycogenolysis. This process is essentially the opposite of glycogenesis with two exceptions: (1) there is no UDP-glucose step, and (2) a different

enzyme, glycogen phosphorylase, is involved. Glucose-1-phosphate is cleaved from glycogen by the enzyme, glycogen phosphorylase, which then can be converted to glucose-6-phosphate as shown below.[36]

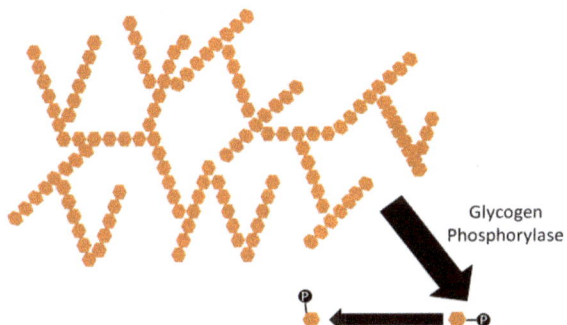

Figure 182. Glycogenolysis

5.2.2.3 Glycolysis

If a person is in a catabolic state or in need of energy, such as during a fast, most glucose-6-phosphate will be used for glycolysis.

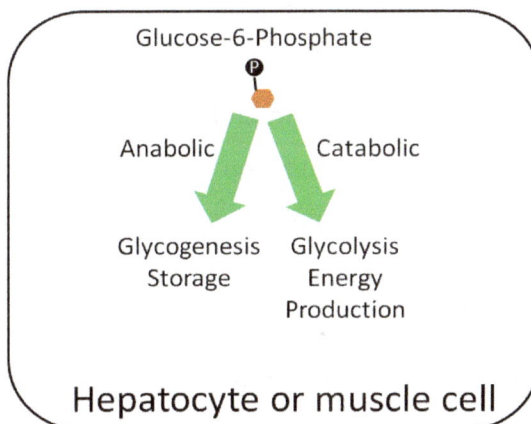

Figure 183. The "fork in the road" for glucose-6-phosphate

Glycolysis is the breaking down of one glucose molecule (6 carbons) into two pyruvate molecules (3 carbons). During the process, a net of two ATPs and two NADHs are also produced.

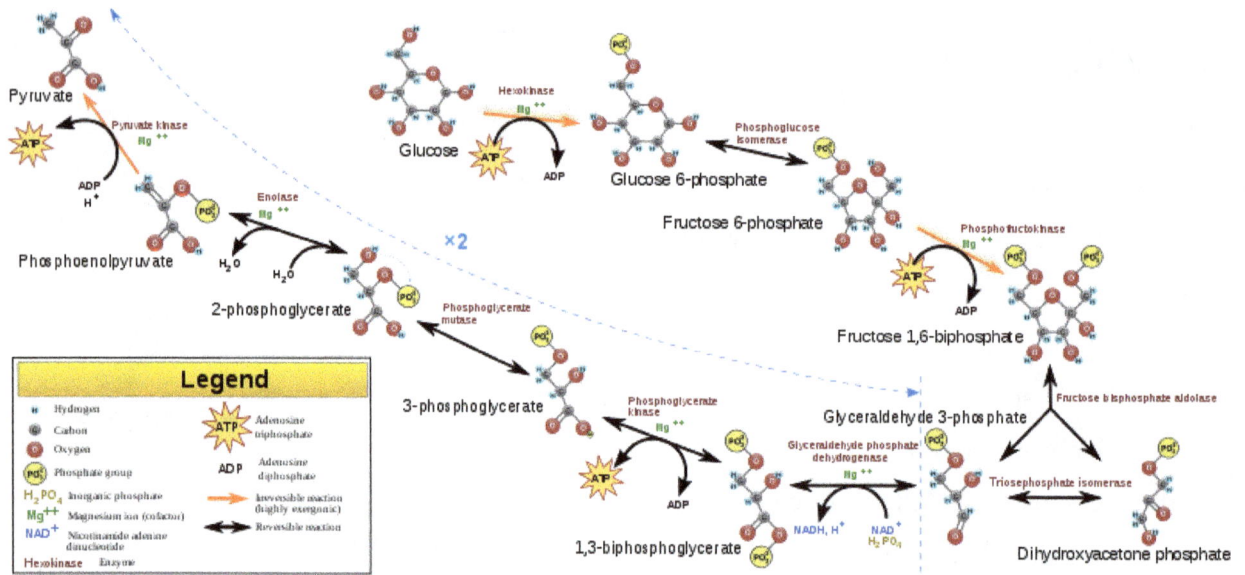

Figure 184. Glycolysis[xxxiii]

5.2.2.4 Stages of Glycolysis

1. Energy investment step - 2 ATP are added to the 6-carbon molecule.

2. Glucose Split - The 6-carbon molecule is split into two 3 carbon molecules.

3. Energy harvesting step - 1 NADH and 2 ATPs are produced from each 3-carbon molecule (there are two 3 carbon molecules formed from each glucose).

Thus, from a molecule of glucose, the harvesting step produces a total of four ATPs and two NADHs. Subtracting the harvesting from the investment step, the net output from one molecule of glucose is two ATPs and two NADHs.

The figure below shows the stages of glycolysis, as well as the transition reaction, citric acid cycle, and electron transport chain that are utilized by cells to produce energy. They are also the focus of the next 3 sections.

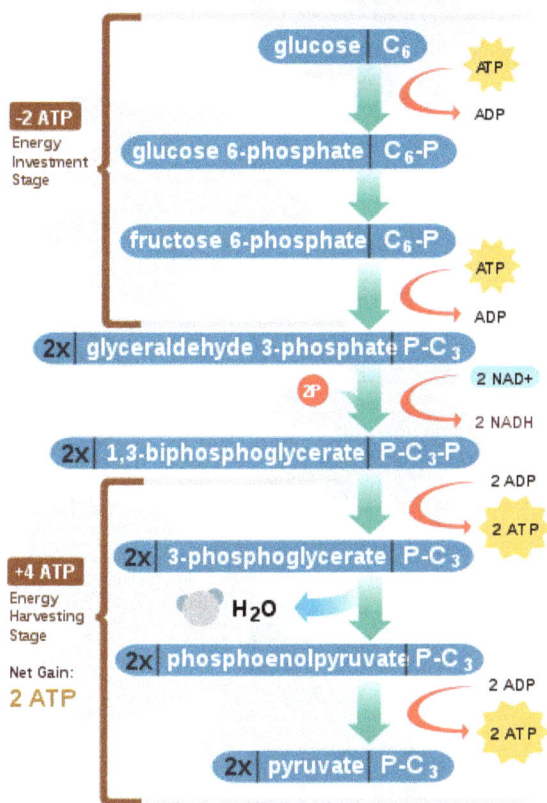
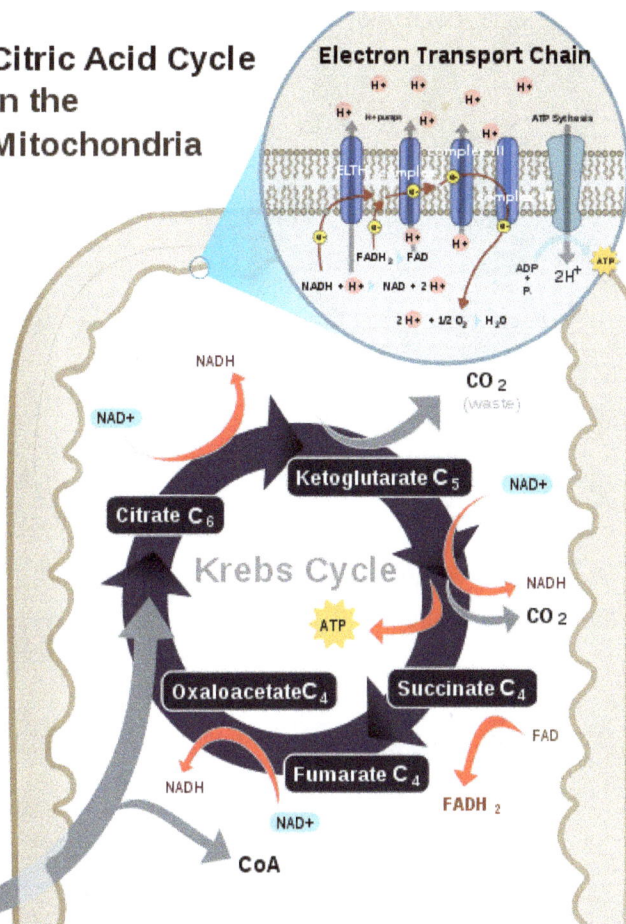

Figure 185. Glycolysis, transition reaction, citric acid cycle, and the electron transport chain[xxxiv]

5.2.3 Transition Reaction

If a person is in a catabolic state, or needs energy, how pyruvate will be used depends on whether adequate oxygen levels are present. If there are adequate oxygen levels (aerobic conditions), pyruvate moves from the cytoplasm, into the mitochondria, and then undergoes the transition reaction. If there are not adequate oxygen levels (anaerobic conditions), pyruvate will instead be used to produce lactate in the cytoplasm. We are going to focus on the aerobic pathway to begin with, then we will address what happens under anaerobic conditions in the anaerobic respiration section.

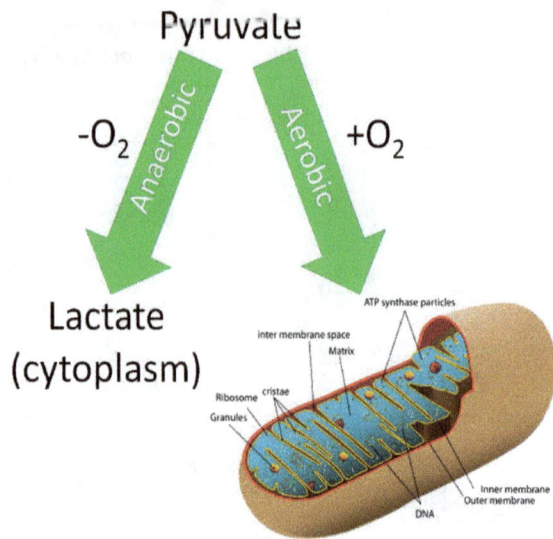

Figure 186. Pyruvate fork in the road. What happens depends on whether it is aerobic or anaerobic respiration

The transition reaction is the transition between glycolysis and the citric acid cycle. The transition reaction converts pyruvate (3 carbons) to acetyl CoA (2 carbons), producing carbon dioxide (CO_2) and a NADH as shown below. The figure below shows the transition reaction with CoA and NAD entering, and acetyl-CoA, CO_2, and NADH being produced.

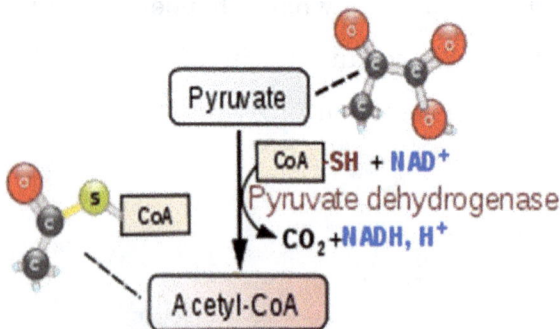

Figure 187. Transition reaction

The acetyl is combined with coenzyme A (CoA) to form acetyl-CoA. The structure of CoA is shown below.

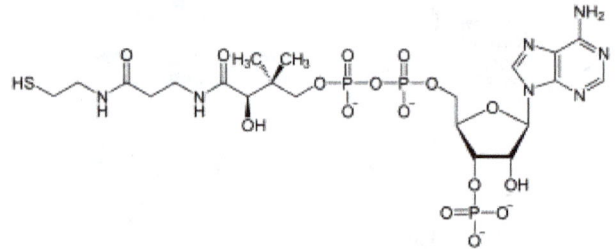

Figure 188. Structure of coenzyme-A

Thus, for one molecule of glucose, the transition reaction produces 2 acetyl-CoAs, 2 molecules of CO_2, and 2 NADHs.

5.2.4 The Citric Acid Cycle

Acetyl-CoA is a pivotal point in metabolism, meaning there are several ways that it can be used. We're going to continue to consider its use in an aerobic, catabolic state (in which there is a requirement for endogenous energy production). Under these conditions, acetyl-CoA will enter the citric acid cycle (also referred to as the Krebs Cycle or TCA Cycle). The following figure shows the citric acid cycle.

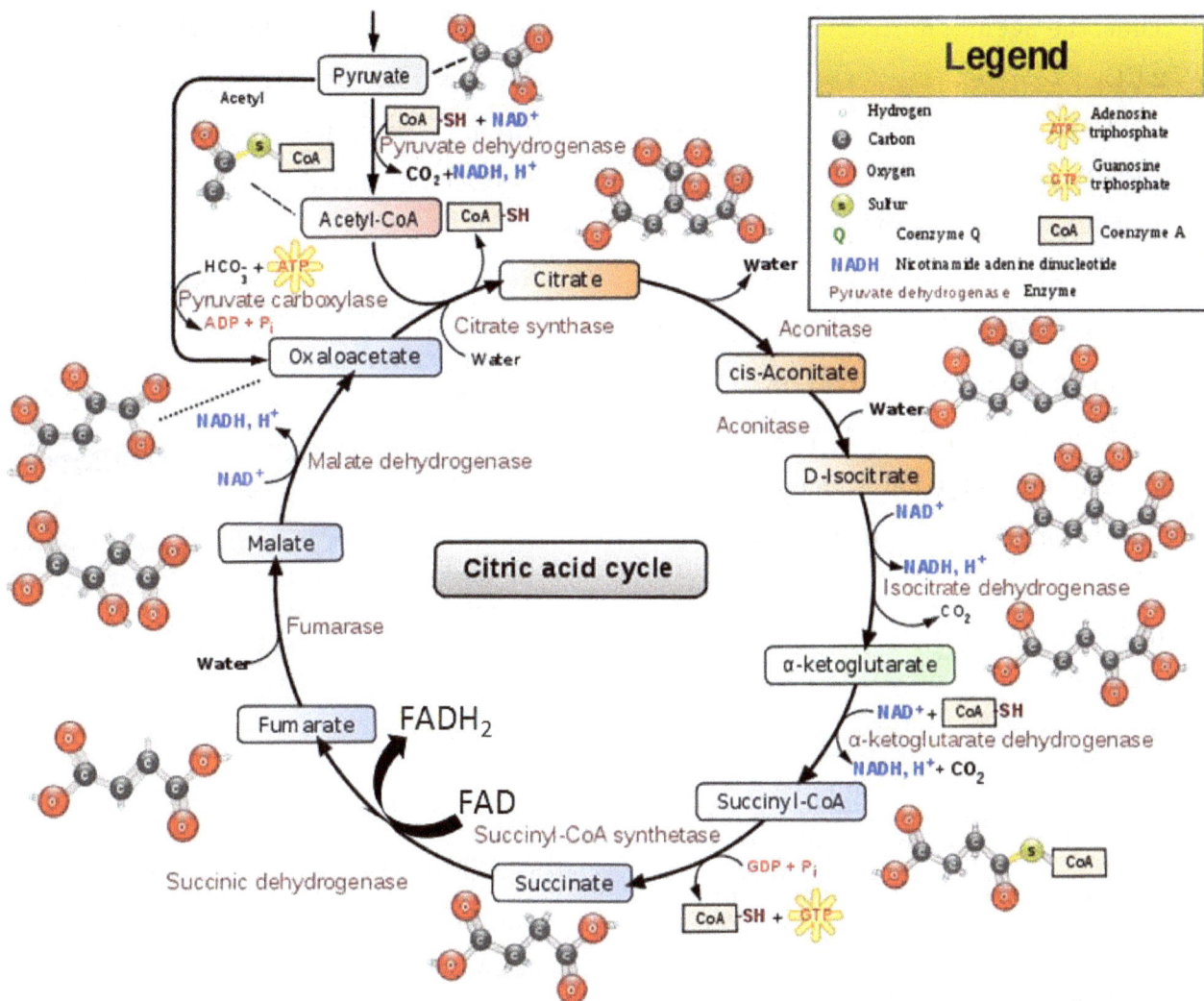

Figure 189. The citric acid cycle[xxxv]

The citric acid cycle begins by acetyl-CoA (2 carbons) combining with oxaloacetate (4 carbons) to form citrate (aka citric acid, 6 carbons). A series of transformations occurs before a carbon is given off as carbon dioxide and NADH is produced. This leaves alpha-ketoglutarate (5 carbons). Another carbon is given off as CO_2 to form succinyl CoA (4 carbons) and produce another NADH. In the next step, one guanosine triphosphate (GTP) is produced as succinyl-CoA is converted to succinate. GTP is readily converted to ATP, thus this step is essentially the generation of 1 ATP. In the next step, an $FADH_2$ is produced along with fumarate. Then, after more steps, another NADH is produced as oxaloacetate is regenerated.

xxxv Released under the GNU Free Documentation License by Narayanese, WikiUserPedia, YassineMrabet, TotoBaggins. https://commons.wikimedia.org/wiki/File:Citric_acid_cycle_with_aconitate_2.svg

Thus, the net output from one cycle is:

2 CO_2

3 NADH

1 $FADH_2$

1 GTP (converted to ATP)

The two carbons that are given off as CO_2 originally came from acetyl-CoA.

There are two acetyl-CoAs produced from one glucose, so the net from one glucose is the amount generated from two cycles:

4 CO_2

6 NADH

2 $FADH_2$

2 GTP (converted to ATP)

Through glycolysis, the transition reaction, and the citric acid cycle, multiple NADH and $FADH_2$ molecules are produced. Under aerobic conditions, these molecules will enter the electron transport chain to be used to generate energy through oxidative phosphorylation as described in the next section.

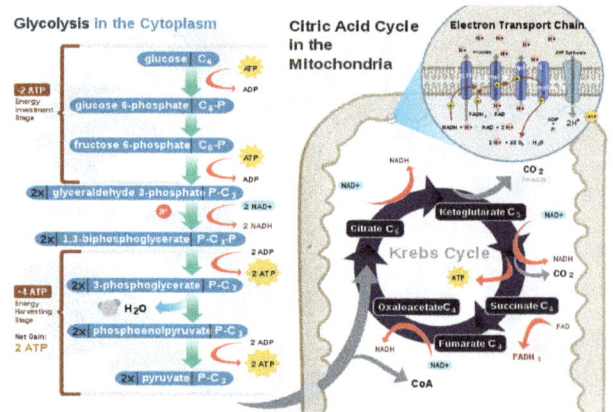

Figure 190. The pathways involved in aerobic respiration

5.2.5 Electron Transport Chain

The electron transport chain is located on the inner membrane of the mitochondria, as shown below.

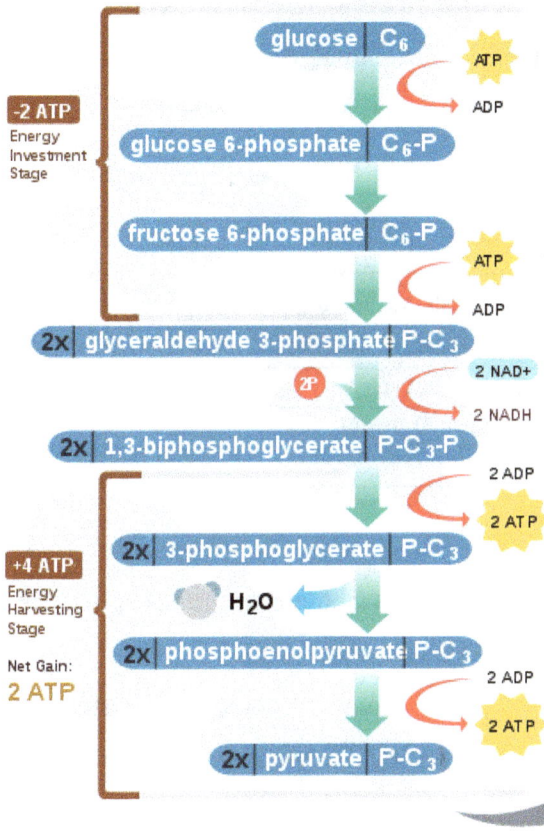

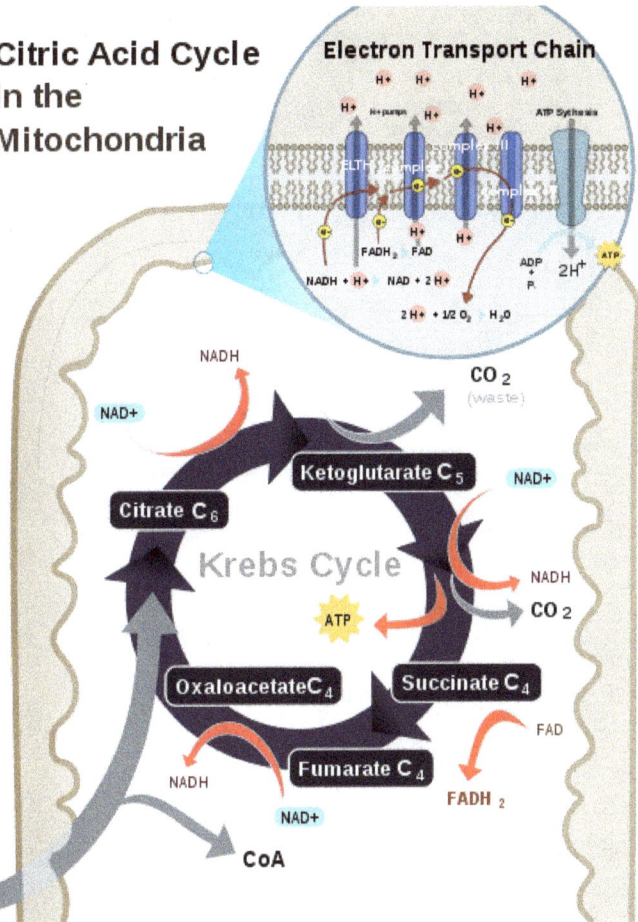

Figure 191. The pathways involved in aerobic respiration

The electron transport chain contains several electron carriers. These carriers take the electrons from NADH and $FADH_2$, pass them down the chain of complexes and electron carriers, and ultimately produce ATP. More specifically, the electron transport chain takes the energy from the electrons on NADH and $FADH_2$ to pump protons (H^+) into the intermembrane space. This creates a proton gradient between the intermembrane space (high) and the matrix (low) of the mitochondria. ATP synthase uses the energy from this gradient to synthesize ATP. Oxygen is required for this process because it serves as the final electron acceptor, forming water. Collectively this process is known as oxidative phosphorylation.

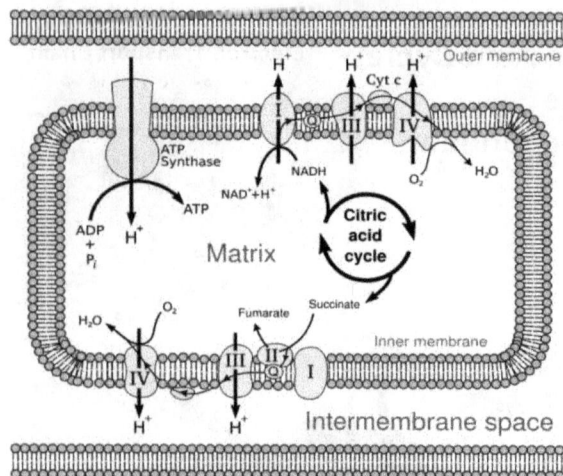

Figure 192. Location of the electron transport chain in the mitochondria

2.5 ATP/NADH and 1.5 ATP/FADH$_2$ are produced in the electron transport chain. Some resources will say 3 ATP/NADH and 2 ATP/FADH$_2$, but these values are generally less accepted now.

For one molecule of glucose, the preceding pathways produce:

Glycolysis: 2 NADH
Transition Reaction: 2 NADH
Citric Acid Cycle: 6 NADH, 2 FADH$_2$
Total   10 NADH, 2 FADH$_2$

Multiply that by the amount of ATP per NADH or FADH2 to yield:
10 NADH X 2.5 ATP/NADH = 25 ATP
  2 FADH$_2$ X 1.5 ATP/FADH$_2$ =   3 ATP
Total   28 ATP

5.2.6   Aerobic Glucose Metabolism Totals

The table below shows the ATP generated from one molecule of glucose in the different metabolic pathways.

Table 24. ATP generated from one molecule of glucose

Metabolic Pathway	ATP Generated
Glycolysis	2
Citric Acid Cycle	2
Electron Transport Chain	28
Total	32

Notice that the clear majority of ATP is generated by the electron transport chain. If we do the math, 28/32 X 100 = 87.5% of the ATP from a molecule of glucose is generated by the electron transport chain. Remember that this is aerobic and requires oxygen to be the final electron acceptor. If 3 ATP/NADH and 2 ATP/FADH$_2$ are used instead of 2.5 ATP/NADH and 1.5 ATP/FADH$_2$ that were used above, total ATP and percentage of ATP produced by the electron transport chain would be different. But the takeaway message remains the same. The electron transport chain by far produces the most ATP from one molecule of glucose.

5.2.7   Anaerobic Respiration

Conditions without oxygen are referred to anaerobic. In this case, the pyruvate will be converted to lactate in the cytoplasm of the cell as shown below.

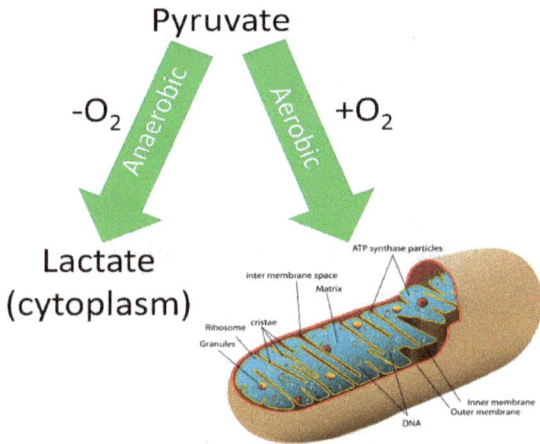

Figure 193. Pyruvate fork in the road, what happens depends on whether it is aerobic or anaerobic respiration

What happens if oxygen isn't available to serve as the final electron acceptor?

As shown in the following video, the ETC becomes backed up with electrons and can't accept them from NADH and $FADH_2$. This leads to a problem in glycolysis because NAD is needed to accept electrons, as shown below. Without the electron transport chain functioning, all NAD has been reduced to NADH and glycolysis cannot continue to produce ATP from glucose.

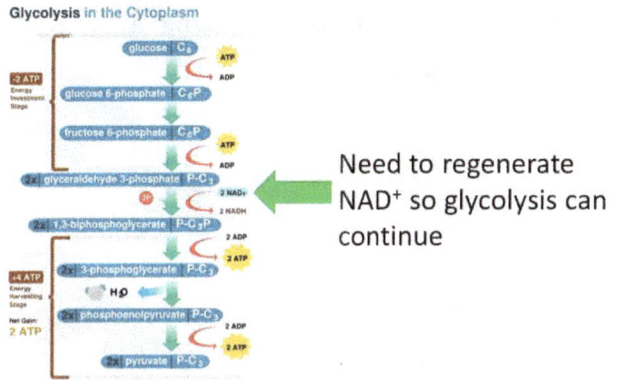

Need to regenerate NAD^+ so glycolysis can continue

Figure 194. Why NAD needs to be regenerated under anaerobic conditions

Thus, there is a workaround to regenerate NAD by converting pyruvate (pyruvic acid) to lactate (lactic acid) as shown below.

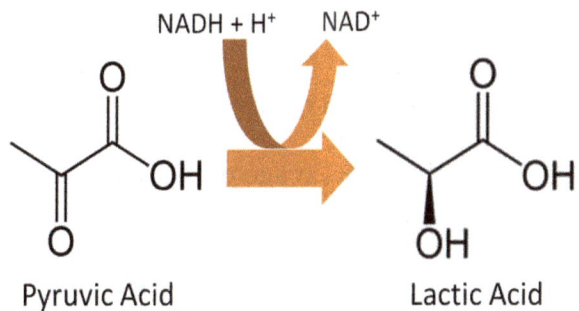

Figure 195. The conversion of pyruvic acid to lactic acid regenerates NAD

However, anaerobic respiration only produces 2 ATP per molecule of glucose, compared to 32 ATP for aerobic respiration. The biggest producer of lactate is the muscle. Through what is known as the Cori cycle, lactate produced in the muscle can be sent to the liver. In the liver, through the process of gluconeogenesis, glucose can be regenerated and sent back to the muscle to be used again for anaerobic respiration forming a cycle as shown below.

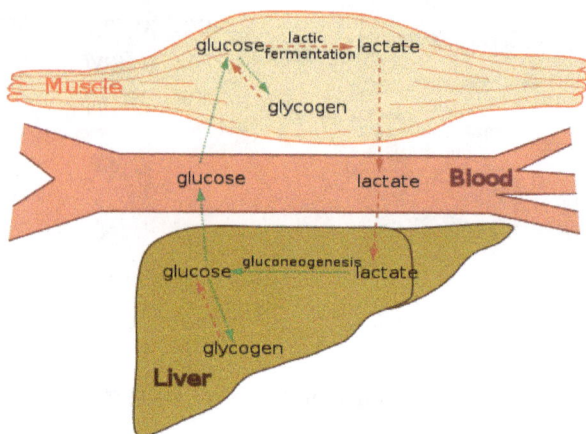

Figure 196. The Cori cycle[xxxvi]

5.3 Lipid Metabolism Pathways

5.3.1 Lipolysis (Triglyceride Breakdown)

Lipolysis is the cleavage of triglycerides to glycerol and fatty acids, as shown below.

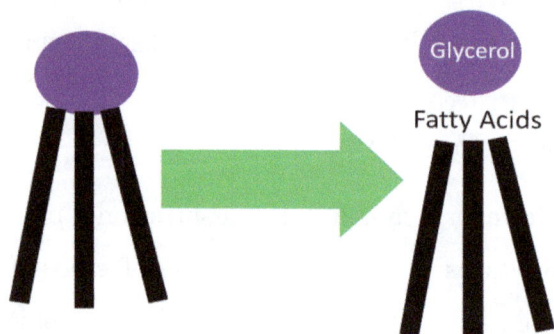

Figure 197. Lipolysis

There are two primary lipolysis enzymes:

1. Lipoprotein lipase (LPL)
2. Hormone-sensitive lipase (HSL)

Despite performing the same function, at the adipose level, the enzymes are primarily active for seemingly opposite reasons. In the fed state, LPL on the endothelium of blood vessels cleaves lipoprotein triglycerides into fatty acids so that they can be taken up into adipocytes for storage. This action of LPL on lipoproteins is shown in the two figures below.

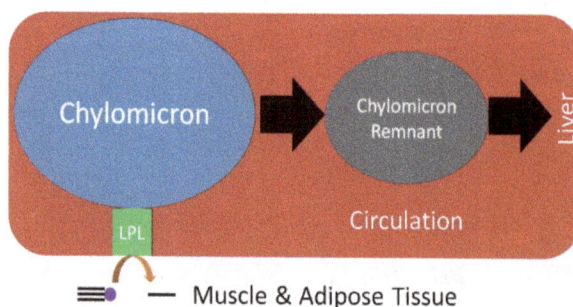

Figure 198. Lipoprotein lipase cleaves fatty acids from the chylomicron, forming a chylomicron remnant

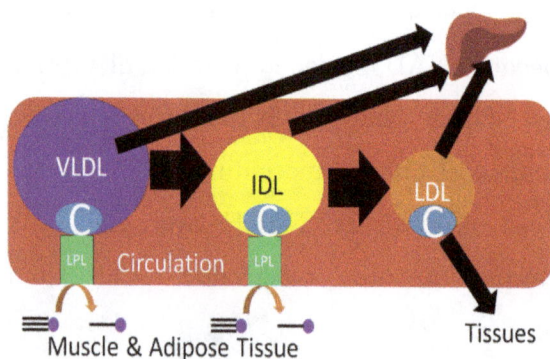

Figure 199. Lipoprotein lipase cleaves triglycerides from VLDL and IDL, forming subsequent lipoproteins (IDL and LDL) that contain less triglyceride

HSL is an important enzyme in adipose tissue, which is a major storage site of triglycerides in the body. The activity of HSL activity is increased by glucagon and epinephrine ("fight or flight" hormones) and decreased by insulin. Thus, in hypoglycaemia (such as during a fast) or a "fight or flight" response, triglycerides in the adipose are cleaved, releasing fatty acids into circulation that then bind with the transport protein albumin. Thus, HSL is important for mobilizing fatty acids so they can be used to produce energy. The figure below shows how fatty acids can be taken up and used by tissues such as the muscle for energy production[15].

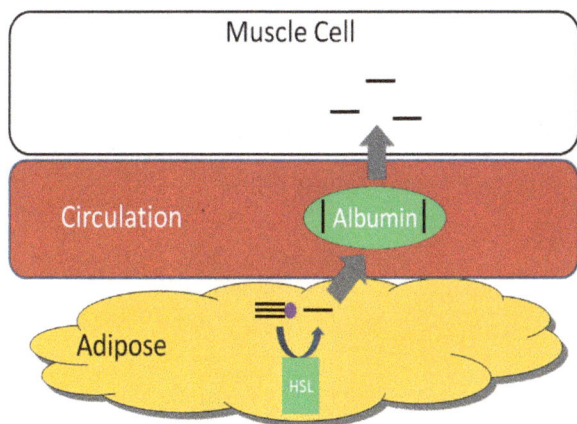

Figure 200. Hormone-sensitive lipase

Glycerol—the 'backbone' of triglycerides has two metabolic fates.

1. It can be broken down in glycolysis

2. It can be used to synthesize glucose (gluconeogenesis)

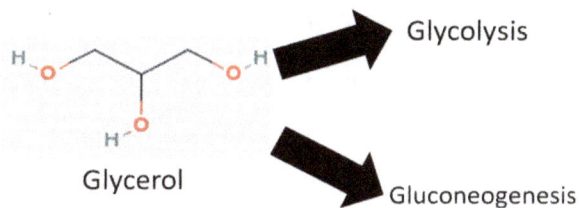

Figure 201. Metabolic fates of glycerol

5.3.2   Fatty Acid Oxidation (Beta-oxidation)

To generate energy from fatty acids, they must be oxidized. This process occurs in the mitochondria, but long chain fatty acids cannot diffuse across the mitochondrial membrane (like absorption into the enterocyte). Carnitine, an amino acid-derived compound, helps shuttle long-chain fatty acids into the mitochondria. The structure of carnitine is shown below.

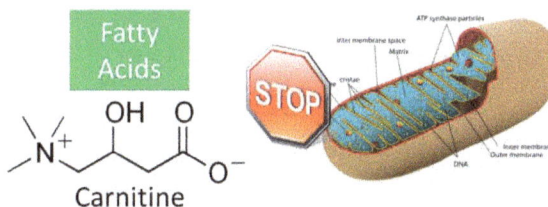

Figure 202. Carnitine shuttles fatty acids into the mitochondria

5.3.2.1 Fatty Acid Shuttling

As shown below, there are two enzymes involved in this process: carnitine palmitoyl transferase I (CPTI) and carnitine palmitoyl transferase II (CPTII). CPTI is located on the outer mitochondrial membrane, CPTII is located on the inner mitochondrial membrane. The fatty acid is first activated by addition of a CoA

117

(forming acyl-CoA), then CPTI adds carnitine. Acyl-Carnitine is then transported into the mitochondrial matrix with the assistance of the enzyme translocase. In the matrix, CPTII removes carnitine from the activated fatty acid (acyl-CoA). Carnitine is recycled back into the cytosol to be used again.

5.3.2.2 Fatty Acid Activation

As shown below, the first step of fatty acid oxidation is activation. A CoA molecule is added to the fatty acid to produce acyl-CoA, converting ATP to AMP in the process. Note that in this step, the ATP is converted to AMP, not ADP. Thus, activation uses the equivalent of 2 ATP molecules[23].

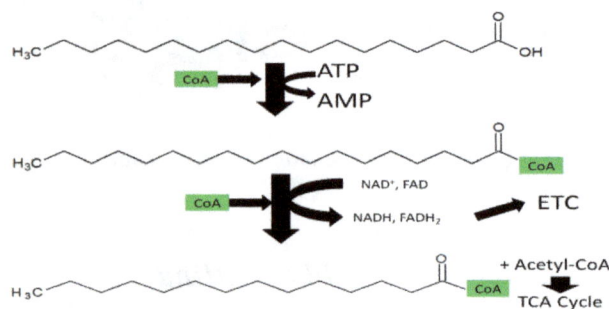

Figure 203. Fatty Acid Oxidation

5.3.2.3 Fatty Acid Oxidation

Fatty acid oxidation is also referred to as beta-oxidation because 2 carbon units are cleaved off at the beta-carbon position (2nd carbon from the acid end) of an activated fatty acid. The cleaved 2 carbon unit forms

acetyl-CoA and produces an activated fatty acid (acyl-CoA) with 2 fewer carbons, acetyl-CoA, NADH, and $FADH_2$.

To completely oxidize the 18-carbon fatty acid above, 8 cycles of beta-oxidation must occur. This will produce:

9 acetyl-CoAs

8 NADH

8 $FADH_2$

Those 9 acetyl-CoAs can continue into the citric acid cycle, where they can produce:

9 GTP

9 $FADH_2$

27 NADH

The products of the complete oxidation of a fatty acid are shown below.

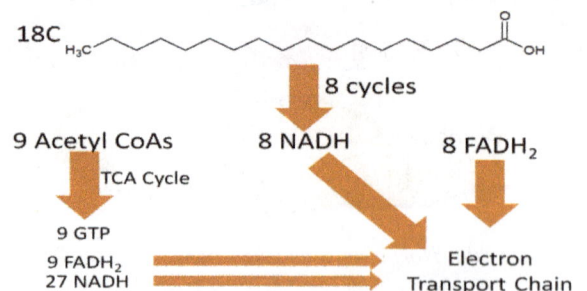

Figure 204. Complete oxidation of an 18 carbon (C) fatty acid

Adding up the NADH & $FADH_2$, the electron transport chain ATP production from beta-oxidation and the citric acid cycle looks like this:

NADH

8 (beta-oxidation) + 27 (TCA) = 35 NADH X 2.5 ATP/NADH = 87.5 ATP

$FADH_2$

8 (beta-oxidation) + 9 (TCA) = 17 $FADH_2$ X 1.5 ATP/$FADH_2$ = 25.5 ATP

GTP

9 GTP = 9 ATP

Total ATP from complete oxidation of an 18-carbon fatty acid:

87.5 + 25.5 + 9 = 122 ATP

Subtract 2 ATP (ATP-->AMP) required for activation of the fatty acid:

122-2 = 120 Net ATP

Compared to glucose (32 ATP) you can see that there is far more energy stored in a fatty acid. This is because fatty acids are in a more reduced form and thus, they yield 9 kcal/g instead of 4 kcal/g like carbohydrates.[4]

5.3.3 De novo Lipogenesis (Fatty Acid Synthesis)

De novo in Latin means "from the beginning." Thus, *de novo* lipogenesis is the synthesis of fatty acids, beginning with acetyl-CoA. Acetyl-CoA must first move out of the mitochondria, where it is then converted to malonyl-CoA (3 carbons).

Malonyl-CoA then is combined with another acetyl-CoA to form a 4-carbon fatty acid (1 carbon is given off as CO_2). The addition of 2 carbons is repeated through a similar process 7 times to produce a 16 carbon fatty acid.[36]

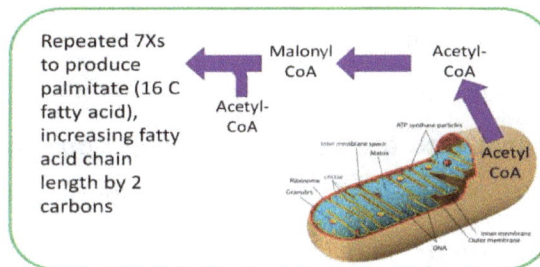

Figure 205. Fatty acid synthesis

Most fatty acids synthesized will be esterified into triglycerides for storage.

5.3.4 Ketone Body Synthesis

Ketone body synthesis occurs always, but we don't notice increased ketones levels in the blood and urine unless there is some degree of carbohydrate restriction. Appreciable levels of ketones are only produced with greater restriction of carbohydrate or during fasting or starvation. A restriction of carbohydrate, either by fasting or by restricting dietary carbohydrate results in reduced insulin levels, thereby reducing lipogenesis and fat accumulation. When glycogen reserves become insufficient to supply glucose necessary for normal fat oxidation (via the provision of oxaloacetate in the Krebs cycle) and for the supply of glucose to the Central Nervous System (CNS), an alternative fuel source is needed. It is commonly suggested that the CNS typically cannot utilise fat for fuel, as the common dietary lipids (long chain fatty acids) are almost always bound to albumin and are unable to cross the blood-brain barrier, although this contention has been drawn into question, for example due to the easy desorption of FAs from albumin[43] and there may be other more subtle reasons as to why neurons, astrocytes and ganglia may be more adapted to using glucose for fuel. Namely that ß-oxidation of fatty acids (FAs) demands more oxygen than the oxidation of glucose, thereby increasing the risk of hypoxia of neurons, ß-oxidation of FAs generates superoxide, causing increased oxidative stress for neurons, and that the rate of ATP generation from fatty acids (as compared to glucose) is slower, and so in times of rapid neuronal firing there may be reduced fuel provision if FAs are the primary energy providing substrate for the brain.[44] This suggests an evolutionary-adaptive advantage to lowering of fatty oxidative capacity of brain cell mitochondria to avoid these challenges and thus favours glucose oxidation in the brain.

Some dietary fats (such as short and medium chain triglycerides) can easily cross the blood-brain barrier (as they are not bound to albumin) and be used extensively by neurons, but their availability is scarce in the typical diet and so the CNS relies primarily on glucose for fuel.

Alternative fatty acid derived fuels 'ketones'; acetoacetate and ß-hydroxybutyric acid (BOHB) and acetone, do not promote the same raft of problems associated with LCFA metabolism in the brain.[44]

Ketone bodies are produced through a process called 'ketogenesis' in the liver to accommodate fuel demands during times of carbohydrate scarcity.

Acetoacetate is the primary ketone body, with BOHB providing the primary circulating ketone. Technically BOHB is not a ketone body (as the ketone moiety has been reduced to a hydroxyl group) however it functions as a primary fuel in the process of ketosis. Some acetoacetate is produced under normal dietary conditions (which include moderate to high intakes of carbohydrate), but this small amount is metabolised readily and rapidly by skeletal and heart tissue, resulting in only minimal levels of circulating ketones. It has been clinically observed that higher fat, moderated carbohydrate diets (such as 'Paleo' and 'Primal' diets), not necessarily of a LCKD nature may result in consistently higher levels of circulating BOHB than would be seen in standard western-style (higher-carbohydrate) diets, yet still under the threshold of what is considered a functional or nutritional ketosis. A dearth of evidence in this area of broad metabolic adaptation to varying macronutrients (especially over a longer term of ingestion) requires further research and elucidation.

When acetoacetate is produced in substantial amounts it can accumulate and be converted into the other ketone bodies (acetone and BOHB) leading to the presence of ketones in the blood and urine (ketonaemia and ketonuria respectively) and in the breath.

Ketones are utilised by tissue as a source of energy. BOHB results in two molecules of acetyl CoA which enter the Krebs cycle. In ketosis blood glucose levels stay within normal physiological limits due to the creation of glucose from glucogenic amino acids and via the liberation of glycerol during fatty oxidation. In silico models further suggest a plausible conversion of fatty acids to glucose [45], more likely to occur in periods of carbohydrate restriction.

All these factors of ketone, fatty-acid and glucose regulation are crucially important as certain cell types, such as red blood cells (RBCs), lacking mitochondria, are only

able to use glucose as a fuel source and thus the preservation of stable glucose levels is critical for survival.

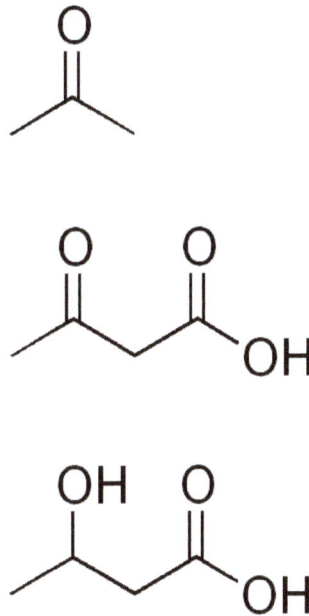

Figure 206. The three ketone bodies from top to bottom (acetone, acetoacetic acid, and beta-hydroxybutyric acid)

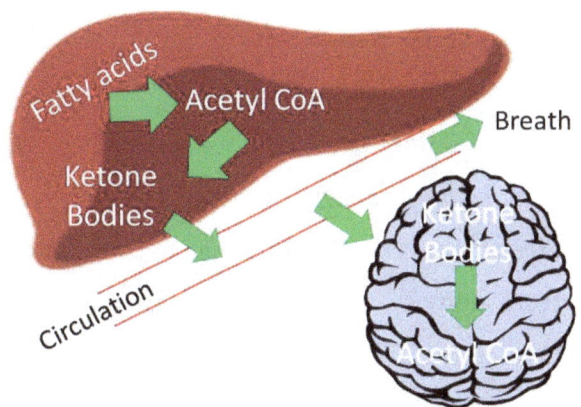

Figure 207. The production, release, use, or exhalation of ketone bodies

121

When a pathology such as diabetes or alcoholism (as compared to the normal state of 'nutritional ketosis'), causes elevated levels of ketones to be secreted, it results in a condition known as ketoacidosis. The elevated level of ketones in the blood decreases the blood's pH, meaning it becomes more acidic. Mild levels of ketosis (< 5mmol/L BOHB) are considered safe and appropriate states of normal human metabolism, however, elevated levels of blood ketones resulting in acidosis cannot be buffered effectively and are both dangerous, and a sign of existing pathology.

5.3.4.1 Differentiating functional, nutritional induced ketosis from DKA and other pathology associated ketosis

Diabetic ketoacidosis (DKA) is a potentially fatal condition characterised by a triad of: hyperglycaemia, increased total body ketone concentration, and metabolic acidosis.[46] DKA results from uncontrolled diabetes mellitus and an inability of peripheral tissue to uptake glucose effectively. There is a release of fatty acids from adipose tissue and an unrestrained production of ketone bodies by the liver.[46] A functional, nutritional ketosis (ketosis absent of pathology) on the other hand is an adaptive response allowing the utilization of ketone bodies (BOHB) by neurons and other tissue and reducing the need for carbohydrate (glucose) as a primary fuel substrate in periods of carbohydrate scarcity. For example, it has been demonstrated that insulin induced hypoglycaemic coma can be reversed by intravenous administration of BOHB[47] and that BOHB and acetoacetate effectively replace glucose as fuel for neurons during starvation[48] and preserves synaptic function even in the presence of glucose deprivation and reduction of glycolysis. Ketosis elicited by dietary intervention has been described variously as 'functional ketosis'[49] or more commonly 'nutritional ketosis'. It has been claimed that Jeff Volek and Stephen Phinney coined the term 'nutritional ketosis' however the term can be found in the medical and scientific literature predating Drs Volek and Phinney, for example in the work of Sargent and colleagues.[50] However in many of the earlier texts, ketosis, even if nutritionally induced (i.e. absent pathological aetiology) ketosis is considered to be a disadvantaged or dangerous state. As early as 1960 Hans Krebs began to elucidate some of the mechanisms of interdependence between fatty acid and carbohydrate metabolism (for instance the effects on fatty acid metabolism and ketone production of reductions in oxaloacetate).[51] This investigation and others began to more aptly differentiate the state of nutritional ketosis versus that of a far greater levels hyperketonaemia seen in pathologies such as diabetic ketoacidosis (DKA). In 1966 Krebs differentiated this 'physiologic' ketosis from pathological ketosis.[52]

Jeff Volek and Stephen Phinney considered the ten-fold physiologic range between 0.5 mmol/L and 5mmol/L as the functional definition for 'nutritional ketosis'. [53, 54] This range has since become a *lingua franca* used in clinical nutrition to define ketosis.

Ketoacidosis may also occur in the alcoholic. In alcoholic ketoacidosis gluconeogenesis is inhibited, creating an 'energy crisis', requiring increased fatty acid metabolism and ketone body formation.

5.4 Cholesterol Synthesis

Acetyl-CoA is also used to synthesize cholesterol. As shown below, there are many reactions and enzymes involved in cholesterol synthesis.

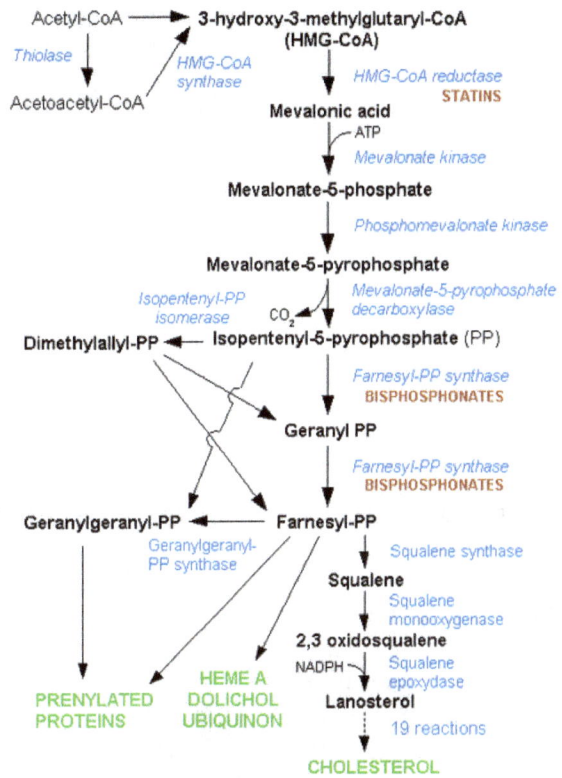

Figure 208. Cholesterol synthesis pathway

Simplifying this, acetyl-CoA is converted to acetoacetyl-CoA (4 carbons) before forming 3-hydroxy-3-methylglutaryl-CoA (HMG-CoA). HMG-CoA is converted to mevalonate by the enzyme HMG-CoA reductase. This enzyme is important because it is the rate-limiting enzyme in cholesterol synthesis.

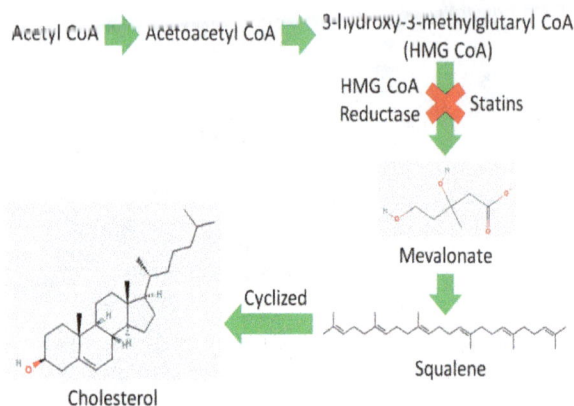

Figure 209. Cholesterol synthesis simplified

A rate-limiting enzyme is like a bottleneck in a highway, as shown below, that determines the flow of traffic past it.

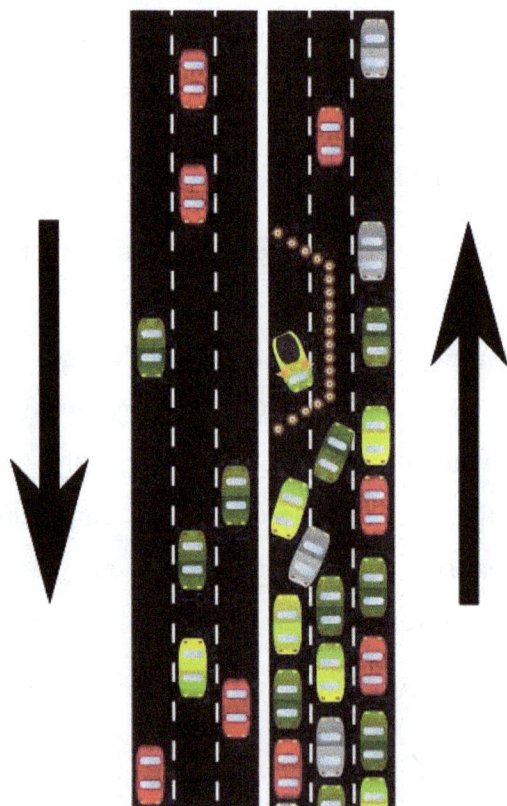

Figure 210. Bottleneck in traffic

Rate-limiting enzymes limit the rate at which a metabolic pathway proceeds. The body synthesizes approximately 1 gram of cholesterol a day. Several tissues synthesize cholesterol, with the liver accounting for ~20% of synthesis. The intestine is believed to be the most active among the other tissues that are responsible for the other 80% of cholesterol synthesis.[36]

5.5 Protein Metabolism

This section will focus on how proteins and amino acids are broken down. There are four protein metabolic pathways that will be covered in this section:

Transamination
  -transfer of an amino group from one amino acid to another
Deamination
  -removal of an amino group, normally from an amino acid.
Gluconeogenesis
  -synthesis of glucose from a non-carbohydrate source.
Protein Turnover/Degradation
  -liberation of amino acids from proteins.

5.5.1 Transamination, Deamination & Ammonia Removal as Urea

The first step in catabolizing, or breaking down, an amino acid is the removal of its amine group ($-NH_3$). Amine groups can be transferred or removed through transamination or deamination, respectively.

5.5.1.1 Transamination

Transamination is the transfer of an amine group from an amino acid to a keto acid (amino acid without an amine group), thus creating a new amino acid and keto acid as shown below.

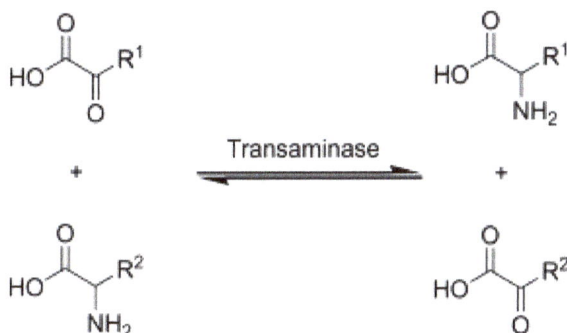

Figure 211. Generic transamination reaction where the top keto acid is converted to an amino acid, while the bottom amino acid is converted to a keto acid

Keto acids and/or carbon skeletons are what remains after amino acids have had their nitrogen group removed by deamination or transamination. Transamination is used to synthesize nonessential amino acids.

5.5.1.2 Deamination

Deamination is the removal of the amine group as ammonia (NH_3), as shown below.

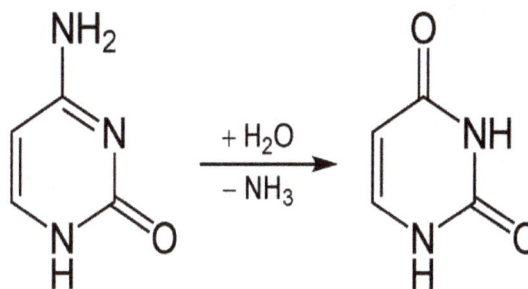

Figure 212. Deamination of cytosine to uracil (nucleotides, not amino acids)

The following animation nicely illustrates the transamination and deamination of amino acids.

The potential problem with deamination is that too much ammonia is toxic, causing a condition known as hyperammonaemia. The symptoms of this condition are shown in the following figure.

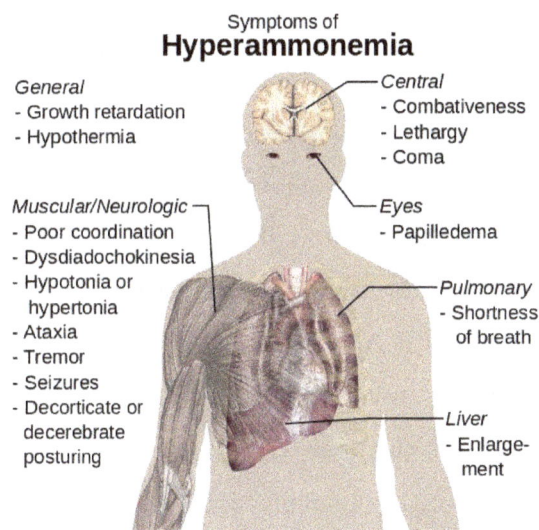

Symptoms of
Hyperammonemia

General
- Growth retardation
- Hypothermia

Central
- Combativeness
- Lethargy
- Coma

Muscular/Neurologic
- Poor coordination
- Dysdiadochokinesia
- Hypotonia or hypertonia
- Ataxia
- Tremor
- Seizures
- Decorticate or decerebrate posturing

Eyes
- Papilledema

Pulmonary
- Shortness of breath

Liver
- Enlargement

Figure 213. Symptoms of hyperammonaemia[xxxvii]

Our body has a method to safely package ammonia in a less toxic form to be

xxxvii Häggström, Mikael (2014). "Medical gallery of Mikael Häggström 2014". *WikiJournal of Medicine* 1 (2). DOI:10.15347/wjm/2014.008. ISSN 2002-4436. Public Domain.

excreted. This safer compound is urea, which is produced by the liver using 2 molecules of ammonia (NH_3) and 1 molecule of carbon dioxide (CO_2). Most urea is then secreted from the liver and incorporated into urine in the kidney to be excreted from the body, as shown below.

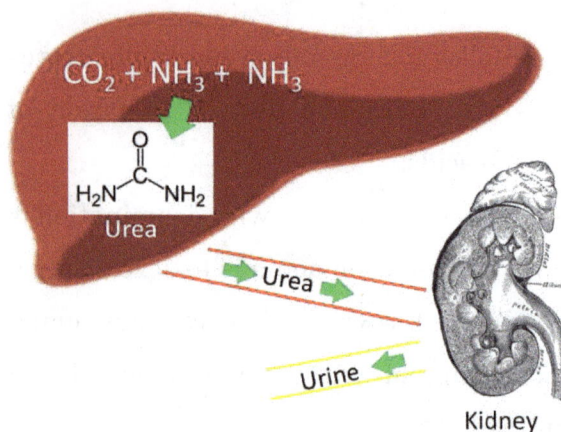

Figure 214. Production of urea helps to safely remove ammonia from the body4

There is a metabolic ceiling for the body to effectively metabolise amino acids via direct oxidation and gluconeogenesis. This condition was dubbed 'rabbit starvation' by early North American explorers due to it occurring when they subsisted almost solely on the lean tissue of rabbit flesh without either enough carbohydrate or fat. This is also one of the reasons that hunter-gatherers choose the fattier parts of an animal to eat in preference to the lean tissue which not only helps to provide the maximum calories (and micronutrition), but perhaps most importantly to avoid the

dire metabolic consequences of protein overconsumption.[55]

Protein overconsumption occurs when over 50% of calories are derived from protein in a diet (or there is an absolute intake of greater than ~300 g) and results in symptoms of: hyperaminoacidaemia, hyperammonaemia, hyperinsulinaemia, diarrhoea and finally death.[56]

5.5.2 Gluconeogenesis

Gluconeogenesis is the synthesis of glucose from non-carbohydrate sources. Many amino acids can be used for this process, and this is particularly relevant for our understanding of metabolic adaptations to diet, hence the reason that this section is included here instead of the carbohydrate metabolism section. Gluconeogenesis is glycolysis in reverse with an oxaloacetate workaround, as shown below. Remember oxaloacetate is also an intermediate in the citric acid cycle.

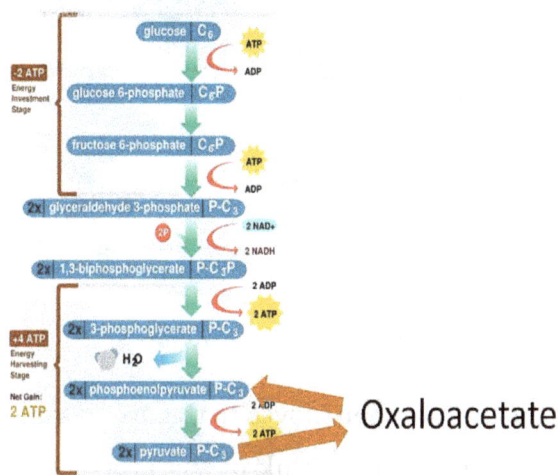

Figure 215. Gluconeogenesis is glycolysis in reverse with an oxaloacetate workaround

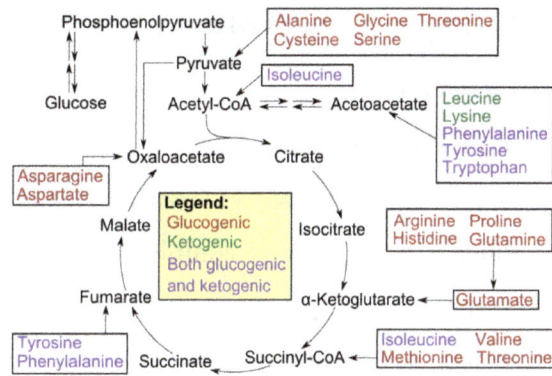

Figure 216. Glucogenic (red), ketogenic (green), and glucogenic and ketogenic amino acids[xxxviii]

Not all amino acids can be used for gluconeogenesis. The ones that can be used are termed glucogenic (red) and can be converted to either pyruvate or a citric acid cycle intermediate. Other amino acids can only be converted to either acetyl-CoA or acetoacetyl-CoA, which cannot be used for gluconeogenesis. However, acetyl-CoA or acetoacetyl-CoA can be used for ketogenesis to synthesize the ketone bodies, acetone and acetoacetate. Thus, these amino acids are instead termed ketogenic (green).

Fatty acids and ketogenic amino acids cannot be used to synthesize glucose. The transition reaction is a one-way reaction, meaning that acetyl-CoA can't be converted back to pyruvate. As a result, fatty acids can't be used to synthesize glucose, because beta-oxidation produces acetyl-CoA. Even if acetyl-CoA enters the citric acid cycle, it will be completely oxidized, and the carbons will be given off as CO_2. Some amino acids can be either glucogenic or ketogenic, depending on how they are metabolized. These amino acids are referred to as glucogenic and ketogenic (pink).

Note: The glycerol 'backbone' of fats can be converted to glucose and in silico evidence has suggested that it may be possible for fatty acids to be converted to glucose,[45] but this has not been demonstrated in vivo.

xxxviii Häggström, Mikael (2014). "Medical gallery of Mikael Häggström 2014". *WikiJournal of Medicine* **1** (2). DOI:10.15347/wjm/2014.008. ISSN 2002-4436. Public Domain

5.5.3 Protein Turnover/Degradation

Proteins serve several functions in the body as structural component. But what happens when these structures (cells, enzymes, etc.) have completed their lifespan?

Proteins are broken down to their constituent amino acids that can be used to synthesize new proteins. There are three main systems of protein degradation:

1. Ubiquitin-proteasome degradation

2. Lysosome degradation

3. Calpain degradation

5.5.3.1 *Ubiquitin-Proteasome Degradation*

Proteins that are damaged or abnormal are tagged with the protein ubiquitin. There are multiple protein subunits involved in the process (E1-E3), but the net result is the production of a protein (substrate) with a ubiquitin tail, as shown below.

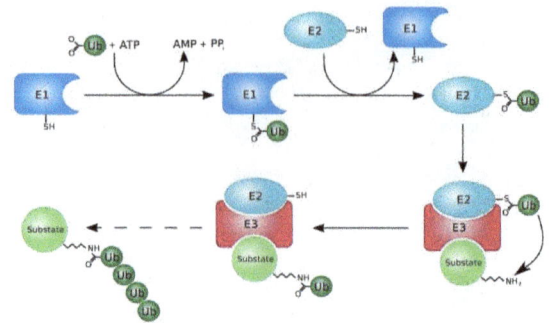

Figure 217. Ubiquitination of a protein[xxxix]

This protein then moves to the proteasome for degradation. Think of the proteasome like a rubbish disposal. The ubiquitinated "rubbish" protein is inserted into the rubbish disposal where it is broken down into its component parts (primarily amino acids).

5.5.3.2 *Lysosome Degradation*

The lysosomes are organelles that are found in cells. They contain several proteases that degrade proteins.

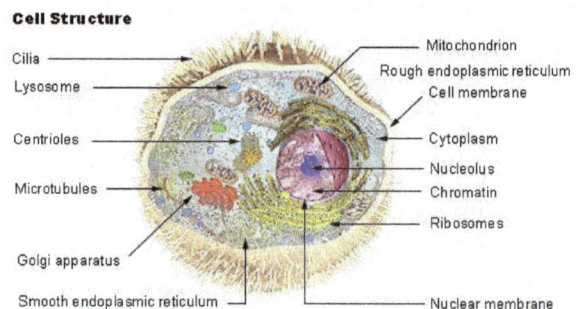

Figure 218. Lysosomes are organelles within the cell[xl]

[xxxix] This file is licensed under the Creative Commons Attribution-Share Alike 3.0 Unported license. Attribution: Rogerdodd

[xl] In the Public Domain (US Gov.) https://training.seer.cancer.gov/anatomy/cells_tissues_membranes/cells/structure.html

5.5.3.3 Calpain Degradation

The last degradation system is the calpain system, which is not as well understood, but does require calcium.

5.6 Alcohol Metabolism

The other energy source is alcohol. The alcohol we consume contains two carbons and is known as ethanol.

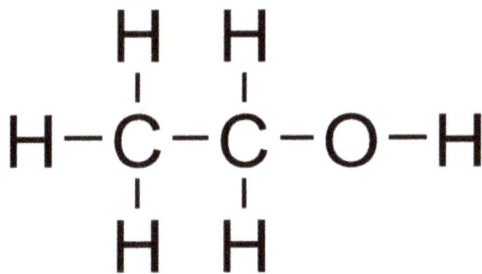

Figure 219. Structure of ethanol

Ethanol is passively absorbed by simple diffusion into the enterocyte. Ethanol metabolism occurs primarily in the liver, but 10-30% is estimated to occur in the stomach.[15] For the average person, the liver can metabolize the amount of ethanol in one standard drink (approximately 10 g of alcohol) per hour.[18] There are three ways that alcohol is metabolized in the body.

1. Catalase—an enzyme that we will cover again in the antioxidants section. Catalase is estimated to metabolize less than 2% of ethanol, so it is not shown below or discussed further.[36]

2. Alcohol dehydrogenase (ADH)—The major ethanol-metabolizing enzyme converts ethanol and NAD to acetaldehyde and NADH, respectively. Aldehyde dehydrogenase (ALDH) uses NAD, CoA, and acetaldehyde to create acetyl-CoA and to produce another NADH. The action of ADH is shown in the figure below.

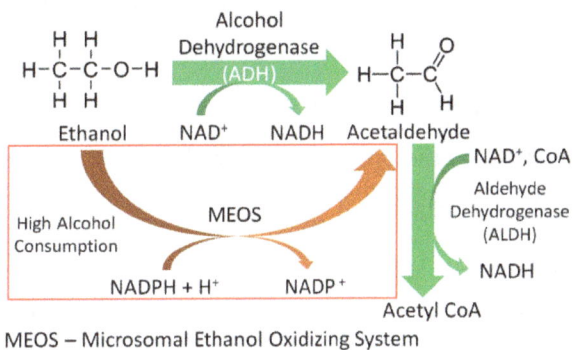

Figure 220. Ethanol metabolism

3. Microsomal ethanol oxidizing system (MEOS)—When a person consumes a large amount of alcohol the MEOS, is the overflow pathway, that also metabolizes ethanol to acetaldehyde. It is estimated that the MEOS metabolizes 20% of ethanol,[3] and it differs from ADH in that it uses ATP to convert reduced nicotinamide adenine dinucleotide phosphate (NADPH + H$^+$) to NADP$^+$. The action of the MEOS is shown in the figure above.

At high intakes or with repeated exposure, there is increased synthesis of MEOS enzymes resulting in more efficient metabolism, also known as increased tolerance. ADH levels do not increase based on alcohol exposure. MEOS also metabolizes a variety of other compounds (drugs, fatty acids, steroids) and alcohol competes for the enzyme's action. This can cause the metabolism of drugs to slow and potentially reach harmful levels in the body.[3]

Females have lower stomach ADH activity and body H_2O concentrations. As a result, a larger proportion of ethanol reaches circulation, thus, in general, females have a lower tolerance for alcohol. Many Asian individuals have low ADH activity. This leads to build up of acetaldehyde and undesirable symptoms such as: flushing, dizziness, nausea, and headaches.[2]

6 Integration of Macronutrient & Alcohol Metabolism

Understanding different metabolic pathways is a crucial step. However, an integrated understanding of the interconnectedness and tissue specificity of metabolism is where this knowledge really becomes powerful. To this end, we will first cover how the different pathways feed into one another and then talk about the metabolic capabilities of the different tissues in the body. We will then discuss what happens metabolically during different conditions or when consuming certain diets.

6.1 Integration of Macronutrient and Alcohol Metabolic Pathways

If you were to draw all the macronutrient and alcohol metabolic pathways covered in chapter 6, hopefully it would look something like the figure below. In this figure:

Carbohydrate pathways are orange

Triglyceride/fatty acid pathways are purple

Protein/amino acid pathways are green

Non-classified pathways are grey

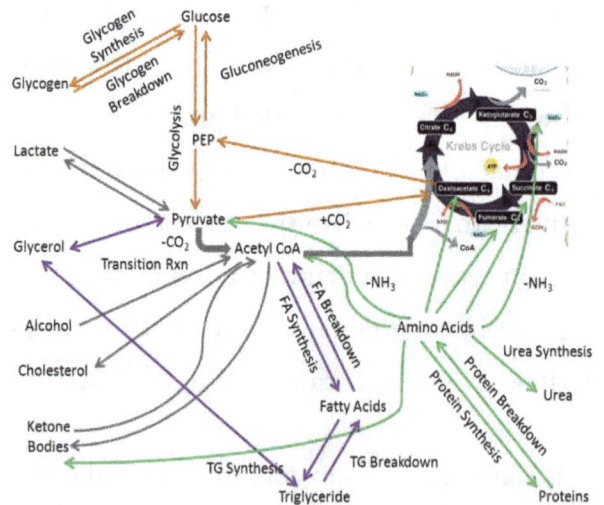

Figure 221. Integrated macronutrient and alcohol metabolism

To simplify, we are going to remove the glycerol and cholesterol pathways so that we can focus on integrating the other pathways in macronutrient and alcohol metabolism.

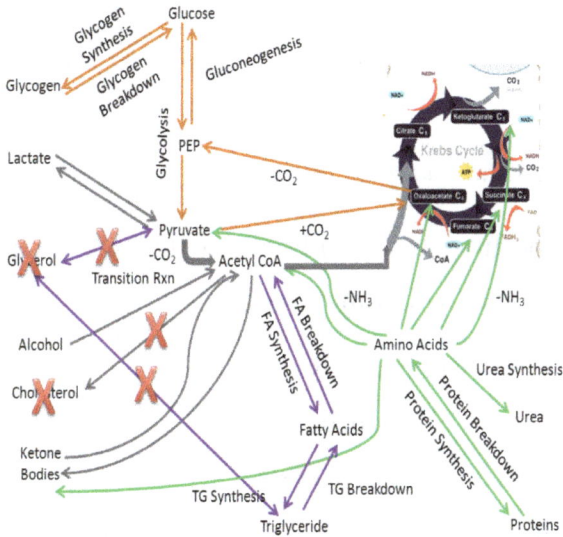

Figure 222. Removal of glycerol and cholesterol pathways

Thus, we are left with the following simplified figure:

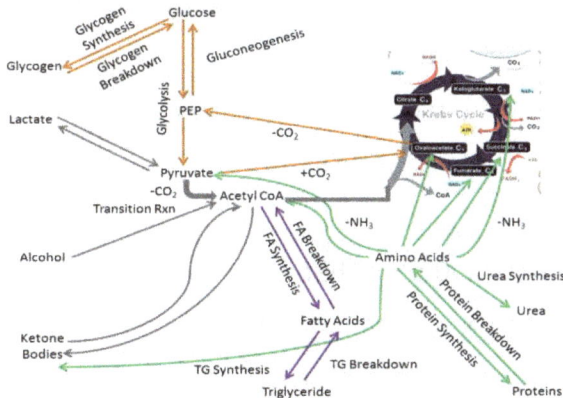

Figure 223. Simplified integrated macronutrient and alcohol metabolism

Notice that acetyl-CoA is the central metabolite in integrated metabolism that connects many different pathways. For example, carbohydrates can be broken down to acetyl-CoA that can then be used to synthesize fats and ultimately triglycerides.

6.2 Liver Macronutrient and Alcohol Metabolism

The liver is the organ that has the greatest macronutrient metabolic capability; there are several metabolic functions that only the liver performs. However, there are two major macronutrient metabolic processes, lactate synthesis and ketone body breakdown, that the liver will not normally perform, as shown in the figure below. Ketone bodies cannot be used by the liver for energy, because the liver lacks the enzyme ß-ketoacyl-CoA transferase, also called thiophorase. Acetone in low concentrations is taken up by the liver and undergoes detoxification through the methylglyoxal pathway which ends with lactate.

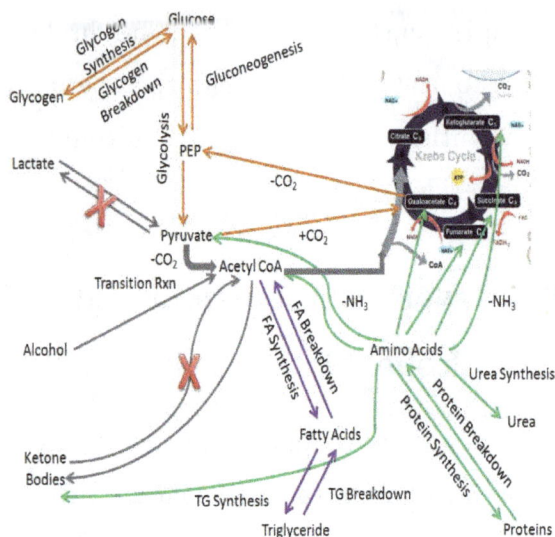

Figure 224. Ketone body breakdown and lactate synthesis are major macronutrient metabolic pathways that the liver does not normally perform

But aside from those two pathways, the liver performs all the other metabolic pathways that we have covered as listed and shown below:

Glycogen synthesis and breakdown

Glycolysis

Gluconeogenesis

Alcohol oxidation

Ketone body synthesis

Fatty acid synthesis and breakdown

Triglyceride synthesis and breakdown

Protein synthesis and breakdown

Urea synthesis

VLDL synthesis

Glucose-6-phosphatase

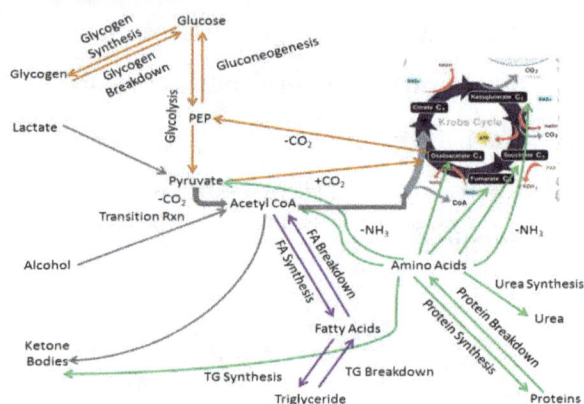

Figure 225. Metabolic capacity of the liver

The liver is the only organ that performs the following functions:

- Ketone body synthesis
- Urea synthesis
- VLDL synthesis

The liver is also the primary, but not exclusive site, of the following functions:

- Alcohol oxidation (also occurs in the stomach)
- Gluconeogenesis (also occurs in the kidney(s))
- Glucose-6-phosphatase activity (also occurs in the kidney(s))

Glucose-6-phosphatase is important because it removes the phosphate from glucose-6-phosphate so that glucose can be released into circulation. Kidneys can perform gluconeogenesis and has glucose-6-phosphatase. However, it is estimated that 90% of glucose formed from gluconeogenesis is produced by the liver;

the remaining 10% is produced by the kidney(s). It is also important to note that muscle tissue does not have this enzyme, so it cannot release glucose into circulation.[22]

6.2.1 Muscle Macronutrient Metabolism

Compared to extrahepatic tissues, in the muscle the following pathways are not performed or are not important:

- Fatty acid synthesis
- Lactate breakdown

These pathways are crossed out in the figure below.

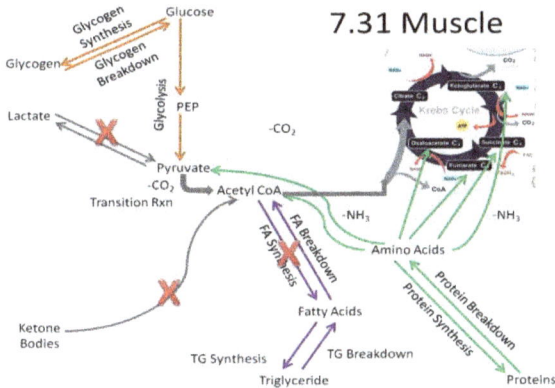

Figure 226. The metabolic pathways that are not performed or important in the muscle, compared to extrahepatic tissues as a whole

Removing those pathways, the following metabolic pathways make up the muscle metabolic capability:

- Glycogen synthesis and breakdown
- Glycolysis
- Protein synthesis and breakdown

- Triglyceride synthesis and breakdown
- Fatty acid breakdown
- Lactate synthesis
- Ketone body breakdown

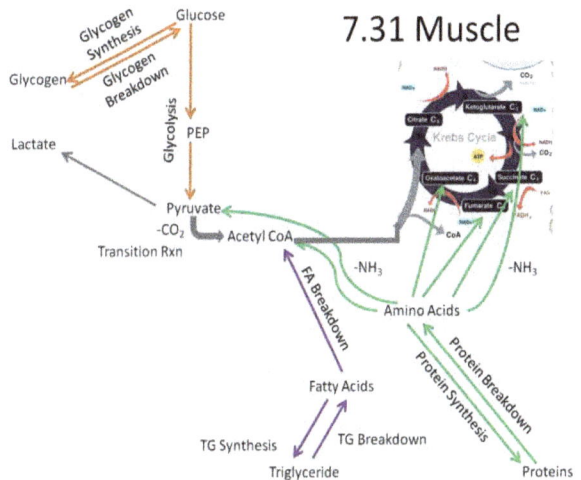

Figure 227. Muscle metabolic capability

Muscle is a major extrahepatic metabolic tissue. It is the only extrahepatic tissue with significant glycogen stores. However, unlike the liver, the muscle cannot secrete glucose after it is taken up (no glucose-6-phosphatase). Thus, you can think of the muscle as being selfish with glucose. It either uses it for itself initially or stores it for its later use.

In times of carbohydrate scarcity, ketone bodies are transported from the liver to other tissues, where acetoacetate and ß-hydroxybutyrate can be reconverted to acetyl-CoA to produce energy via the citric acid cycle.

Acetone in high concentrations due to prolonged fasting or a ketogenic diet is absorbed by cells other than those in the liver and enters a different pathway via 1,2-propanediol. Though the pathway follows a different series of steps requiring ATP, 1,2-propanediol can be turned into pyruvate. The heart (a specific type of muscle) preferentially utilizes fatty acids for energy under normal physiologic conditions. However, under ketotic conditions, the heart can effectively utilize ketone bodies for energy.

6.2.2 Adipose Macronutrient Metabolism

It probably does not surprise you that the major function of the adipose is to store energy as triglycerides. Compared to extrahepatic tissues, in the adipose the following pathways are not performed or are not important:

- Glycogen synthesis and breakdown
- Lactate production
- Ketone body breakdown
- Fatty acid breakdown
- Protein synthesis and breakdown
- Citric acid cycle (not much since it is not as active and doesn't have the energy requirement of other tissue types.)

These pathways are crossed out in the figure below.

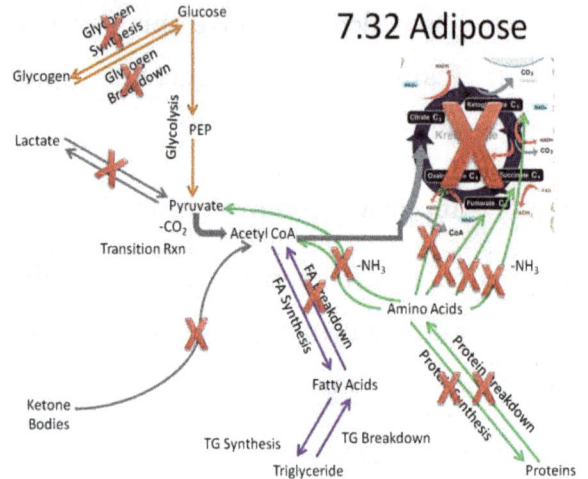

Figure 228. The metabolic pathways that are not performed or important in the adipose, compared to extrahepatic tissues as a whole

Removing those pathways, we are left with metabolic capabilities listed below.

- Glycolysis
- Fatty acid synthesis
- Triglyceride synthesis and breakdown

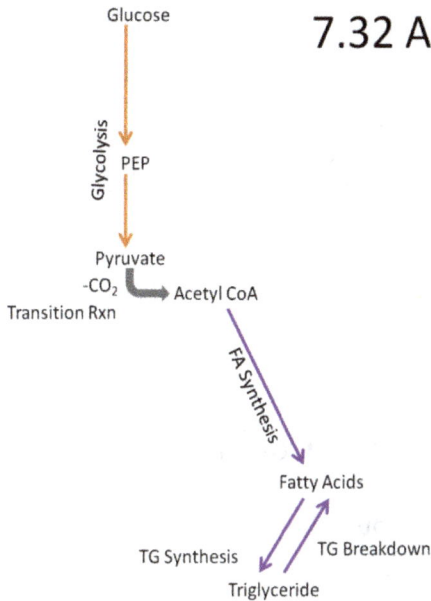

Figure 229. *Adipose metabolic capability*

Fatty acid synthesis only occurs in the adipose and liver. In the adipose, fatty acids are synthesized and most will be esterified into triglycerides to be stored. In the liver, some fatty acids will be esterified into triglycerides to be stored, but most triglycerides will be incorporated into VLDL so that they can be used or stored by other tissues.

6.2.3 Brain Macronutrient Metabolism

Compared to the extrahepatic tissues, in the brain the following pathways are not performed or are not important:

- Glycogen synthesis and breakdown
- Lactate synthesis and breakdown
- Fatty acid synthesis and breakdown
- Triglyceride synthesis and breakdown
- Protein synthesis and breakdown

These pathways are crossed out on the figure below.

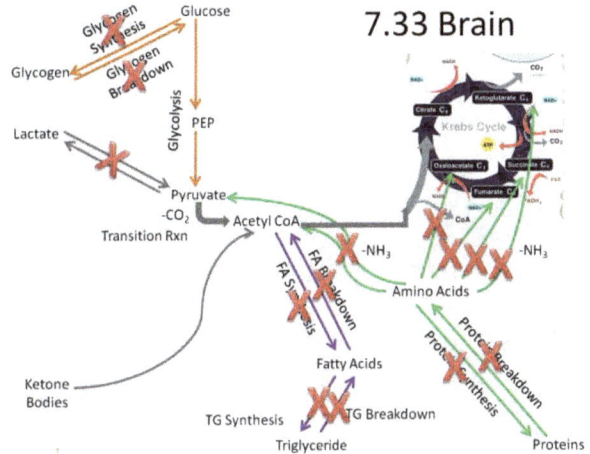

Figure 230. *The metabolic pathways that are not performed or important in the brain compared to extrahepatic tissues as a whole*

Low activity of an enzyme in the beta-oxidation pathway limits the activity of this pathway.[2]

By removing those pathways, the only pathways left are:

- Glycolysis
- Ketone body breakdown

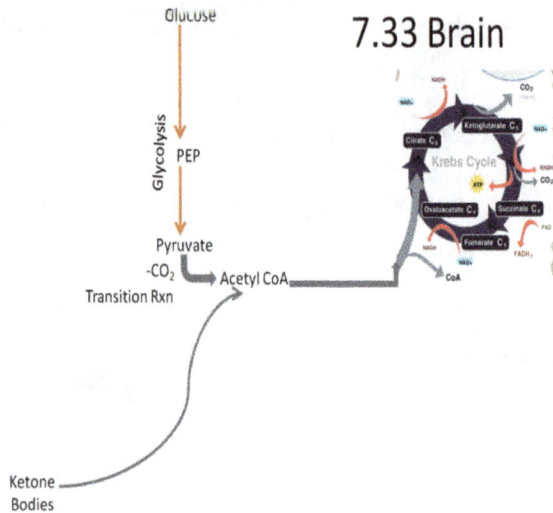

Figure 231. Brain metabolic capability

Thus, due to its limited metabolic capabilities, the brain needs to receive either glucose or ketone bodies to use as an energy source.

6.2.3.1 Fats and the brain

ß-oxidation of fatty acids (FAs) demands more oxygen than the oxidation of glucose, thereby increasing the risk of hypoxia of neurons of the brain and central nervous system (CNS), ß-oxidation of FAs generates superoxide, causing increased oxidative stress for neurons, and that the rate of ATP generation from fatty acids (as compared to glucose) is slower, and so in times of rapid neuronal firing there may be reduced fuel provision if FAs are the primary energy providing substrate for the brain.[44] This suggests an evolutionary-adaptive advantage to lowering of fatty oxidative capacity of brain cell

mitochondria to avoid these challenges and thus favours glucose oxidation in the brain. The ketone bodies (acetoacetate and ß-hydroxybutyric acid (BOHB) and acetone), do not promote the same raft of problems associated with fatty acid metabolism in the brain.[44]

6.3 Metabolic Conditions

Now that you should understand the glycaemic response and macronutrient metabolism, you should be able to understand the broader effects of insulin and glucagon that are summarized in the following tables. Knowing which hormones and enzymes are elevated under different conditions helps understand the metabolism that will therefore occur.

Table 25. Insulin's effects on targets in tissues

Effect	Tissue	Target
↑ Glucose Uptake	Muscle, Adipose	↑ GLUT4
↑ Glucose Uptake	Liver	↑ Glucokinase
↑ Glycogen Synthesis	Liver, Muscle	↑ Glycogen Synthase
↓ Glycogen Breakdown	Liver, Muscle	↓ Glycogen Phosphorylase
↑ Glycolysis, ↑ Transition Reaction	Liver, Muscle	↑ Phosphofructokinase-1 ↑ Pyruvate Dehydrogenase Complex
↑ Fatty Acid Synthesis	Liver	↑ Fatty Acid Synthase

↑ Triglyceride Synthesis	Adipose	↑ Lipoprotein Lipase

Table 26. Glucagon's effects on targets in tissues

Effect	Tissue	Target
↑ Glycogen Breakdown	Liver	↑ Glycogen Phosphorylase
↓ Glycogen Synthesis	Liver	↓ Glycogen Synthase
↑ Gluconeogenesis	Liver	Multiple Enzymes
↓ Glycolysis	Liver	↓ Phosphofructokinase-1
↑ Ketone Body Synthesis	Liver	↑ Acetyl-CoA Carboxylase
↑ Triglyceride Breakdown	Adipose	↑ Hormone-Sensitive Lipase

6.3.1 Fasting

In this condition a person has been fasting for an extended period. This would typically be longer time-frames than our normal night-time fast of 8-10 hours. So generally, we would consider fasting to be periods of >12 hours without taking food. Because of fasting, the person is in a catabolic state, with lowered blood glucose levels, which causes the pancreas to secrete glucagon.

The liver will break down glycogen and secrete glucose for other tissues to use until its stores are exhausted. Amino acids and lactate from muscle will be used for gluconeogenesis to synthesize glucose that will also be secreted. Glycolysis will be reduced to spare glucose for use by other tissues. From the breakdown of amino acids, there will be an increase in the synthesis and secretion of urea from the liver to safely rid the body of ammonia from the amino acids. Fatty acids that are received from adipose tissue will be broken down to acetyl-CoA and used to synthesize ketone bodies that are secreted for tissues, such as the brain, that cannot directly (or at best, inefficiently) use fatty acids as a fuel.

The muscle will break down glycogen to glucose until glycogen stores are exhausted, and receive glucose from the liver that enters glycolysis, forming pyruvate. Glucose will be used for anaerobic (lactate) and aerobic (pyruvate) respiration. Pyruvate will enter the transition reaction to form acetyl-CoA. The acetyl-CoA will then enter the citric acid cycle, and NADH and $FADH_2$ enter the electron transport chain to generate ATP. Once there isn't enough glucose for the muscle to use, fatty acids taken up from the adipose and from breakdown of muscle triglyceride stores will be broken down to acetyl-CoA. The acetyl-CoA will then enter the citric acid cycle, and NADH and $FADH_2$ enter the electron transport chain to generate ATP. Amino acids from protein breakdown and lactate (Cori Cycle) will be secreted to be used by the liver for gluconeogenesis.

The adipose tissue will break down triglycerides to fatty acids and release these for use by the muscle and the liver. It is not going to be taking up anything.

6.3.2 Very-Low Carbohydrate Diets

In this condition, assume a person just started into a ketogenic diet. He/she has just consumed a meal of all protein and fat with no carbohydrates. As a result, this person is in an anabolic state, but blood glucose levels are low, meaning the pancreas will secrete glucagon.

Liver glycogen stores will be broken down to secrete glucose for other tissues. Glycolysis will not occur to any great extent, to spare glucose for other tissues. Using amino acids from digestion and lactate from muscle, gluconeogenesis will synthesize glucose that will also be secreted. From the breakdown of amino acids, there will be an increase in the synthesis and secretion of urea from the liver to safely rid the body of ammonia from the amino acids. Amino acids will also be used for protein synthesis. Some triglycerides from chylomicron remnants will be broken down to fatty acids. These will then be broken down to acetyl-CoA and used to synthesize ketone bodies that

are secreted for tissues, such as the brain, that cannot directly use fatty acids as a fuel. Other triglycerides will be packaged into VLDL and secreted from the liver.

The muscle is going to break down glycogen to glucose, and receive glucose from the liver that enters glycolysis, forming pyruvate. Glucose will be used for anaerobic (lactate) and aerobic (pyruvate) glycolysis. Pyruvate will enter the transition reaction to form acetyl-CoA. The acetyl-CoA will then enter the citric acid cycle, and NADH and $FADH_2$ will enter the electron transport chain to generate ATP. Once there isn't enough glucose for the muscle to use, the fatty acids will be taken up from chylomicrons, chylomicron remnants, VLDL, IDL, and LDL and broken down to acetyl-CoA. The acetyl-CoA will then enter the citric acid cycle, and NADH and $FADH_2$ will enter the electron transport chain to generate ATP. Amino acids will be taken up to use for protein synthesis, and lactate will be secreted for the liver to use for gluconeogenesis (Cori cycle).

In the adipose, fatty acids that are cleaved from chylomicrons, chylomicron remnants, VLDL, IDL, and LDL are also going to be taken up. These fatty acids will be used to synthesize triglycerides for storage. With glucagon levels high in this condition hormone-sensitive lipase would be active.

However, since this is an anabolic state the net effect would be uptake of fatty acids after cleavage by lipoprotein lipase. The adipose won't be secreting anything under this condition.

6.3.3 High-Carbohydrate Diet (i.e. Ornish or Pritikin Diet)

In this condition, assume a person is on a very high carbohydrate, low fat diet, and just consumed a meal containing carbohydrates, with minimal but adequate amount of protein and very little fat. As a result, this person is in an anabolic state with high blood glucose levels, meaning the pancreas will secrete insulin.

The liver will take up glucose and synthesize glycogen until its stores are filled. After these stores are full, glucose can be broken down through glycolysis to pyruvate, then form acetyl-CoA in the transition reaction. Because we are in the fed or anabolic state, acetyl-CoA will be used for fatty acid synthesis, and the fatty acids will be used for triglyceride synthesis.

This synthesis, or creation of, triglycerides (fats) is called 'de novo lipogenesis' (DNL). The contention has been made that de novo lipogenesis does not appreciably occur in humans or that when it occurs it does not result in any appreciable change in total fat balance. However, it has been observed that overfeeding, with a high (approximately 85%) carbohydrate diet causes appreciable de novo lipogenesis (approximately 150g of lipid created per day)[57] as does total parenteral nutrition featuring 75% calories from glucose as compared to a lipid-based formula featuring only 15% calories from glucose. Those with insulin resistance and fatty-liver disease also exhibit higher levels of de novo lipogenesis.

There are increases in de novo lipogenesis in relation to overconsumption of carbohydrate, sugars, and excess calories. However, it is unclear whether carbohydrate, fructose and other sugars consumed at typical levels, affect hepatic lipogenesis and NAFLD pathogenesis in humans independently of excess energy. Long-term states of metabolic disorder and obesity are characterised by an excess of calorie intake though, and it is likely that overconsumption of carbohydrate and sugars will lead to increased DNL and contribute to the milieu of causes, effects and co-factors associated with increasing metabolic disorder.

These triglycerides, consisting predominantly of palmitic, myristic and oleic acids, will be packaged into VLDL and secreted from the liver. Amino acids will also be taken up and used for protein synthesis as needed. Because there is plenty of glucose, gluconeogenesis and ketone body synthesis will not be operating to any great extent.

The muscle will take up glucose and synthesize glycogen until those stores are filled. Some glucose will go through glycolysis to produce pyruvate, then form acetyl-CoA in the transition reaction. The acetyl-CoA will enter the citric acid cycle, and NADH and FADH$_2$ will enter the electron transport chain to generate ATP. Fatty acids that are cleaved from VLDL, IDL, and LDL are also going to be taken up. These fatty acids will be used to synthesize triglycerides for storage. Whatever amino acids are taken up will be used for protein synthesis. The muscle will not be secreting anything in this condition. The adipose is going to take up glucose that will enter glycolysis, where pyruvate will be produced, then acetyl-CoA will be produced in the transition reaction. Because we are in the fed or anabolic state, the acetyl-CoA will be used for fatty acid synthesis, and the fatty acids will be used for triglyceride synthesis. Fatty acids that are cleaved from VLDL, IDL, and LDL are going to be taken up and primarily used to synthesize triglycerides for storage. The adipose won't be secreting anything under this condition.

The brain will have plenty of glucose available for use, so the production of ketone bodies is not required.

7 Micronutrients Overview & Dietary Reference Intakes (DRIs)

Micronutrients consist of essential vitamins and minerals and non-essential and conditionally essential compounds that are helpful for the body. In this chapter, an overview of vitamins and minerals will be presented followed by a description of the dietary reference intakes (DRIs), which are used as benchmarks of micronutrient intake.

7.1 Vitamins

The name vitamin comes from Casimir Funk, who in 1912 thought vital amines (NH_3) were responsible for preventing what we know now are vitamin deficiencies. He coined the term 'vitamines' to describe these compounds. Eventually it was discovered that these compounds were not amines and the 'e' was dropped to form the modern word vitamins.[58]

Vitamins are classified as either fat-soluble or water-soluble. The fat-soluble vitamins are: Vitamins A, D, E, and K.

The water-soluble vitamins are vitamin C and the B vitamins, which are shown in the table below.

Table 27. The B vitamins and their common names

Vitamin	Common Name
B_1	Thiamin
B_2	Riboflavin
B_3	Niacin
B_5	Pantothenic Acid
B_6*	Pyridoxines
B_7	Biotin
B_9	Folates
B_{12}*	Cobalamins

*Normally used instead of common name

A common question about vitamins is: *"Why are there so many B vitamins"* and *"Why are there missing numbers?"*

Before they even knew that vitamins existed, a scientist named E.V. McCollum recognized that a deficiency in what he called 'fat-soluble factor A' resulted in severe ophthalmia (inflammation of the eye). In addition, a deficiency in 'water-soluble factor B' resulted in beriberi (a deficiency discussed more later).[58]

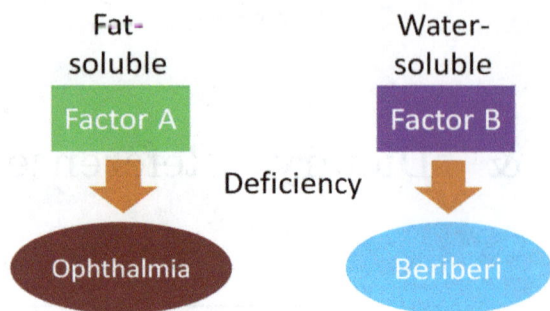

Figure 232. Factor A deficiency led to ophthalmia, factor B deficiency led to beriberi

Factor A is what we now know as vitamin A. However, researchers soon realized that factor B consisted of two factors that they termed B_1 and B_2. Then they realized that there are multiple components in B_2, and

they began identifying the wide array of B vitamins that we know today.[58]

You might be thinking "but the numbers on the B vitamins still do not add up."

You are right, vitamins B_4, B_8, B_{10}, and B_{11} were 'discovered' and then removed, usually because they were undefined, or were found to not actually be either vitamins or essential at all.

Relative to other scientific milestones, the discovery of vitamins is a recent occurrence, as shown in the table below.

Table 28. Vitamin, year proposed, isolated, structure determined, and synthesis achieved up to 1944[58]

Vitamin	Year Proposed	Isolated	Structure Determined	Synthesis Achieved
Thiamin	1901	1926	1936	1936
Vitamin C	1907	1926	1932	1933
Vitamin A	1915	1939	1942	-
Vitamin D	1919	1931	1932	1932
Vitamin E	1922	1936	1938	1938
Niacin	1926	1937	1937	1867*
Biotin	1926	1939	1942	1943
Vitamin K	1929	1939	1942	1943
Pantothenic Acid	1931	1939	1939	1940
Folate	1931	1939	-	-
Riboflavin	1933	1933	1934	1935
Vitamin B_6	1934	1936	1938	1939

* Was established long before it was known to be a vitamin

Several B vitamins serve as cofactors/coenzymes. The following table lists the cofactors/coenzymes formed from B vitamins that will be discussed in more detail in the following subsections.

Table 29. Cofactors/coenzymes formed from B vitamins

Vitamin	Cofactors/Coenzymes
Thiamin	Thiamin Pyrophosphate (TPP)
Riboflavin	Flavin Adenine Dinucleotide (FAD),

Niacin	Flavin Mononucleotide (FMN)
	Nicotine Adenine Dinucleotide (NAD), Nicotine Adenine Dinucleotide Phosphate (NADP)
Pantothenic Acid	Coenzyme A
Vitamin B$_6$	Pyridoxal Phosphate (PLP)
Biotin	-
Folate	Tetrahydrofolate (THF)
Vitamin B$_{12}$	Adenosylcobalamin, Methylcobalamin

B$_{15}$	Pangamic Acid	Considered unsafe by US Food and Drug Administration
B$_{16}$	Dimethylglycine	
B$_{17}$		
B$_{20}$	L-carnitine	

7.1.1   The missing B vitamins

It is important to mention the 'missing' B vitamins because they are still often promoted as health remedies and tonics in various forms by certain practitioners. Some of these are dangerous though, and so, it is important for practitioners to understand just a little more about them.

Table 30. 'Missing' B vitamins and reason for omission

Former B vitamin number	Common Name	Reason for omission
B$_4$	Either adenine, carnitine or choline	Undefined, not true vitamins
B$_8$	Adenosine monophosphate, Inositol	Undefined, not true vitamins
B$_{10}$	PABA	No essential requirement in the human body, not a vitamin
B$_{11}$	Pantothenic Acid	
B$_{13}$	Orotic Acid	
B$_{14}$		

7.2   Minerals

Minerals are elements that are essential for body functions that can't be synthesized in the body. Some people refer to them as elements instead of minerals, and the names can be used interchangeably. However, in the nutrition community, they are more commonly referred to as minerals. Minerals can be divided up into three categories:

- Macrominerals
- Trace Minerals (aka Microminerals)
- Ultratrace Minerals

There is not an exact, agreed on definition for how the categories are defined, but in general they are defined by the amount required and found in the body such that:

Macrominerals > Trace Minerals > Ultratrace Minerals

Table 31. Alphabetical listing of the 20 minerals and their chemical symbols

Macrominerals	Trace Minerals	Ultratrace Minerals
Calcium (Ca)	Chromium (Cr)	Arsenic (Ar)
Chloride (Cl)[a]	Copper (Cu)	Boron (B)
Magnesium (Mg)	Fluoride (F)	Nickel (Ni)
Phosphorus (P)[b]	Iodine (I)	Silicon (Si)
Potassium (K)	Iron (Fe)	Vanadium (V)
Sodium (Na)	Manganese (Mn)	
	Molybdenum (Mo)	
	Selenium (Se)	
	Zinc (Zn)	

[a] Chlorine ion, Cl⁻

[b] Phosphate in body, PO₄

Minerals are elements. The figure below shows the distribution of minerals in the periodic table which you should be familiar with from your chemistry education.

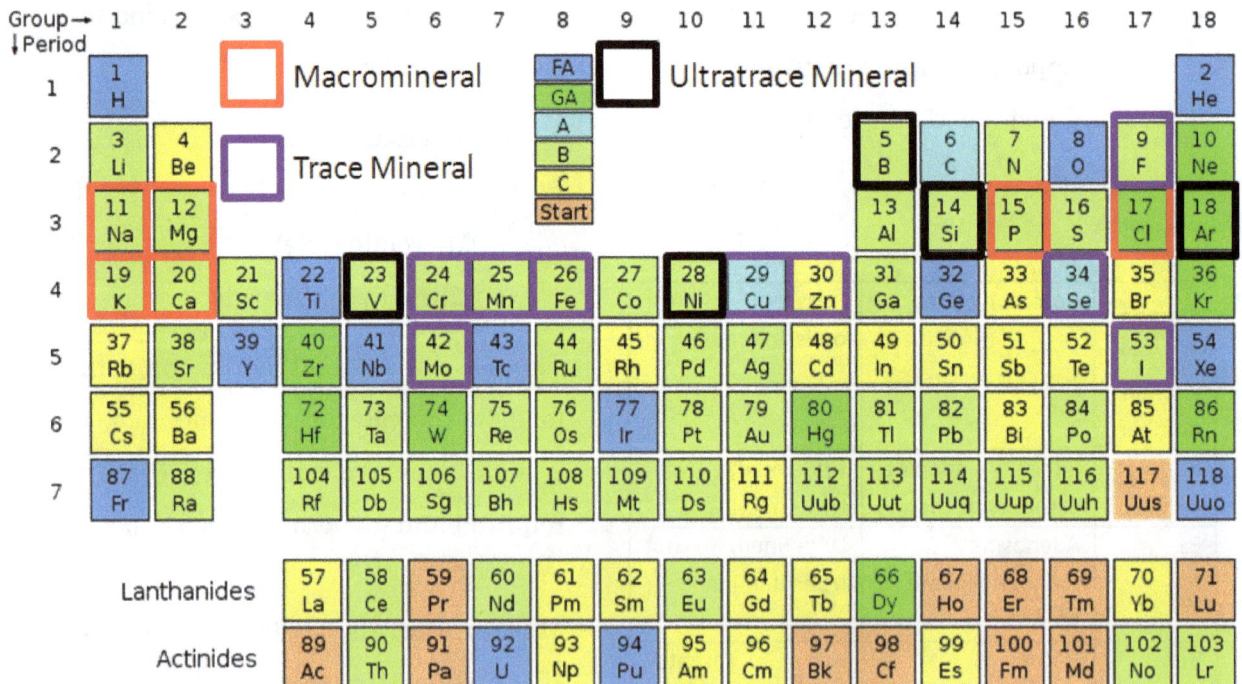

Figure 233. Minerals are elements

7.3 Covering Vitamins & Minerals

There are two common ways to teach about vitamins and minerals in nutrition classes. The traditional way is to start with fat-soluble vitamins and go down through the vitamins alphabetically (i.e. vitamin A, vitamin D, vitamin E, vitamin K). However, this method leads students to learn about vitamins and minerals more individually instead of how they work together. For instance, it makes sense to cover calcium with vitamin D, and iron with copper and zinc. We are going to cover vitamins and minerals based on their function rather than covering them by whether they are a water-soluble vitamin or trace mineral. The hope is that you will gain a more integrative understanding of vitamins and minerals from this approach. Here are the different functional categories that we are going to cover. Notice that some micronutrients fit into more than one functional category. Each vitamin and mineral will be covered only in one section with some mention of its overlap in other section(s) in certain cases.

Table 32. Micronutrients and their major targets or roles in the body

Antioxidants	Macronutrient Metabolism	1-Carbon Metabolism	Blood	Bones & Teeth	Electrolytes
Vitamin E	Thiamin	Folate	Vitamin K	Vitamin D	Sodium
Vitamin C	Riboflavin	Vitamin B_{12}	Iron	Calcium	Potassium
Selenium	Niacin	Vitamin B_6	Vitamin B_6	Vitamin K	Chloride
Iron	Pantothenic Acid		Folate	Phosphorus	Phosphorus
Copper	Vitamin B_6		Vitamin B_{12}	Magnesium	Magnesium
Zinc	Biotin		Copper	Fluoride	
Manganese	Vitamin B_{12}		Calcium	Vitamin A	
Riboflavin	Vitamin C			Iron	
	Iodine			Copper	
	Manganese			Zinc	
	Magnesium				

7.4 Dietary Reference Intakes (DRIs)

Dietary Reference Intakes (DRIs) are more than numbers in the table, even though that is often how many people view them.

Most of you are probably familiar with Dietary Guidelines for Health. DRIs and Dietary Guidelines provide different information for different audiences.

Dietary Guidelines provide **qualitative** advice to the public about diet and chronic disease prevention and maintaining health.

DRIs provide **quantitative** advice to professionals about amounts of nutrients or food components to be of benefit.

DRIs are a collective term to refer to these components:

- Estimated Average Requirement (EAR)
- Recommended Dietary Allowance (RDA) or Intake (RDI)
- Adequate Intake (AI)
- Tolerable Upper Intake Level (UL)

Many people refer to the UL as simply the "upper limit", leaving off "tolerable".

The RDA is the measure that professionals use to assess the quality of people's diets. It is the requirement estimated to meet the needs of 97.5% of the population. But the RDA is calculated using the EAR. Therefore, the EAR needs to be set before an RDA can be set. There must be applicable research to set an EAR. An EAR is the estimated requirement for 50% of the population (hence the average in its name) as shown in the figure below. On the left vertical axis is the risk of inadequacy, and on the bottom of the figure is the observed level of intake that increases from left to right. We will talk about the right axis label in a later figure. Notice that for the

EAR, the risk for inadequacy is 0.5 (50%) whereas the RDA the risk of inadequacy is 0.025 (2.5%).

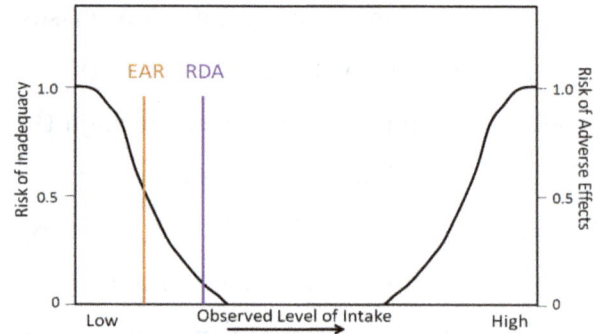

Figure 234. The EAR meets the needs of 50% of the population, RDA 97.5% of the population

The figure below shows the EAR on the normal distribution and splits out the different standard deviations as percent. Notice that for 50% of population, their adequate intake is below the EAR and 50% of the population their adequate intake is above the EAR.

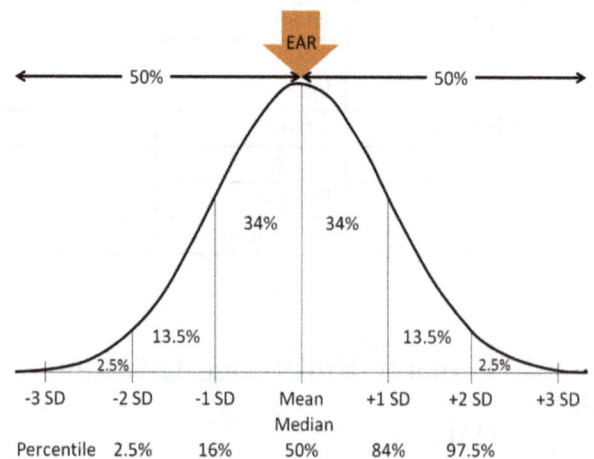

Figure 235. The EAR meets the needs of 50% of the population as depicted in this normal distribution. SD - standard deviation

If an EAR is set, the formula for setting the RDA is:

EAR + 2 Standard Deviations = RDA

The following figure shows the distribution and how the percentages and standard deviation changes from the EAR. For the RDA, only 2.5% of people's intake for the chosen outcome will be above RDA.

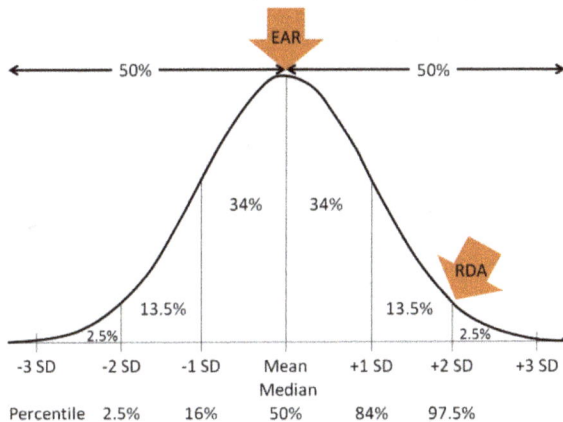

Figure 236. The RDA meets the needs for 97.5% of the population

For nutrients lacking the research evidence needed to set an EAR, an AI is set instead. An AI is a level that appears to be adequate in a defined population or subgroup. As you can see, the EAR is adequate for 50% (0.5) of the population and is lower than the RDA. The RDA is adequate for 97.5% (0.025) of the population, and higher than the EAR. The AI level of intake is believed to be between the EAR/RDA and the UL, but since it is not research-based, it is not exactly known where this level falls as shown below.

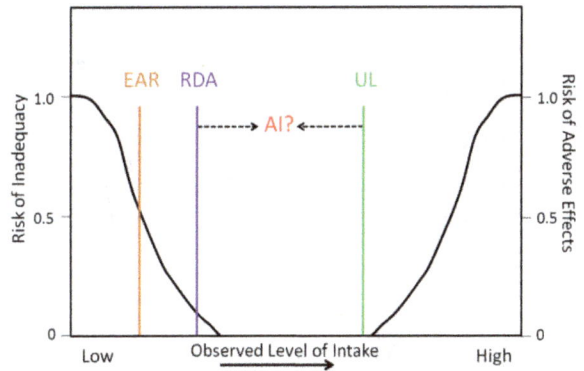

Figure 237. The AI compared to the other DRI components

The last of the DRIs is the Tolerable Upper Intake Level (UL). This is the highest level of daily nutrient intake that is unlikely to pose risk of adverse health effects to almost all individuals in the population. To set this, the committee first sets a no observed adverse effect level (NOAEL) and/or the lowest observed adverse effect level (LOAEL). The UL is then set lower based on several uncertainty/safety factors off the NOAEL or LOAEL as shown below. The right vertical axis is used to represent the risk of an adverse event. Notice the NOAEL at the point where no adverse effects have been reported. The LOAEL is somewhere above the NOAEL. The UL is set at a level where it is believed that people will not experience the selected adverse effect.

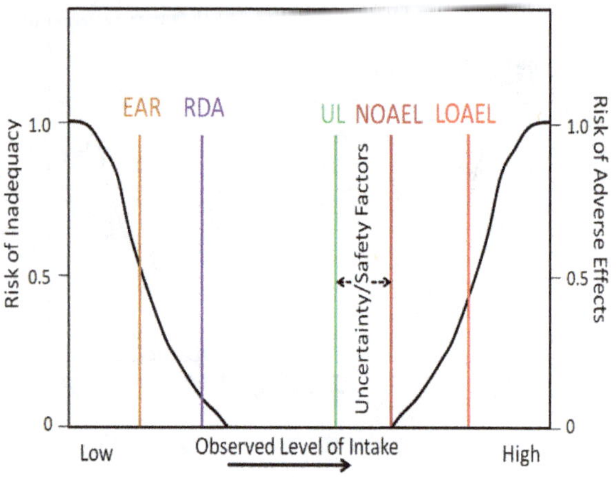

Figure 238. Upper limits compared to EAR and RDA

The US population is a well-studied one that gives us indications of nutrient sufficiency in 'developed' nations.

So, how are Americans doing in meeting the DRIs?

The following figure shows the percentage of Americans that are not meeting the EAR for some of the earlier micronutrients that had DRIs set. Keep in mind that the EAR is lower than the RDA.

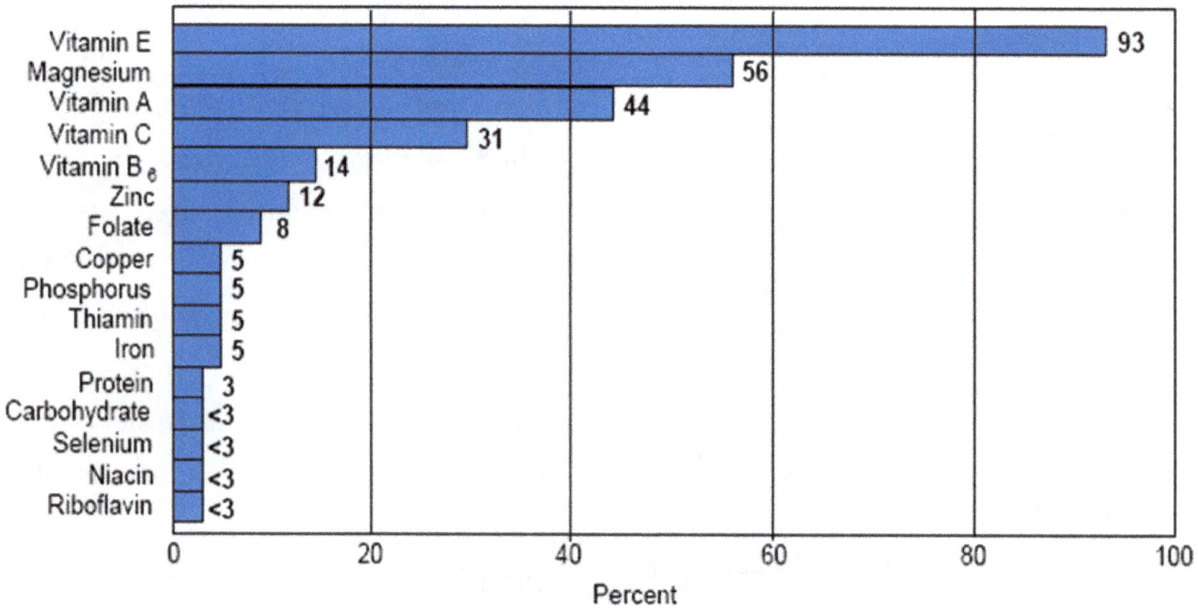

Figure 239. Percent of Americans not meeting EAR from food.[xli]

As you can see, a sizable percentage of Americans don't meet the EAR for vitamin E, magnesium, vitamin A, and vitamin C. Also, keep in mind that this also does not include micronutrients that have AI instead of EARs and RDAs.

[xli] https://www.ars.usda.gov/ARSUserFiles/80400530/pdf/0102/usualintaketables2001-02.pdf

8 Antioxidant Micronutrients

In this chapter we describe antioxidants before discussing the three major antioxidant micronutrients: vitamin E, vitamin C and selenium.

8.1 Antioxidants

The antioxidant vitamins and minerals are:

- Vitamin E
- Vitamin C
- Selenium
- Iron
- Copper
- Zinc
- Manganese
- Riboflavin

In this section, we are going to cover vitamin E, vitamin C, and selenium in detail because being an antioxidant is their primary function. Iron, copper, zinc, and manganese are cofactors for the antioxidant enzymes catalase and superoxide dismutase, as shown below.

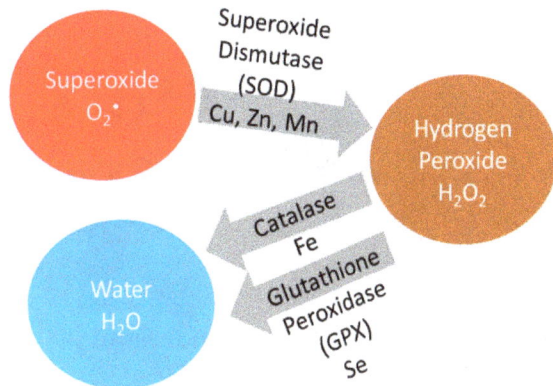

Figure 240. Antioxidant enzymes that use minerals as cofactors

Superoxide dismutase converts superoxide into hydrogen peroxide. Catalase converts hydrogen peroxide into water. Iron, copper, and zinc will be covered in greater detail in the blood, bones, and teeth chapter (chapter 11). Manganese will be covered in the macronutrient metabolism chapter.

Riboflavin, in the cofactor NAD, is an important cofactor for several antioxidant enzymes, but it will be covered in more depth in the macronutrient metabolism micronutrients chapter (Chapter 9).

8.1.1 Free Radicals & Oxidative Stress

As you have learned already, oxidation is the loss of an electron as shown below.

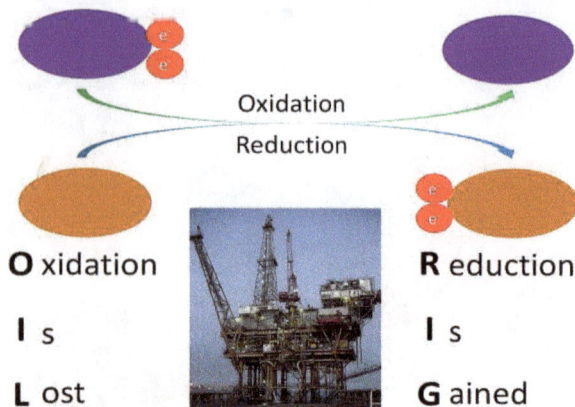

Figure 241. The purple compound is oxidized; the orange compound is reduced

Some important terms to understand:

Free Radical—a molecule with an unpaired electron in its outer orbital.

The following example shows normal oxygen losing an electron from its outer orbital and thus, becoming an oxygen free radical.

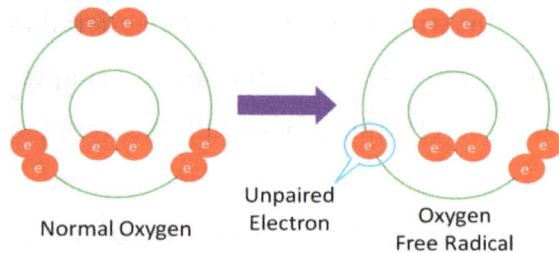

Figure 242. Normal oxygen is converted to an oxygen free radical by losing one electron in its outer orbital, leaving one unpaired electron

Free radicals are highly reactive because they actively seek an electron to stabilize the molecule.

Reactive Oxygen Species (ROS)—an oxygen-containing, free radical species.

Some of the most common ROS are:

- Superoxide ($O_2\bullet$)
- Hydroxyl Radical ($\bullet OH$)
- Hydrogen Peroxide Radical ($HO_2\bullet$)
- Peroxyl Radical ($ROO_2\bullet$)
- Alkoxyl Radical ($RO\bullet$)
- Ozone (O_3)
- Singlet Oxygen ($^1O_2$)
- Hydrogen Peroxide (H_2O_2)

$\bullet$ after the name symbolises radical

Oxidative Stress—the imbalance between the production of ROS and the body's ability to quench them.

The following figure shows that inflammation caused by hitting your thumb with a hammer, exposure to UV light, radiation, smoking, and air pollution are all sources of free radicals.

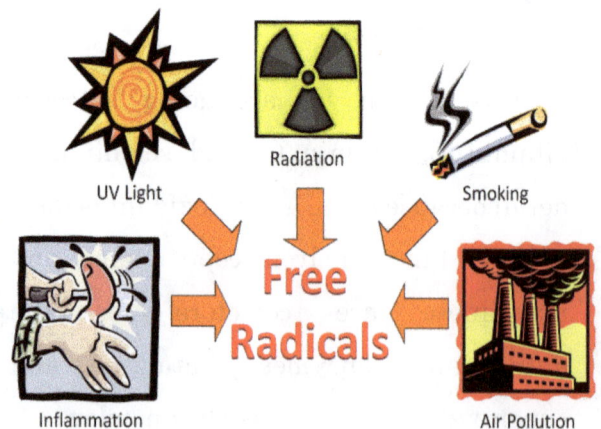

Figure 243. Some sources of free radicals

Free radicals can be generated by a variety of sources that can be classified as endogenous (within the body) and exogenous sources (outside the body).

So, we have these free radicals searching for an electron, what's the big deal?

The problem arises if the free radicals oxidize LDL, proteins, or DNA as shown below.

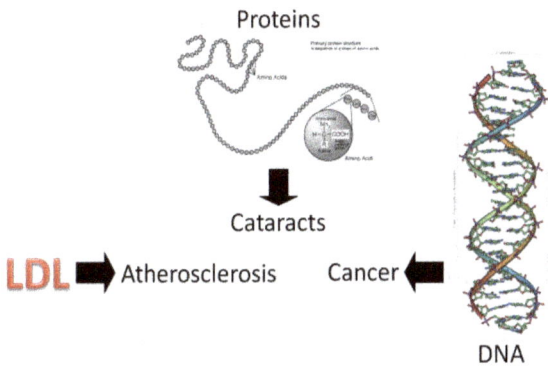

Figure 244. Free radicals can attack LDL, proteins, and DNA

Oxidized LDL is more atherogenic, meaning it is more likely to contribute to atherosclerosis (hardening of the arteries) than normal LDL. Protein oxidation is believed to be involved in the development of cataracts. Cataracts are the clouding of the lens of the eye.

If a nucleotide in DNA is attacked, it can result in a mutation. A mutation is a change in the nucleotide or base pair sequence of DNA. Mutations are a common occurrence in cancer.

8.1.2   What is an Antioxidant?

We are ready to move on to antioxidants, which as their name indicates, combat free radicals, ROS, and oxidative stress.

But it's not quite that simple. You have probably heard the saying "take one for the team." Instead of taking one for the team, antioxidants "give one for the team." The 'giving' is the donation of an electron from the antioxidant to a free radical, to regenerate a stable compound, as shown below.

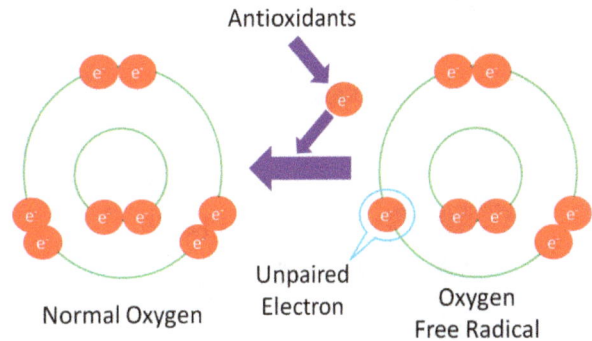

Figure 245. Regeneration of normal oxygen from oxygen free radical by the donation of an electron from an antioxidant

Donating an electron is how vitamins act as antioxidants. Minerals, on the other hand, are not antioxidants themselves. Instead, they act as cofactors for antioxidant enzymes.

These antioxidant enzymes include:

- Superoxide dismutase (SOD): uses copper, zinc, and manganese as cofactors (there is more than one

SOD enzyme); convert superoxide to hydrogen peroxide and oxygen.[36]

- Catalase: uses iron as a cofactor; converts hydrogen peroxide to water.[36]

- Glutathione peroxidase (GPX): is a selenoenzyme that converts hydrogen peroxide to water. It can also convert other ROS to water.[36]

The action of these enzymes is shown below.

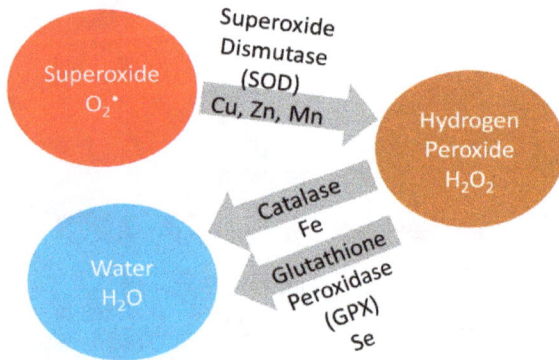

Figure 246. Antioxidant enzymes that use minerals as cofactors

Antioxidants are thought to work in concert with one another, forming what is known as the antioxidant network. An example of the antioxidant network is shown below. Alpha-tocopherol (major form of vitamin E in our body) is oxidized, forming an alpha-tocopherol radical. This donation of an electron stabilizes reactive oxygen species. Ascorbate (vitamin C) is then oxidized, forming dehydroascorbate to regenerate (reduce) alpha-tocopherol.

Ascorbate is then regenerated by the selenoenzyme thioredoxin reductase. Thus, this demonstrates how antioxidants can function as a network to regenerate one another so they can continue to function as antioxidants.

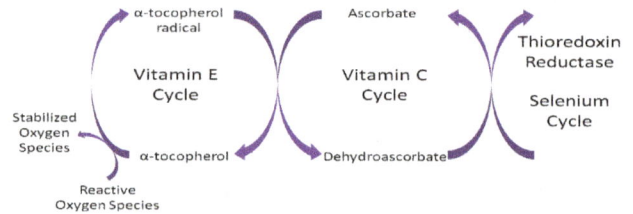

Figure 247. The theorized antioxidant network[59]

8.1.3 Meaningful Antioxidant(s)

There is a lot of confusion among the public on antioxidants. For the most part, this is for good reason. Many food companies put antioxidant numbers on the packages that sound good to consumers, who have no idea how to interpret them. Thus, it is increasingly important to understand what a meaningful antioxidant is.

A meaningful antioxidant has two characteristics:

1. There is a sufficient amount of the antioxidant at the right location
2. It is not redundant

What does this mean?

Let's consider the example of lycopene and vitamin E (alpha-tocopherol), which are both fat-soluble antioxidants. *In vitro* antioxidant assays have found that lycopene is 10-fold more effective in quenching singlet oxygen than alpha-tocopherol.[1] However, when you look at the concentrations found in the body, there is far more alpha-tocopherol than lycopene. For example, LDL on average contain 11.6 molecules of alpha tocopherol and 0.9 molecules of lycopene. Thus, if we divide alpha tocopherol by lycopene 11.6/0.9 we find that there is on average 12.9 times more alpha-tocopherol than lycopene.[1] Other examples in the body:

- Prostate—162-fold higher alpha-tocopherol than lycopene concentrations
- Skin—17 to 269-fold higher alpha-tocopherol than lycopene concentrations
- Plasma—53-fold higher alpha tocopherol than lycopene concentrations[60]

Thus, even though lycopene is a better antioxidant *in vitro*, since the concentration of alpha-tocopherol is so much higher in tissues (locations of need), it is likely the more meaningful antioxidant. In addition, if lycopene and alpha-tocopherol have similar antioxidant functions (fat-soluble antioxidants), lycopene's potential antioxidant action is redundant to alpha-tocopherol's antioxidant function and thus, also less

likely to be a meaningful antioxidant. Indeed, further examination of the literature has not suggested that lycopene can act as an antioxidant *in vivo*, even though it is a good one *in vitro*.[60]

You may be wondering *"What about the in vitro antioxidant assays, like the oxygen radical absorbance capacity (ORAC) assay that some food and supplement companies are including on their labels?"*

This is an example of how some companies/businesses use ORAC values to market their product(s). However, the USDA removed its table of ORAC values "due to mounting evidence that the values indicating antioxidant capacity have no relevance to the effects of specific bioactive compounds, including polyphenols on human health.[2]"

However, going back to the two characteristics of meaningful antioxidants, there really is no evidence that shows that a high ORAC score leads to any benefit *in vivo*. This is because the measure also doesn't consider characteristics such as bioavailability. Bioavailability is the amount of a compound that is absorbed or reaches circulation. Many of these purported super antioxidants have not been shown to be absorbed or maintained in the body in a way that would suggest that they would be meaningful antioxidants.

8.1.4 Too Much of a Good Thing? Antioxidants as Pro-oxidants

Chapter 1 described a clinical trial that found that high-dose beta-carotene supplementation increased lung cancer risk in smokers. This is an example of findings that support that high doses of antioxidants may be "too much of a good thing", causing more harm than benefit. The parabolic, or U-shaped figure, below displays how the level of nutrient concentration or intake (x-axis) relates to an antioxidant measure (y-axis). The lowest level of antioxidant intake or tissue concentration results in nutrient deficiency if the antioxidant is essential (vitamins and minerals). Intake levels above deficient, but less than optimal, are referred to as low suboptimal. Suboptimal means the levels are not optimal. Thus, low suboptimal and high suboptimal sandwich optimal. The high suboptimal level is between optimal and where the nutrient becomes toxic.

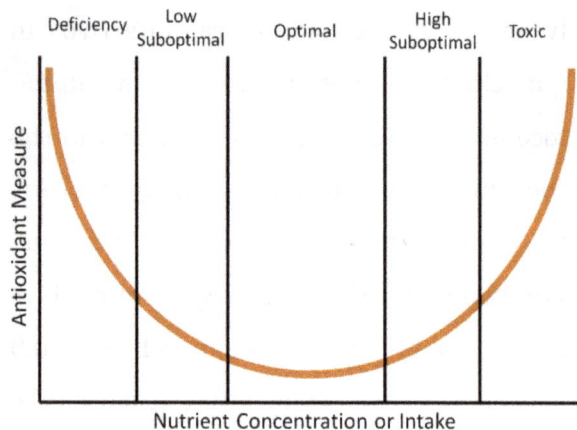

Figure 248. How the levels of nutrient concentration or intake alters antioxidant measures in the body (Adapted from [61])

An example of where this phenomenon has been shown to occur is in the dog prostate with toenail selenium concentrations, which are a good indicator of long-term selenium status.[1] Researchers found that when they plotted prostate DNA damage (antioxidant measure) against toenail selenium status (nutrient concentration or intake) that it resulted in a U-shaped curve like the one shown above.[61]

Thus, it is good to have antioxidants in your diet, but too much can be counterproductive.

8.2 Vitamin E

There are eight different forms of vitamin E: four tocopherols and four tocotrienols. The difference between tocopherols and tocotrienols is that the former has saturated tails, while the latter have unsaturated tails. Within tocopherols and tocotrienols, the difference between the different forms is the position of the methyl groups on the ring. The four different forms within the tocopherol and tocotrienols are designated by the Greek letters: alpha, beta, gamma, and delta. The difference in these structures is shown in the figures below.

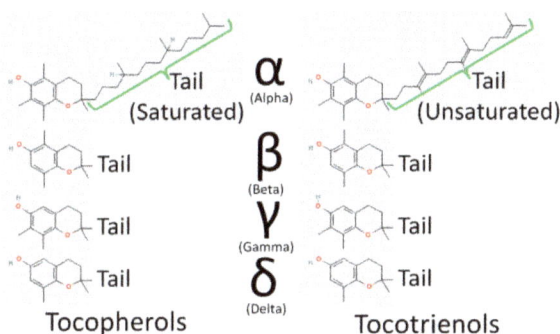

Figure 249. Structures of the different forms of vitamin E

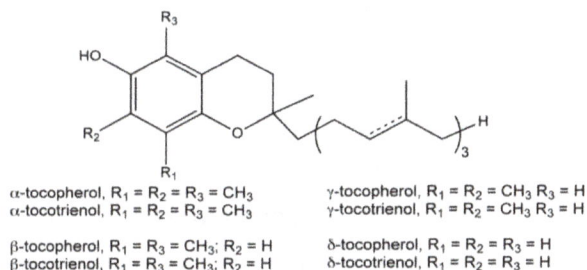

α-tocopherol, $R_1 = R_2 = R_3 = CH_3$
α-tocotrienol, $R_1 = R_2 = R_3 = CH_3$

β-tocopherol, $R_1 = R_3 = CH_3$; $R_2 = H$
β-tocotrienol, $R_1 = R_3 = CH_3$; $R_2 = H$

γ-tocopherol, $R_1 = R_2 = CH_3$ $R_3 = H$
γ-tocotrienol, $R_1 = R_2 = CH_3$ $R_3 = H$

δ-tocopherol, $R_1 = R_2 = R_3 = H$
δ-tocotrienol, $R_1 = R_2 = R_3 = H$

Figure 250. Structures of different forms of vitamin E

The primary form of vitamin E found in the body is alpha-tocopherol and for a long time this was considered to be the only

bioactive form. However, all the tocopherols and tocotrienols are beginning to demonstrate important actions for health, including increased antioxidant activity and reductions in cancer formation and overloading with alpha-tocopherol alone may reduce levels of the other health-promoting forms of Vitamin E in the body.[62]

Much of what we know about the antioxidant actions of Vitamin E comes from alpha-tocopherol and this is the major antioxidant form. When it serves as an antioxidant it forms an alpha-tocopherol radical, as shown below.

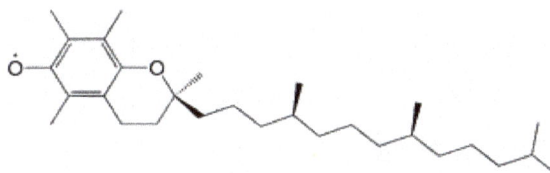

Figure 251. Alpha-tocopherol radical

Alpha-tocopherol is believed to be the first part of an antioxidant network (shown below) where it is oxidized to donate an electron to stabilize reactive oxygen species. Alpha-tocopherol radical can then be reduced by the donation of an electron from ascorbate.

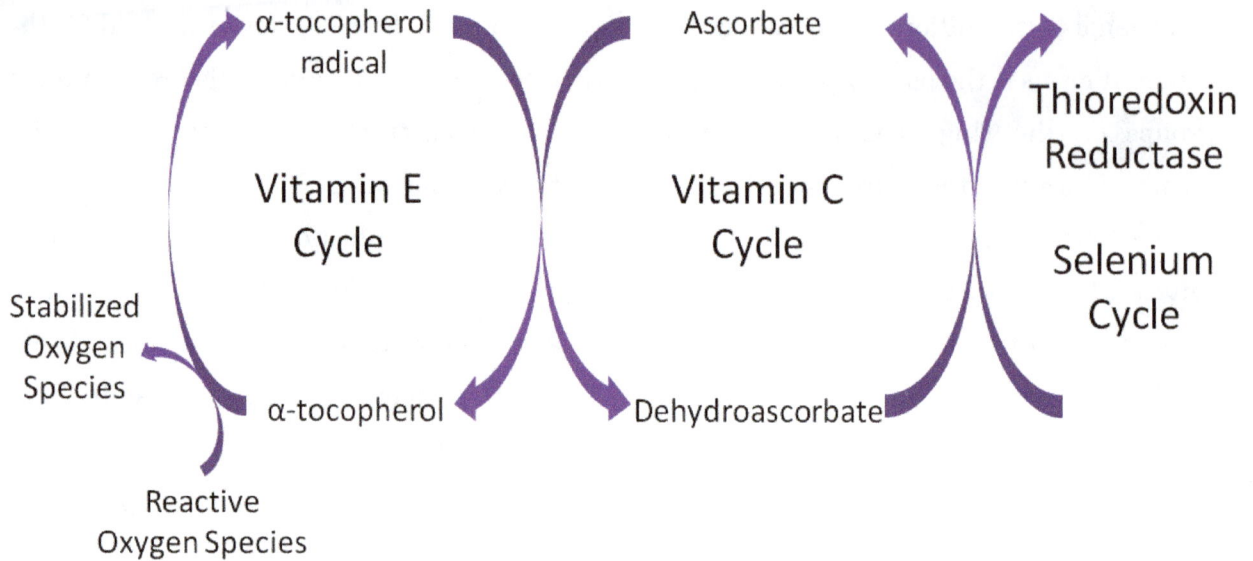

Figure 252. The theorized antioxidant network[59]

To help protect the antioxidant function of alpha-tocopherol (by preventing the formation of alpha-tocopherol radical) in foods and during digestion, some manufacturers have added compounds to this site of alpha-tocopherol through ester bonds. These are referred to as alpha-tocopherol derivatives or alpha-tocopherol esters. The most common forms are alpha-tocopherol acetate, alpha-tocopherol succinate, and alpha-tocopherol phosphate (Ester-E®). The figures below show the structure of alpha-tocopherol acetate, and the structure of succinic acid.

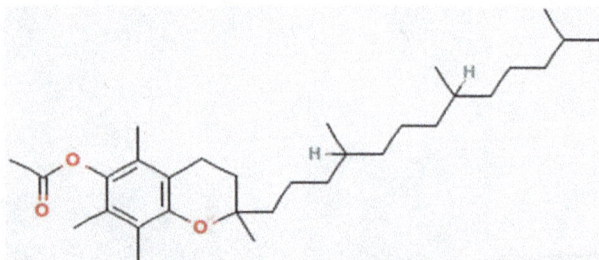

Figure 254. Succinic acid

Alpha-tocopherol derivatives, such as acetate in alpha-tocopherol acetate, are cleaved prior to absorption in the small intestine by esterases, meaning that alpha-tocopherol is absorbed, not the alpha-tocopherol derivative.

8.2.1 Alpha-Tocopherol: Natural vs. Synthetic

In addition to being found naturally in foods, alpha-tocopherol can also be synthesized. It is important to know whether alpha-tocopherol is natural or synthetic because the stereochemistry

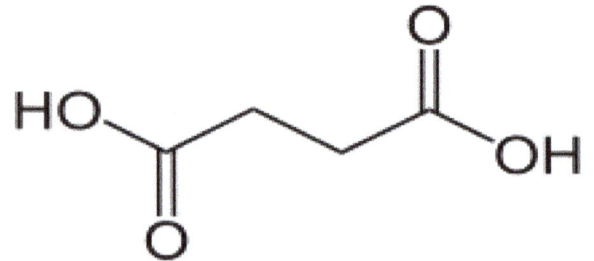

Figure 253. Alpha-tocopherol acetate

differs between these forms. Alpha-tocopherol contains three chiral centres (non-superimposable mirror images) designated as R or S.

The three chiral centres in alpha-tocopherol are located at the 2 ,4, and 8 positions. The numbers do not make sense if you count the carbons, but this is how they are numbered for some reason.[1]

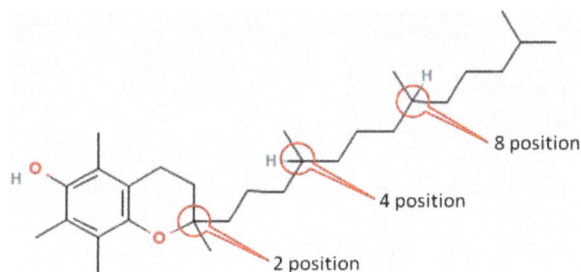

Figure 255. The 2, 4, and 8 positions of alpha-tocopherol are chiral centres

In natural alpha-tocopherol, all 3 chiral centres are in the R configuration. Thus, it is designated RRR-alpha-tocopherol. The R's represent the 2, 4, and 8 positions of alpha-tocopherol, respectively, as shown below.[1]

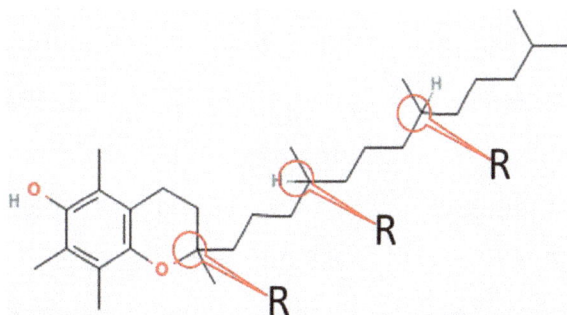

Figure 256. Natural alpha-tocopherol 2, 4, and 8 positions are in the R conformation

Synthetic alpha-tocopherol is a racemic (equal) mixture of all the different

stereochemical possibilities at the three chiral centres. These are:

RRR

RRS

RSS

RSR

SRR

SSR

SSS

SRS

The two forms of alpha-tocopherol are designated (these are placed before alpha-tocopherol to indicate whether it is natural or synthetic) as listed below:

1. Natural

New designation: RRR-alpha-tocopherol (because all 3 positions are RRR)

Old designation: d-alpha-tocopherol

2. Synthetic

New designation: all-rac-alpha-tocopherol (because it is a racemic mixture)

Old designation: dl-alpha-tocopherol

The old d and dl designations were describing the chemical structure that are sometimes still used. Keep in mind the 'natural' and 'synthetic' are describing the stereochemistry of alpha-tocopherol and not whether it naturally derived. For example, there are natural alpha-tocopherol derivatives where the derivatives are added through synthetic procedures, i.e. they are produced in a lab, but they are still chemically 'natural'.

8.2.2 Vitamin E Absorption, Metabolism, & Excretion

The slight change in stereochemistry between the natural (or RRR or d-alpha) and synthetic (mixed or dl-alpha) form, makes a significant difference in how alpha-tocopherol is maintained in the body.

All forms of vitamin E (tocopherols, tocotrienols) are absorbed equally. Fat-soluble vitamins are handled like lipids and thus are incorporated into chylomicrons that have triglycerides removed by lipoprotein lipase. The chylomicron remnants containing the different forms of vitamin E are then taken up by the liver. The figure below shows the absorption, metabolism, and excretion of vitamin E.

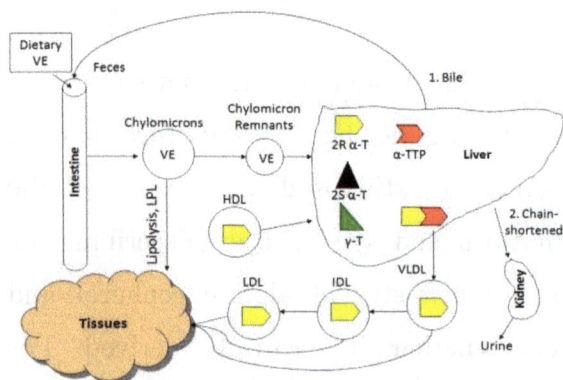

Figure 257. The absorption, metabolism, and excretion of vitamin E

The liver contains a protein called alpha-tocopherol transfer protein (alpha-TTP), which is responsible for maintaining higher levels of alpha-tocopherol in the body. Alpha-TTP preferentially binds to 2R alpha-tocopherol and helps facilitate its incorporation into VLDL. 2R means any form of alpha-tocopherol in which the 2 position is in the R conformation. The following table summarizes the forms of alpha-tocopherol that bind well to alpha-TTP, and those that don't bind well to alpha-TTP.

Table 33. Alpha-tocopherol isomers and binding to alpha-TTP

Do not bind well to alpha-TTP	Bind well to alpha-TTP
SRR	RRR
SSR	RRS
SSS	RSS
SRS	RSR

Other forms of vitamin E (gamma-tocopherol, tocotrienols) also don't bind well to alpha-TTP and thus, are found in lower levels than alpha-tocopherol in the body. The following graph shows plasma vitamin E levels from a study in which subjects were given 150 mg each of RRR-alpha-tocopherol, all-rac-alpha-tocopherol, or gamma-tocopherol.[63]

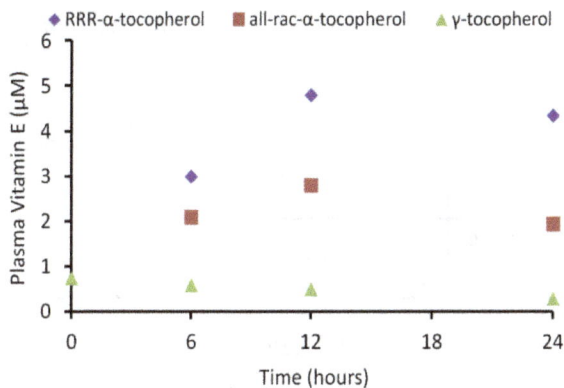

Figure 258. Plasma vitamin E concentrations in response to a 150 mg dose of RRR-alpha-tocopherol, all-rac-alpha-tocopherol, or gamma-tocopherol

As you can see in the figure, there was a greater rise in the plasma alpha-tocopherol levels after receiving RRR-alpha-tocopherol vs. all-rac-alpha-tocopherol. This is not a surprise because approximately 50% of all-rac-alpha-tocopherol is 2R alpha-tocopherol that binds well with alpha-TTP. You can also see that the plasma gamma-tocopherol concentration is much lower than either natural or synthetic alpha-tocopherol.

From VLDL and subsequent lipoproteins, vitamin E reaches tissues, with most vitamin E in the body being found in the adipose tissue. There are two main routes of vitamin E excretion. The major route of excretion is through bile that is then excreted in faeces. The second route is in the urine after vitamin E is chain-shortened in a process like beta-oxidation to make them more water-soluble.

8.2.3 Dietary Vitamin E & Amounts Found in Body

The best food sources of vitamin E are primarily oils and nuts. As you can see below, the forms of vitamin E that nuts and oils contain varies, with the two major forms being alpha and gamma-tocopherol. Soybean, corn, and flaxseed oils are good sources of gamma-tocopherol. Palm and canola oils contain almost equal amounts of alpha-tocopherol and gamma-tocopherol. Safflower oil, almonds, sunflower oil, and wheat germ oil are good sources of alpha-tocopherol. Beta-tocopherol and delta-tocopherol are found in lower levels in foods. Tocotrienols, for the most part, are not found in high levels in the diet. The amount of tocopherols in different nuts and oils are shown in the figure below.

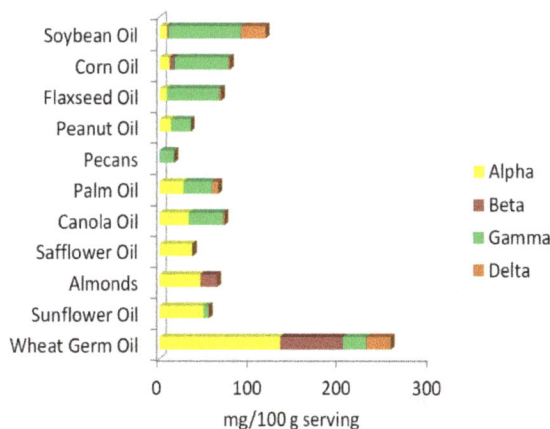

Figure 259. Tocopherol distribution in plant products[64]

Three-fourths of the oil that Americans consume is soybean oil. As a result, it is

159

estimated that they consume 2-4 times more gamma-tocopherol than alpha-tocopherol. Europeans consume more olive, sunflower, and canola oil and thus are believed to consume at least 2 times more alpha-tocopherol than gamma-tocopherol.[64]

Despite Americans' higher intake of gamma tocopherol compared to other countries, serum concentrations do not differ much, as illustrated in the table below.

Table 34. International serum gamma-tocopherol and alpha-tocopherol concentrations (uM/L) [64]

Location	Gamma-tocopherol	Alpha-tocopherol
USA 1*	2-7	15-20
USA 2	5.4	22.3
USA 3	2.5	21.8
Costa Rica	2.7	28.6-31.8
France	1.05-1.28	26.7
Ireland	1.74-1.87	26.3
The Netherlands	2.3	23.9-25.5
Spain	0.88-1.14	27.4-28.3
Italy	1.29	24.3
Sweden	3.2	23.8
Lithuania	1.64	21.7
Austria	1.48	21.1

Note: Several studies with differing results have reported serum levels in the United States.

Tissue concentrations, for the most part, also indicate a greater accumulation of alpha-tocopherol than gamma-tocopherol as shown in the table below.

Table 35. Tissue gamma-tocopherol and alpha-tocopherol concentrations (nM/g) [64]

Tissue	Gamma-tocopherol	Alpha-tocopherol
Skin	180	127
Adipose	176	440
Muscle	107	155

8.2.4   Vitamin E Deficiency & Toxicity

Vitamin E deficiency is extremely rare. Depletion studies require years on a vitamin E-deficient diet to cause deficiency.[1] Deficiency primarily occurs in people with lipid malabsorption problems or Ataxia with Isolated Vitamin E Deficiency (AVED). Individuals with AVED have a mutation in their alpha-TTP that prevents it from functioning correctly. The primary symptoms of vitamin E deficiency are neurological problems.

Elevated levels of vitamin E intake does not result in a noted toxicity. However, higher levels of intake are associated with decreased blood coagulation. Haemorrhagic stroke has been linked to high vitamin E levels.

It is believed that this increased bleeding risk is due to a vitamin E metabolite that has anti-vitamin K activity. This potential antagonism will be described more in the vitamin K section.

8.2.5 Vitamin E DRI & IUs

Before 2001, all forms of vitamin E counted towards the RDA, using a measure called alpha-tocopherol equivalents. In 2001, the Dietary Reference Intake (DRI) committee decided only 2R forms of alpha-tocopherol should be used to estimate the requirement, because these forms bind to alpha-TTP. Thus, other forms of vitamin E (gamma-tocopherol, tocotrienols etc.) do not count towards the requirement and the unit is now mg of alpha-tocopherol. As a result, soybean, corn, and flaxseed oils, which are reliable sources of gamma-tocopherol, are no longer considered to be useful sources of vitamin E. There is some debate as to whether this should be reinvestigated with respect to emerging evidence for the benefits of other forms of vitamin E. The figure below is a reminder of the tocopherol content of different nuts and oils.

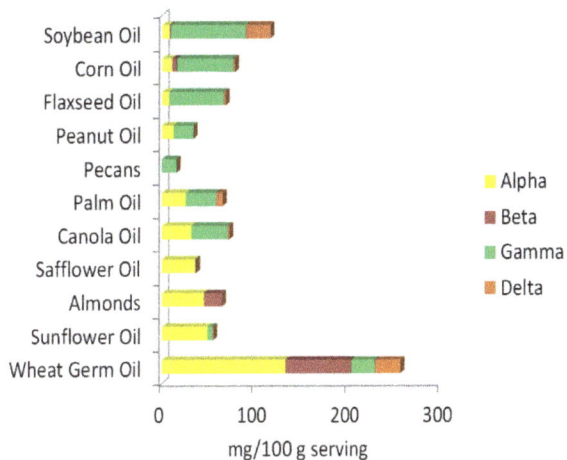

Figure 260. Only the yellow bars count towards the 2001 DRI requirement

Another level of complexity is added by the introduction of international units (IU). IUs are a unit that are used to describe the bioactivity of different compounds, including 4 vitamins: A, D, E, and C. It would be less confusing if these units were not used. However, most supplements use IUs. IUs are not as common on food items. For vitamin E, IUs are specific for alpha-tocopherol and adjusted for the molecular weight of the different forms (alpha-tocopherol acetate etc.). The conversion factors for converting IU to mg of alpha-tocopherol are:

- 0.67 for RRR-alpha-tocopherol (and its esters)
- 0.45 for all-rac-alpha-tocopherol (and its esters)

Here are some example calculations showing how to use these conversion factors:

Example 1. For a supplement containing 100 IU of RRR-alpha tocopherol:

100 IU X 0.67 = 67 mg alpha-tocopherol

Example 2. For a supplement containing 100 IU of all-rac-alpha tocopherol:

100 IU X 0.45 = 45 mg alpha-tocopherol[2,3]

8.3 Vitamin C

Vitamin C is well-known for being a water-soluble antioxidant. Humans are one of the few mammals that don't synthesize vitamin C, making it an essential micronutrient. Other mammals that don't synthesize vitamin C include primates, guinea pigs, and other less prevalent species.[22]

Vitamin C's scientific names are ascorbic acid or ascorbate and the oxidized form is dehydroascorbic acid or dehydroascorbate. The structure of vitamin C is shown below.

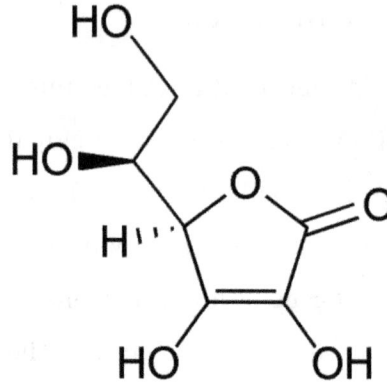

Figure 261. Structure of ascorbic acid

When ascorbic acid is oxidized, it forms semidehydroascorbate (1 degree of oxidation) and then dehydroascorbate (2 degrees of oxidation). The structure of dehydroascorbic acid is shown below.

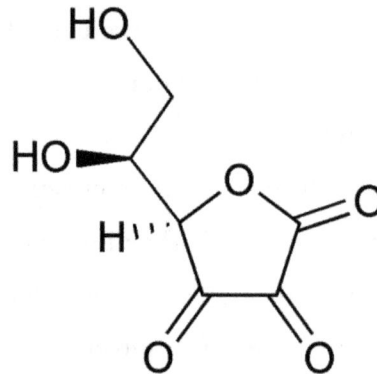

Figure 262. Structure of dehydroascorbic acid

The figure below shows the reaction through which ascorbic acid can stabilize or quench two free radicals. The two circled hydrogens are lost and replaced by double bonds when ascorbic acid is oxidized to dehydroascorbic acid. Reducing dehydroascorbic acid back to ascorbic acid is the opposite reaction.

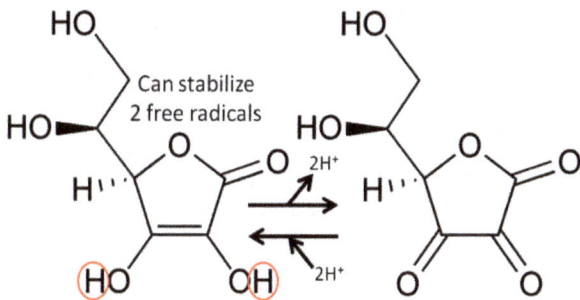

Figure 263. The oxidation-reduction reaction between ascorbic acid (left) and dehydroascorbic acid (right)[xlii]

Ascorbic acid is believed to be a part of an antioxidant network (shown below) where it is oxidized to reduce alpha-tocopherol radical. Dehydroascorbic acid can be reduced by thioredoxin reductase, a selenoenzyme, to regenerate ascorbic acid.

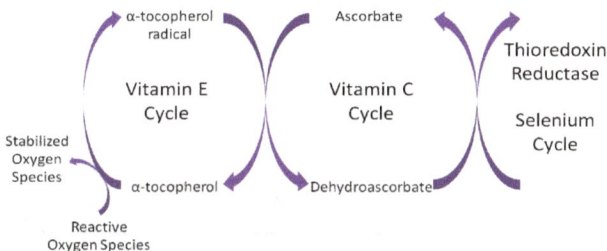

Figure 8.34 The theorized antioxidant network[59]

8.3.1 Vitamin C Absorption & Tissue Accumulation

Vitamin C is found in foods primarily as ascorbic acid (80-90%), but dehydroascorbic acid (10-20%) is also present. The bioavailability of vitamin C is high at lower doses as shown below but drops to less than 50% at higher doses.[35]

Table 36. Bioavailability of vitamin C

Dose (mg)	% Bioavailability
200	112
500	73
1250	49

Ascorbic acid is actively absorbed by sodium vitamin C cotransporter (SVCT) 1. This active transport is driven by the sodium electrochemical gradient created by sodium-potassium ATPase. Ascorbic acid then diffuses into the capillary and ultimately enters general circulation. Vitamin C generally circulates as ascorbic acid.

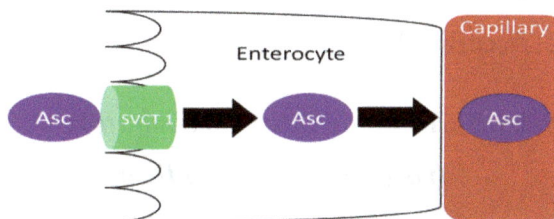

Figure 264. Ascorbic acid (Asc) absorption

8.3.1.1 Accumulation

Most water-soluble vitamins are not stored in the body. Vitamin C is not stored, but is accumulated in certain tissues in the body where it can be 5-100 times higher than found in the plasma.[22] The table below shows the concentrations of vitamin C in different tissues and fluids.[35]

Table 37. Human tissue & fluid ascorbic acid concentrations

Organ	Vitamin C Concentration*	Organ	Vitamin C Concentration*
Pituitary Gland	40-50	Lungs	7
Adrenal Gland	30-40	Skeletal Muscle	3-4
Eye Lens	25-31	Testes	3
Liver	10-16	Thyroid	2
Brain	13-15	Cerebrospinal Fluid	3.8
Pancreas	10-15	Plasma	0.4-1
Spleen	10-15	Saliva	0.1-9.1
Kidneys	5-15		

* mg/100 g wet tissue, mg/100 mL for fluids

How does the body accumulate such high levels of vitamin C?

There are 2 primary mechanisms:

1. Ascorbic Acid (Ascorbate) uptake using sodium-dependent vitamin C transporter (SVCT) 1 or

2. Ascorbic Acid (Ascorbate) Recycling

8.3.1.2 Ascorbic Acid (Ascorbate) transport using sodium-dependent vitamin C transporter (SVCT) 1 or 2

As shown below, SVCT 1 and SVCT 2 transport ascorbic acid or ascorbate into the cell against the concentration gradient (represented by orange wedge in the figure below). Like absorption, this uptake is driven by the action of sodium-potassium ATPase. This mechanism is saturable, meaning that at high concentrations it reaches a threshold where it cannot take up ascorbic acid any faster. Thus, there is

a limit to how much can be taken up through this mechanism.[65]

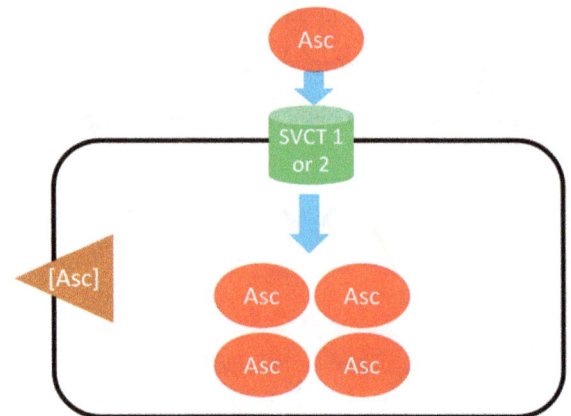

Figure 265. Ascorbic acid uptake using SVCT 1 and 2 against the ascorbic acid concentration gradient

8.3.1.3 Ascorbic Acid (Ascorbate) Recycling

In ascorbic acid recycling, ascorbic acid is oxidized to dehydroascorbic acid (DHA). DHA is then transported into the cell down its concentration gradient using GLUT1 or 3. Once inside the cell, DHA is reduced back to ascorbic acid, thus maintaining the

DHA gradient. As a result, the cell can accumulate high levels of ascorbic acid.[65, 66]

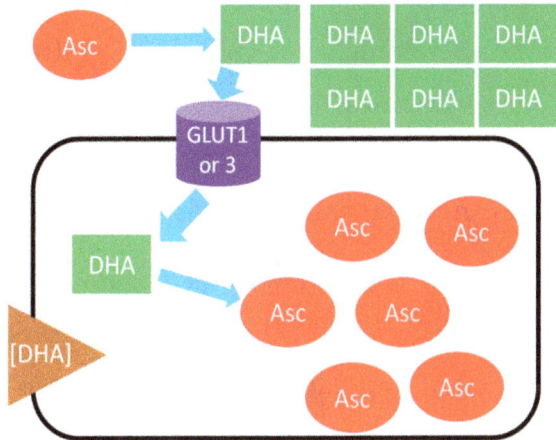

Figure 266. Ascorbic acid recycling

8.3.2 Enzymatic Functions

In addition to its antioxidant function, vitamin C is also a cofactor for several enzymes. The enzymes proline hydroxylase and lysyl hydroxylase are important in the formation of the protein collagen. Hydroxylase means that the enzymes add alcohol (hydroxyl, -OH) to the amino acids proline and lysine, as shown below.

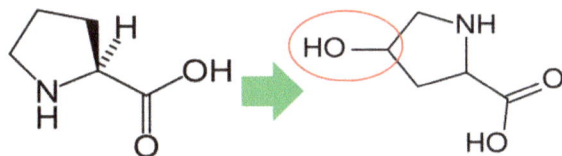

Figure 267. Proline hydroxylase adds an alcohol group (circled) to proline forming hydroxyproline

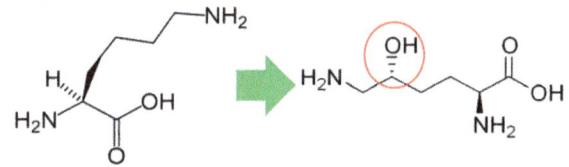

Figure 268. Lysyl hydroxylase adds an alcohol group (circled) to lysine forming hydroxylysine

As shown below, proline and lysyl hydroxylases require ferrous iron (Fe^{2+}) to function. But while the hydroxylating proline or lysine, ferrous iron (Fe^{2+}) is oxidized to ferric iron (Fe^{3+}). Ascorbic acid is required to reduce Fe^{3+} to Fe^{2+}, forming semidehydroascorbic acid in the process. With Fe^{2+}, the enzyme is then able to continue to hydroxylate proline and lysine.

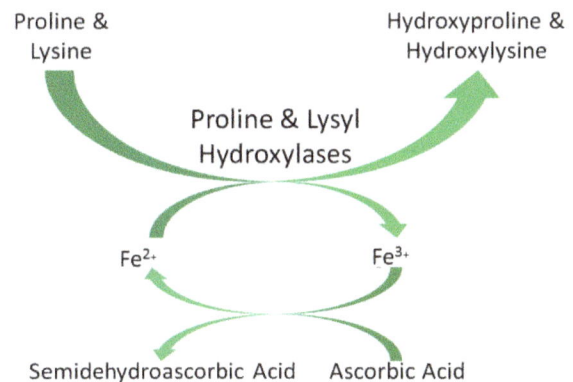

Figure 269. Ascorbic acid reduces iron so that it can continue to serve as a cofactor for proline and lysyl hydroxylases

Why should you care about collagen formation?

Because collagen is estimated to account for 30% or more of total body proteins.[67] Collagen contains a number of hydroxylated prolines that are needed for collagen strands to properly cross-link.

This cross-linking is important for collagen to wind together like a rope, forming the strong triple helix known as tropocollagen.

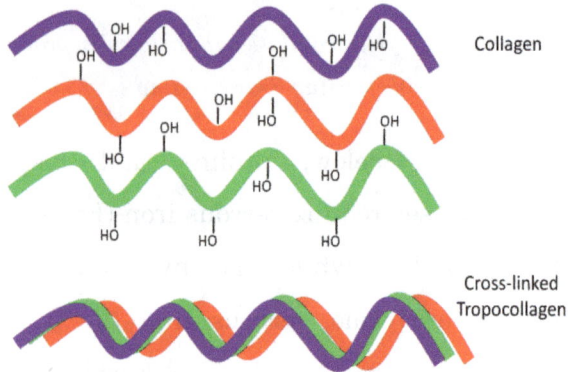

Figure 270. Production of cross-linked tropocollagen in the presence of adequate vitamin C

But if there isn't enough ascorbic acid available, the collagen strands are under-hydroxylated and instead of forming strong tropocollagen, the under-hydroxylated collagen is degraded as shown below.

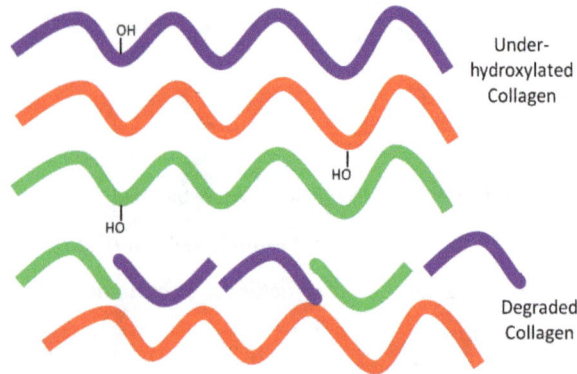

Figure 271. Production of under-hydroxylated collagen

This weak collagen then results in the symptoms seen in the vitamin C deficiency, scurvy, that will be discussed in the next subsection.

Ascorbic Acid is also needed for:

- Carnitine synthesis
- Tyrosine synthesis and catabolism
- Serotonin (neurotransmitter) synthesis
- Other hormone and neurotransmitter synthesis[36]

The figure below shows how ascorbic acid is needed for dopamine hydroxylase, which ultimately produces the hormone epinephrine.

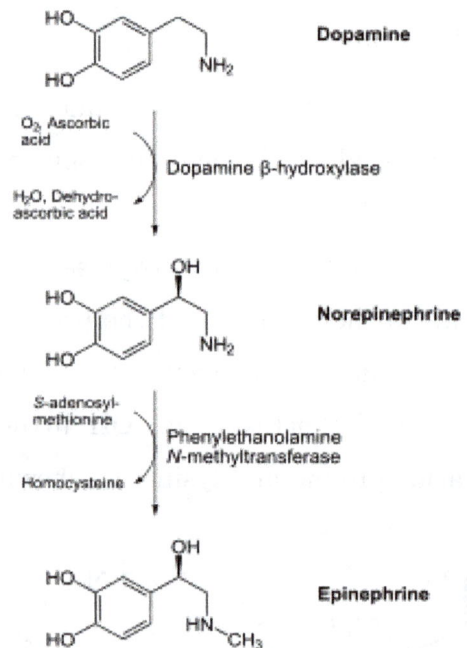

Figure 272. Dopamine beta-hydroxylase requires ascorbic acid to produce norepinephrine

8.3.3 Vitamin C Deficiency (Scurvy)

Why should you care about the functions of vitamin C?

Because they explain the symptoms of vitamin C deficiency, known as 'scurvy'.

While it is rare nowadays, scurvy was a major cause of mortality. In fact, more people died in the Crusades from scurvy than warfare, and on long ocean voyages up until the 1800s it was commonly expected for half of the sailors to die from scurvy. The symptoms of scurvy are a result of weak collagen, that in turn, weakens connective tissue throughout the body. Symptoms of scurvy include bleeding gums, pinpoint haemorrhages, and corkscrew hairs as shown in the figure and below.

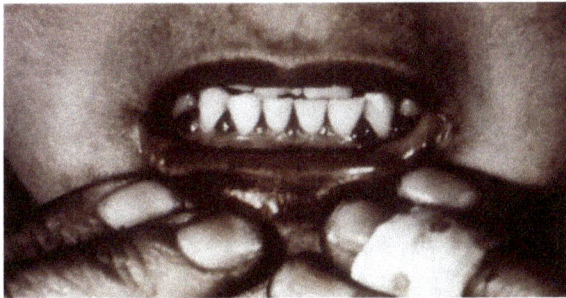

Figure 273. Bleeding gums resulting from scurvy[xliii]

Additional symptoms include impaired wound and fracture healing, easy bruising, and loose or decaying teeth. Scurvy can be fatal if not treated. Subclinical deficiencies are considered to cause some of these symptoms in people without a frank deficiency.[36]

Scurvy was the first discovered nutritional deficiency, in 1746 by James Lind, who is shown below.

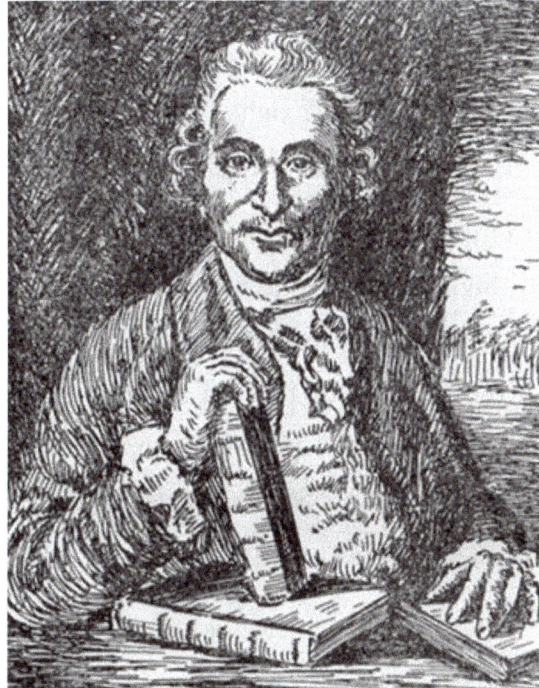

Figure 274. Dr James Lind discovered that scurvy was caused by a nutrition deficiency[xliv]

Lind was a surgeon on a British navy ship. Frequently during voyages, the sailors would develop scurvy for reasons that weren't understood at the time. It was known that citrus fruits could cure or prevent scurvy, but it was believed this was due to their acidity. Lind performed clinical trials comparing citrus juice to dilute sulfuric acid and vinegar and found that only citrus juice caused the sailors to recover. As a result of the discovery, the

---

British sailors became known as "Limeys", now a common slang term for an Englishman, because they would drink this juice to prevent the development of the disease.[58]

8.3.4 Vitamin C Toxicity, Linus Pauling & the Common Cold

Vitamin C doesn't have a toxicity per se, but high doses (usually greater than 2 grams/day) can lead to diarrhoea and gastrointestinal distress. In addition, high intake of vitamin C increases excretion of uric acid (urate) and oxalic acid (oxalate). The structure of these two compounds are shown below.

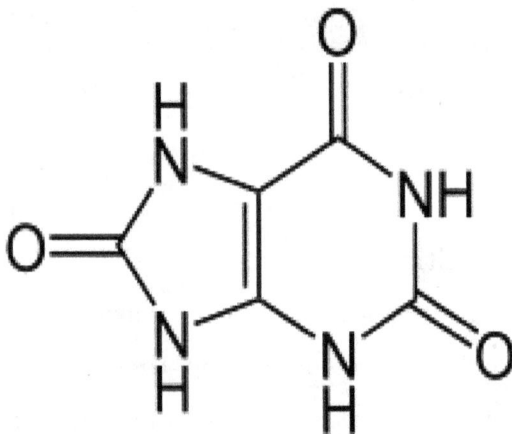

Figure 276. Structure of calcium oxalate

These compounds are the primary components of two types of kidney stones. The figures below show the most common sites of pain in someone with kidney stones.

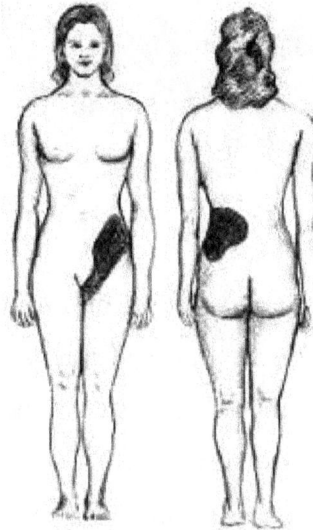

Figure 275. Structure of uric acid

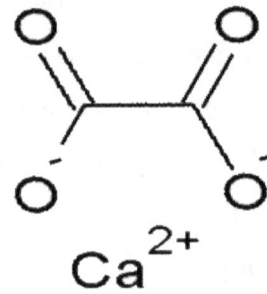

Figure 277. Kidney stones normally cause pain in the shaded areas[xlv]

Calcium oxalate is one of the primary forms of kidney stones with uric acid stones being rarer. However, a link

---

between excretion of these compounds and actual stone formation hasn't been established. Nevertheless, high-dose vitamin C supplementation should be approached with some caution, since it not clear whether it increases the risk of forming kidney stones.[68]

8.3.4.1 Linus Pauling and the common cold

The person who popularized taking mega doses of vitamin C was Linus Pauling. Dr Pauling was a chemist and is the only person to receive two unshared Nobel Prizes. The Nobel Prize is a prestigious award, and Dr Pauling was very close to solving the structure of DNA. This would have likely netted him another Nobel prize, but Watson and Crick beat him to it.

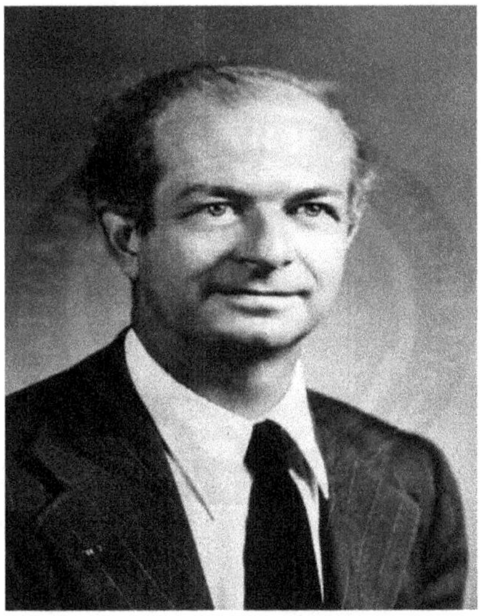

Figure 278. Linus Pauling[xlvi]

Later in his life, Pauling became convinced that mega doses of vitamin C could prevent the common cold. In 1970 his book *Vitamin C and the Common Cold* was released and became a bestseller. Later he came to believe that vitamin C could prevent cardiovascular disease, cancer, and combat aging.[7] However, critics of his beliefs countered that all megadose supplementation was doing was creating “expensive urine”. This refers to the fact that the RDA is only 75-90 mg/day for adults and Pauling recommended taking 1-2 grams of vitamin C daily.[8]

Pauling may have been at least partially vindicated. A Cochrane database review of the evidence suggests that regular Vitamin C supplementation, with higher than ‘normal’ doses, although not preventing colds and flu, can reduce the length and severity of the common cold.[65]

8.4 Selenium

Selenium can be divided into two categories: organic and inorganic. The organic forms contain carbon, while the inorganic forms do not. The primary inorganic forms of selenium are selenite (SeO_3) and selenate (SeO_4). Selenite and selenate are not commonly found alone in

[xlvi] http://en.wikipedia.org/wiki/File:Linus_Pauling_NIH.jpg

nature; they are usually complexed with sodium to form sodium selenite (Na_2SeO_3) and sodium selenate (Na_2SeO_4)[22].

Selenomethionine is the most common organic form of selenium. The structure of selenomethionine is shown above the structure of the amino acid methionine in the figure below.

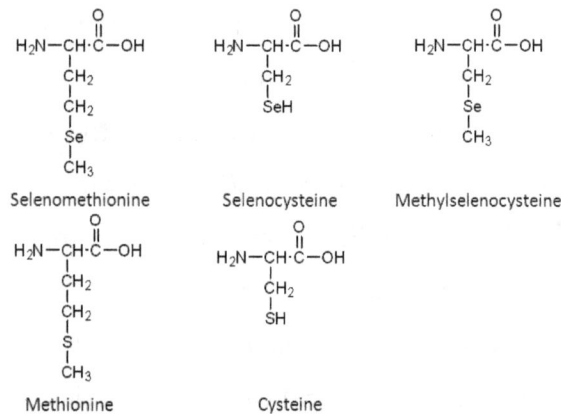

Figure 279. Structures of organic forms of selenium & similar sulphur-containing amino acids

In comparing the structures of selenomethionine or methionine, you can see that the only difference is that selenium has been substituted for the sulphur (S) atom in methionine. Selenocysteine is considered the 21st amino acid by some, because there is a codon that directs its insertion into selenoproteins. Like selenomethionine vs. methionine, the only difference between selenocysteine and cysteine is the substitution of selenium for sulphur. The last organic form is methylselenocysteine (aka Se-methylselenocysteine). Notice that its structure is like selenocysteine, but with a methyl group added (like the name suggests).

The selenium content of plants is dependent on the soil where they are grown.

Inorganic forms of selenium are commonly used in supplements. Selenomethionine is the most common organic form of selenium in supplements and food. It is found in cereal grains such as wheat, corn, and rice as well as soy. Yeast are typically used to produce selenomethionine for supplements. It should be noted that selenomethionine accumulates at much higher levels in the body than other forms of selenium. This is because it can be non-specifically incorporated into body proteins in place of methionine. However, despite accumulating at higher levels, selenomethionine is less effective than the methylselenocysteine in decreasing cancer incidence or growth in animal models.[69] However, it is not common to find methylselenocysteine supplements because methylselenocysteine is a form that plants accumulate to prevent selenium from becoming toxic to themselves.

8.4.1 Selenoproteins

As mentioned earlier, selenium's antioxidant function is not due to the mineral itself, but a result of selenoproteins. This is illustrated in the figure below, where the different coloured circles represent amino acids in the crescent shaped enzyme. In most enzymes, the mineral is a cofactor that is external to the enzyme, as shown on the left. Selenoenzymes contain selenocysteine as an amino acid in the active site of the enzyme. Thus, in selenoenzymes, selenium does not serve as a cofactor, which is different than most minerals required for enzyme function.

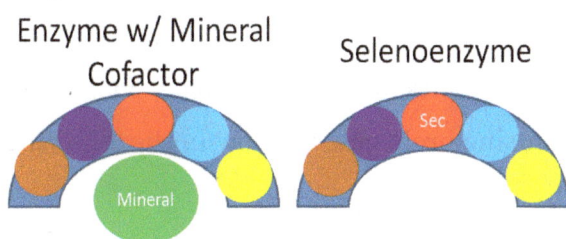

Figure 280. Enzyme with a mineral cofactor versus a selenoenzyme

25 human selenoproteins, containing the amino acid selenocysteine, have been identified. The following table lists these selenoproteins along with their function.

Table 38. The 25 Human Selenoproteins

Selenoprotein	Function
Glutathione peroxidase 1 (GPX1)	Antioxidant enzyme
Glutathione peroxidase 2 (GPX2)	Antioxidant enzyme
Glutathione peroxidase 3 (GPX3)	Antioxidant enzyme
Glutathione Peroxidase 4 (GPX4)	Antioxidant enzyme
Glutathione Peroxidase 6 (GPX6)	Antioxidant enzyme
Iodothyronine 5'-deiodinase-1 (DI1)	Plasma T3 production
Iodothyronine 5'-deiodinase-2 (DI2)	Local T3 production
Iodothyronine 5'-deiodinase-3 (DI3)	T3 degradation
Thioredoxin Reductase (TR1)	Antioxidant enzyme
Thioredoxin Reductase (TR2)	Antioxidant enzyme
Thioredoxin Reductase (TR3)	Antioxidant enzyme
Selenophosphate synthetase 2 (SPS2)	Selenophosphate synthesis
Selenoprotein 15 (Sep15)	Unknown
Selenoprotein H (SepH)	Unknown
Selenoprotein I (SepI)	Unknown
Selenoprotein K (SepK)	Unknown
Selenoprotein M (SepM)	Unknown
Selenoprotein N (SepN)	Unknown
Selenoprotein O (SepO)	Unknown
Selenoprotein P (SepP)	Unknown
Selenoprotein R (SepR)	Unknown
Selenoprotein S (SepS)	Unknown
Selenoprotein T (SepT)	Unknown
Selenoprotein V (SepV)	Unknown
Selenoprotein W (SepW)	Unknown

Hopefully, from looking at the table, you see that the glutathione peroxidase enzymes and thioredoxin reductases are antioxidant enzymes. The iodothyronine 5'-deiodinases are involved in the metabolism of thyroid hormones, which will be discussed further in the iodine section. The function of the majority of other selenoproteins isn't known, so they were named selenoprotein and given a letter. As described earlier and shown below, glutathione peroxidase converts hydrogen peroxide into water.

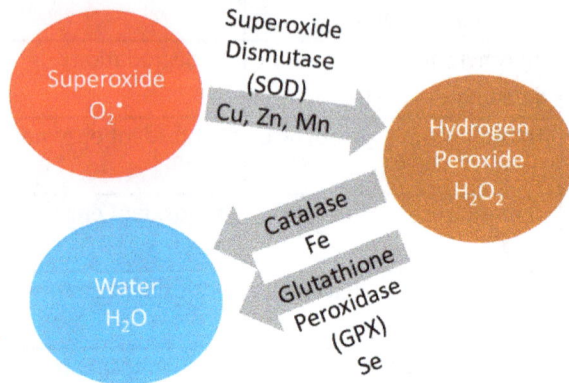

Figure 281. Antioxidant enzymes that use minerals as cofactors

Remember that thioredoxin reductase can regenerate ascorbate from dehydroascorbate in the theorized antioxidant network (shown previously, and below).

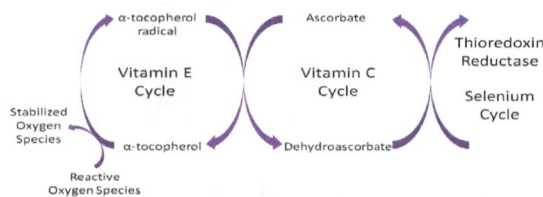

Figure 282. The theorized antioxidant networks

8.4.2 Selenium Absorption, Excretion, Toxicity & Its Questionable Deficiency

Selenium is highly absorbed. Thus, selenium levels in the body are not regulated by absorption, but rather by urinary excretion. Organic selenium forms may be absorbed slightly better than inorganic forms, as one study found that 98% of a dose of selenomethionine was absorbed, compared to 84% of selenite.[22]

Selenium is primarily excreted in the urine, but at elevated levels it can be expired, producing garlic odour breath—a primary sign of overload and potential toxicity.

Selenium toxicity can be a problem, especially for animals living in or around a body of water in an area with high soil selenium levels. This is because runoff from the soil causes selenium to collect in the water in elevated levels and then starts working its way up the food chain and causing problems, as show in the following link.

In humans, the initial symptoms are nausea, fatigue, and diarrhoea. If continued, the person may develop hair and nail brittleness, rash or skin lesions, and nervous system abnormalities.

The questionable selenium deficiency is Keshan disease. This disease occurred primarily in the mountainous regions of China, causing heart lesions. However, sodium selenate supplementation failed to totally eradicate Keshan disease like you would expect if it was a selenium deficiency. The incidence of Keshan disease also fluctuated seasonally and annually, which is unusual for a deficiency and more consistent of an infectious disease. Research found Coxsackie virus in the heart of Keshan disease victims. They isolated this virus and used it to perform the experiment illustrated below.

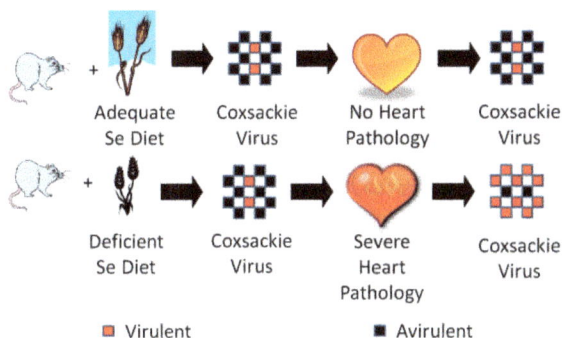

Figure 283. Keshan disease experiment

One group of mice was fed an adequate selenium diet and another group a deficient selenium diet. They were then infected with Coxsackie virus that was mostly avirulent, but also contained some virulent virus. A virulent virus is one that causes a disease, and an avirulent virus is one that doesn't cause a disease (some vaccines use avirulent viruses). After a period, they found that the selenium deficient animals developed severe heart pathology, while the selenium adequate animals did not develop heart pathology. They then isolated the virus from the hearts of the mice from both groups and found that the Coxsackie virus from the deficient animal's hearts had become mostly virulent. They then took it one step further as shown in the figure below.

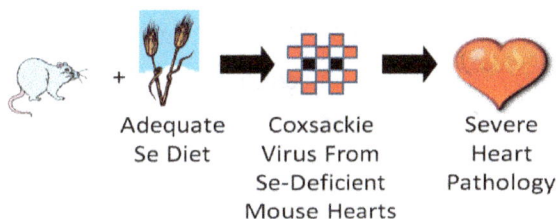

Figure 284. Keshan disease experiment continued

They took the isolated virus from the selenium-deficient mouse hearts and infected selenium adequate animals with it. The selenium adequate animals developed the severe heart pathology like the selenium-deficient animals had previously.

What's going on?

They found mutations in the virus from the selenium-deficient animals that they believe caused it to become virulent. They believe that high oxidative stress in these animals leads to mutations in the virus, causing it to become virulent.

Who cares?

Research has found comparable results with vitamin E. Researchers are also examining the effects on other viruses such as influenza (flu) and HIV. If they find a similar phenomenon occurring in other viruses, it means that you and your friend who eats a horrible diet (eats no fruit and vegetables) could be exposed to a virus. You don't know you were exposed because your immune system fights off the virus. However, your friend gets sick. He/she can serve as a host in which the virus mutates

173

Edited and revised by Cliff Harvey. Derived from the Flexbook by Brian Lindshield

making it more virulent, which when
you're exposed a second time, may make
you sick.

9 Macronutrient Metabolism Micronutrients

The macronutrient metabolism vitamins and minerals are:

- Thiamin
- Riboflavin
- Niacin
- Pantothenic Acid
- Vitamin B$_6$
- Biotin
- Vitamin B$_{12}$
- Vitamin C
- Iodine
- Manganese
- Magnesium

All but three of these will be covered in this section. Vitamin B$_{12}$ will be covered in the one-carbon metabolism chapter, vitamin C was covered in the antioxidant chapter, and magnesium is going to be covered in the electrolyte chapter. We're left with iodine, manganese, and many of the B vitamins. We'll cover the two minerals followed by the B vitamins.

9.1 Iodine

Iodine's only major, yet critical, function is that it is required for thyroid hormone synthesis. The thyroid gland is a butterfly-shaped organ found in the neck. The parathyroid glands are also found within the thyroid gland.

Thyroid and Parathyroid Glands

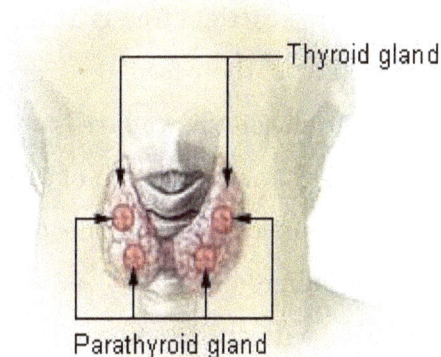

Figure 285. Location of the thyroid and parathyroid glands[xlvii]

Iodine is found in foods primarily as iodide (I$^-$), while some bread dough has iodate (IO$_3^-$) added to help with gluten cross-linking,[36] although this is not commonly used now. Like selenium, iodide concentrations in soil vary greatly between different regions, causing food

---

xlvii https://training.seer.cancer.gov/anatomy/endocrine/glands/thyroid.html

concentrations to greatly fluctuate. Sea water is high in iodine, thus foods of marine origin, such as seaweed and seafood, are good dietary sources of iodine. Dairy products, in countries with high factory-farming rates, also tend to be good sources of iodide because it is added to cattle feeds, iodine-containing medications, and iodide-containing sanitizing solutions used in dairy facilities.[16, 18] In countries like New Zealand however, where cattle is free-pastured, there are lower iodine contents in dairy. In some areas this can be mitigated by cattle free-grazing on seaweed as part of their feed.

Most iodine in the diet nowadays is derived from iodised salt. Consumption of juts one half teaspoon of iodised salt meets RDA amounts for iodine.

Salt is iodized with either potassium iodide (KI) or potassium iodate (KIO_3). The positives of each are:

Potassium iodide

+ Less expensive

+ Higher iodine content (76% vs. 59% for KIO_3)

+ More soluble

Potassium Iodate

+ More stable

Table 39. Compound & level used for salt iodization in different countries

Country	Compound	Level Used (mg I/kg salt)
Australia	KIO_3	65
Cameroon	KIO_3	50
Canada	KI	77
China	KIO_3	40
Ecuador	KI	40
Germany	KIO_3	25
India	KIO_3	30
Indonesia	KIO_3	25
Kenya	KIO_3	100
Nigeria	KIO_3	50
Panama	KIO_3/KI*	67-100
USA	KI	77
Zimbabwe	KIO_3	50 (at point of entry)
New Zealand	KIO_3	25-65

* If KI is used it must be guaranteed that there is no significant iodine loss

With people now consuming non-iodised salt there may be a greater risk of relative iodine deficiency occurring. Likewise, the reduction in salt, suggested by dietary guidelines over the past four decades is likely to have reduced iodine status and may be increasing rates of goitre and thyroid dysfunction. Iodised salt has played a key role in reducing iodine deficiency and goitre in New Zealand. But dietary exposure to iodine has steadily decreased since 1982,[70, 71] due mainly to the implementation of low-salt guidelines. Some dietary compounds interfere with thyroid hormone production or utilization. These compounds are known as goitrogens.[72] However, it is not believed that goitrogens are of clinical importance unless there is a coexisting iodine deficiency. Some examples of foods that contain goitrogens are Cassava root, millet, cruciferous vegetables like broccoli, cabbage and Brussels sprouts, onions, garlic, and some legumes like soybeans and peanuts.

9.1.1 Iodised Salt vs 'Natural' Salt

There is considerable talk in the natural health media about the virtues of 'natural' salts (such as Himalayan salt, rock salt, and Celtic sea salt) and the perceived dangers of iodised table salt.

While there are some nutritional advantages (other ancillary minerals) from the 'natural' salts, a significant disadvantage is that they may be markedly lower in iodine. It is worth remembering that most available table salt is simply sea salt, typically with the addition of an iodine compound and an anti-caking agent (such as '554' sodium aluminosilicate).

9.1.2 Thyroid Hormone

The thyroid is like a net that 'catches' most of the absorbed iodine, keeping it for use in synthesizing thyroid hormone. The two primary forms of thyroid hormone are triiodothyronine (T_3) and thyroxine (T_4).

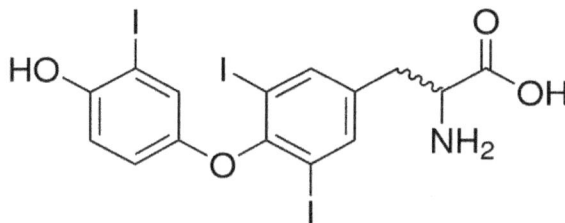

Figure 286. The structure of triiodothyronine (T3)

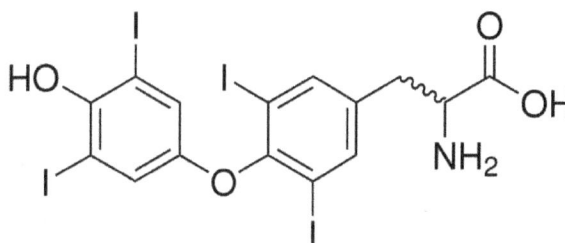

Figure 287. The structure of thyroxine (T4)

T_4 is the primary circulating form and is really a prohormone that is converted to the active T_3 form. The enzymes that metabolize thyroid hormone are known as deiodinases. There are three deiodinases (Type I, Type II, Type III) that are selenoenzymes whose location and function are summarized in the table below.

Table 40. Location and function of the three deiodinases

Enzyme	Tissues	Function
Deiodinase Type I (DI1)	Liver, kidney, thyroid gland	Plasma T_3 production
Deiodinase Type II (DI2)	Brain, pituitary, brown adipose	Local T_3 production
Deiodinase Type III (DI3)	Brain, placenta	T_3 degradation

Thyroid hormone regulates the basal metabolic rate and is important for growth and development. Thyroid hormone is

177

particularly important for brain development, but hypothyroidism (low thyroid hormone) also leads to decreased muscle mass and skeletal development.[22]

9.2 Iodine Deficiency & Toxicity

There are two iodine deficiency disorders (IDD); goitre and cretinism. Goitre is a painless deficiency condition that results from the enlargement of the thyroid to help increase its ability to take up iodine. A couple of pictures of goitre are shown below.

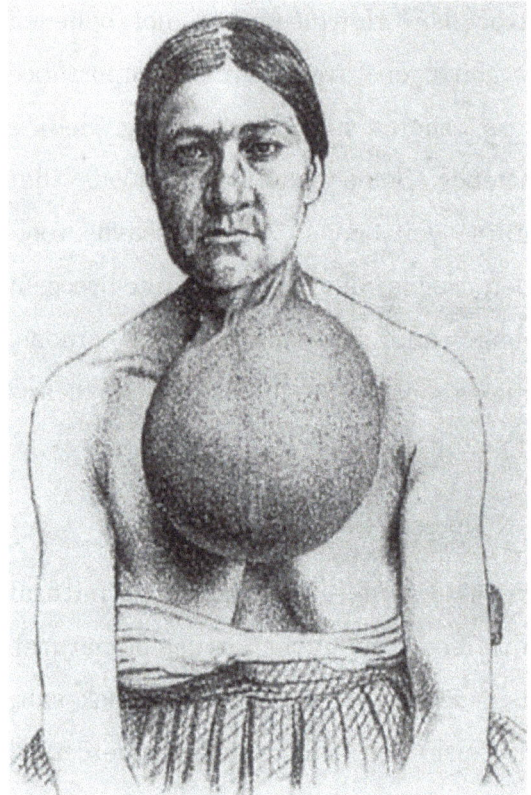

Figure 289. Illustration of a woman with a goitre[xlix]

A more serious consequence of iodine deficiency occurs during pregnancy to the foetus. Iodine deficiency during this time can lead to the severe mental and physical retardation known as cretinism. This condition is characterized by severe hypothyroidism, stunted growth, speech loss, and paralysis.[22, 35]

Iodine toxicity is rare, but like iodine deficiency, it can result in thyroid enlargement, and hypothyroidism or hyperthyroidism. Acute toxicity results in

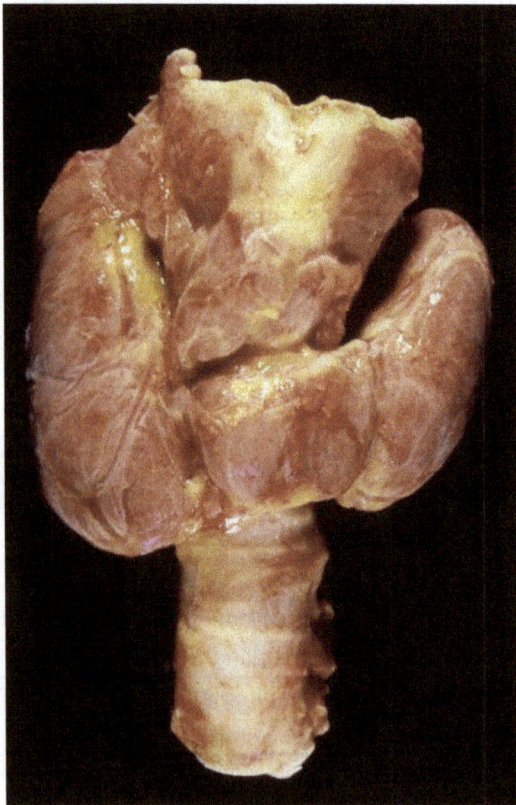

Figure 288. Hyperplasia of the thyroid gland[xlviii]

xlix E. Theodor Kocher: *Zur Pathologie und Therapie des Kropfes.* Deutsche Zeitschrift für Chirurgie 1874; 4, 417

gastrointestinal irritation, abdominal pain, nausea, vomiting, and diarrhea.[36]

9.3 Manganese

We know far less about manganese than many other minerals. Like most minerals it serves as a cofactor for several enzymes that are discussed in more detail below.

The enzyme superoxide dismutase uses manganese as a cofactor to convert superoxide to hydrogen peroxide as shown below.

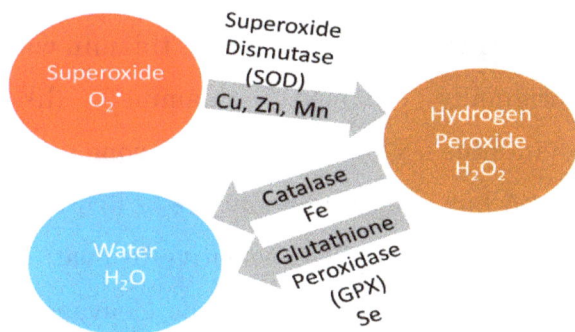

Figure 290. Antioxidant enzymes that use minerals as cofactors

In addition, both the enzymes involved in the gluconeogenesis-oxaloacetate workaround use manganese as cofactors as shown below.

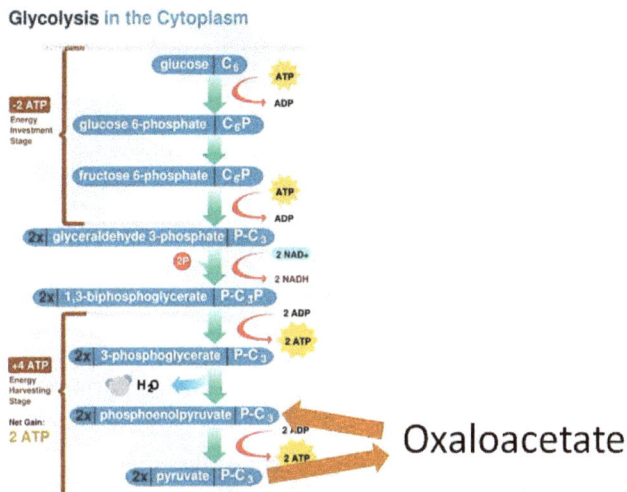

Figure 291. Both enzymes of the oxaloacetate workaround in gluconeogenesis use manganese as cofactors

One enzyme in the urea cycle uses manganese as a cofactor.

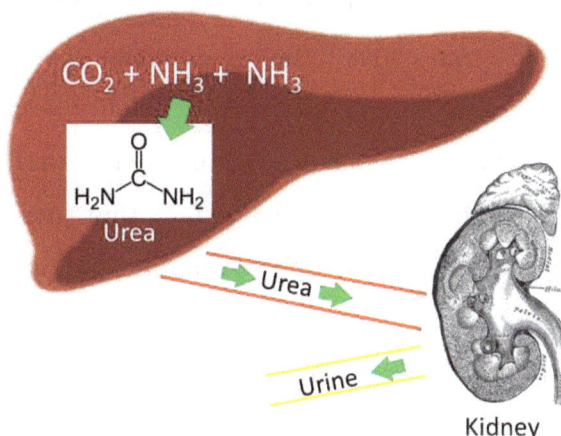

Figure 292. Production of urea helps to safely remove ammonia from the body

Enzymes critical to the production of proteoglycans, which are essential components of cartilage and bone, use manganese as a cofactor.[36]

179

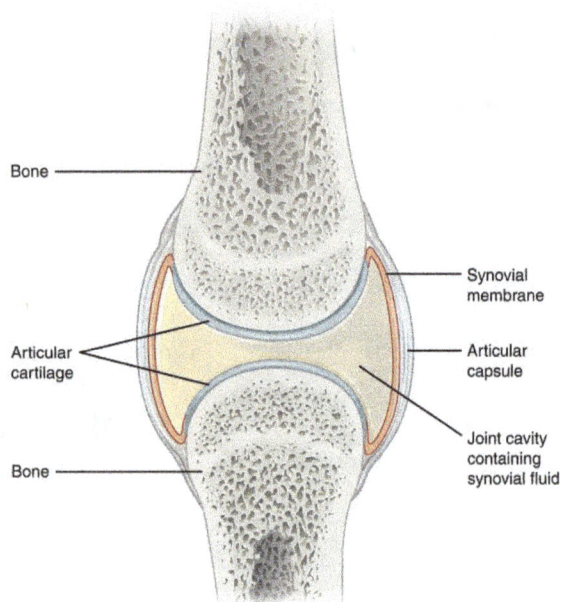

Figure 293. Synovial joint anatomy[l]

Absorption of manganese is not well understood but is believed to be low (<5%). The main route (90%) of excretion is via bile excreted in faeces.[36] Deficiency and toxicities of manganese are extremely rare. The deficiency is so rare in fact, that there is little information available on the symptoms of the condition. Symptoms in those who were deliberately made deficient include vomiting, dermatitis, changes in hair colour, & skeletal defects.[36]

Toxicity symptoms include neurological disorders similar to schizophrenia and Parkinson's disease. In Chilean miners exposed to Mn-containing dust the toxicity was named Manganese Madness.[22, 35]

9.4 Thiamin

Thiamin (Vitamin B$_1$) structurally consists of two rings that are bridged together as shown below.

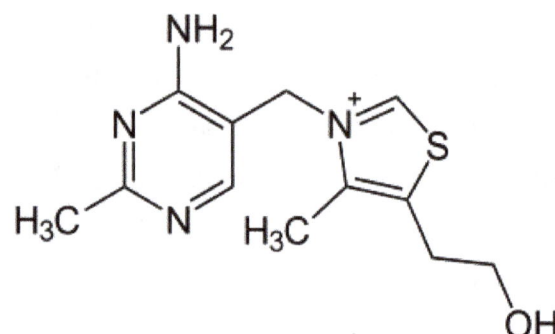

Figure 294. Structure of thiamin

One of the original vitamins, thiamin was originally named thiamine (like 'vitamine'). This spelling is still sometimes used but more commonly the -e has been dropped. Thiamin is sensitive to heat; so prolonged heating causes the cleavage of thiamin between the two rings rendering it inactive.[16]

Like most of the B vitamins, thiamins primary function is as a cofactor for enzymes. It is not thiamin alone that serves as a cofactor but instead thiamin diphosphate (thiamin + 2 phosphates), which is more commonly referred to as thiamin pyrophosphate (TPP). The structure of thiamin pyrophosphate is shown below.

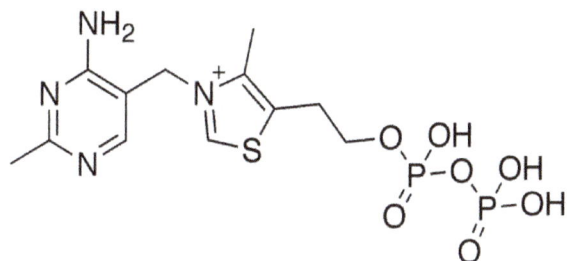

Figure 295. Structure of thiamin pyrophosphate (aka thiamin diphosphate

In plants, thiamin is found in its free form, but in animals it is mostly thiamin pyrophosphate. These phosphates must be cleaved before thiamin is taken up into the enterocyte.[36]

Thiamin uptake and absorption is believed to be an efficient process that is passive when thiamin intake is high and active when thiamin intakes are low.[36] This helps to ensure that we receive the appropriate amount of thiamine from the diet. There are two thiamin transporters (THTR), THTR1 and THTR2, that are involved in thiamin uptake and absorption. THTR1 is found on the brush border and basolateral membrane, while THTR2 is only found on the brush border membrane.[73]

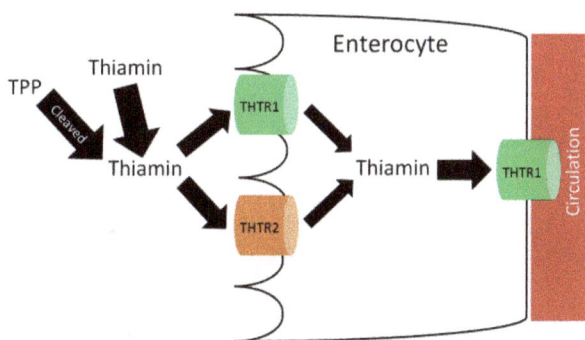

Figure 296. Thiamin uptake and absorption

Figure 9.33

Like most water-soluble vitamins there is little storage of thiamin.

9.4.1 Thiamin Functions

There are three major functions of thiamin[36]:

1. Cofactor for decarboxylation reactions (TPP)
2. Cofactor for the synthesis of pentoses (5-carbon sugars) and NADPH (TPP)
3. Membrane and nerve conduction (Not as a cofactor)

9.4.1.1 Decarboxylation Reactions

A decarboxylation reaction is one that results in the loss of carbon dioxide (CO_2) from the molecule as shown below.

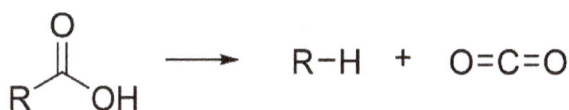

Figure 297. Decarboxylation reaction

The transition reaction and one reaction in the citric acid cycle are decarboxylation reactions that use TPP as a cofactor. The figure below shows the transition reaction and citric acid cycle.

181

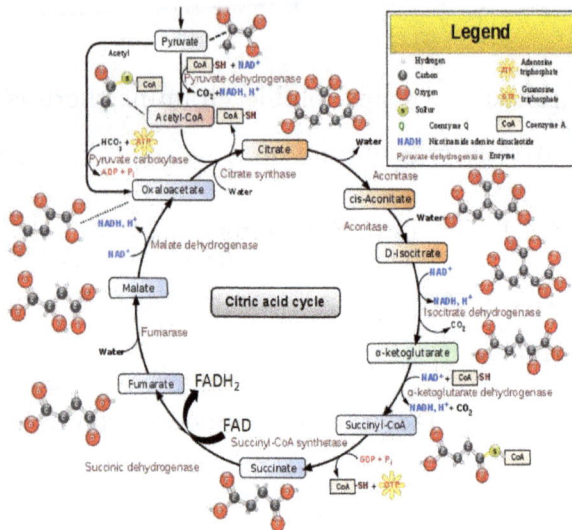

Figure 298. The transition reaction and citric acid cycle

As shown below the conversion of pyruvate to acetyl CoA in the transition reaction is a decarboxylation reaction that requires TPP as a cofactor. CO_2 (circled) is produced because of this reaction.

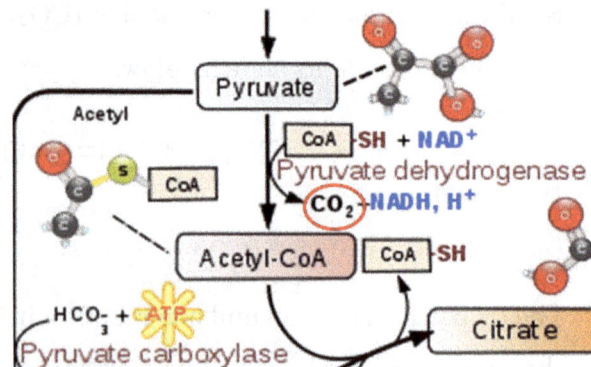

Figure 299. The transition reaction requires TPP as a cofactor

A similar TPP decarboxylation reaction occurs in the citric acid cycle converting alpha-ketoglutarate to succinyl-CoA. CO_2 (circled) is given off because of this reaction.

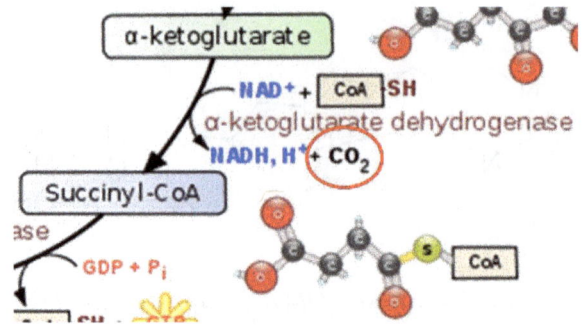

Figure 300. Alpha-ketoglutarate dehydrogenase requires TPP as a cofactor

TPP also functions as a cofactor for the decarboxylation of valine, leucine, and isoleucine (branched-chain amino acids).[36]

9.4.1.2 Synthesis of Pentoses and NADPH

TPP is a cofactor for the enzyme transketolase. Transketolase is a key enzyme in the pentose phosphate (aka hexose monophosphate shunt) pathway. This pathway is important for converting 6-carbon sugars into 5-carbon sugars (pentose) that are needed for synthesis of DNA, RNA, and NADPH. In addition, pentoses such as fructose are converted to forms that can be used for glycolysis and gluconeogenesis.[22] Transketolase catalyses multiple reactions in the pathway as shown below.

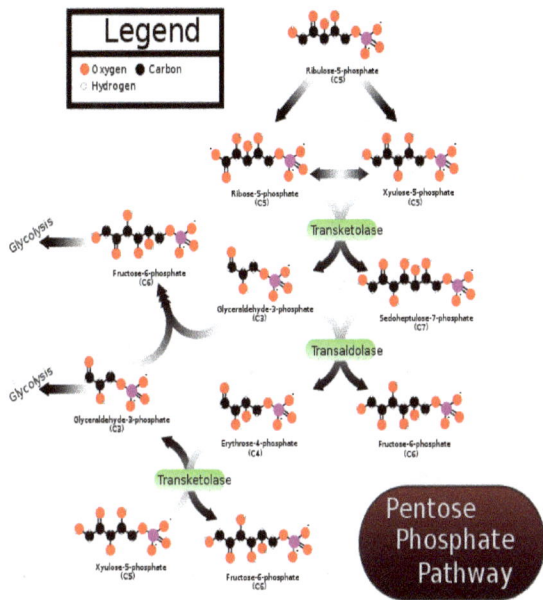

Figure 301. Transketolase in the pentose phosphate pathway uses TPP as a cofactor

9.4.1.3 Membrane and Nerve Conduction

In addition to its cofactor roles, thiamin, in the form of thiamin triphosphate (TTP, 3 phosphates), is believed to contribute to nervous system function.[36]

9.4.2 Thiamin Deficiency & Toxicity

Thiamin deficiency is rare in developed countries, but still occurs in poorer countries where white or 'polished' rice is a staple food. During the polishing process which removes the husk and outer, nutrient-rich layers of the rice grain, thiamin and many other nutrients, are removed. Some people may also have a mutation in the THTR1 gene that causes

them to become thiamin deficient.[1] Thiamin deficiency is known as beriberi, which translated means "I can't, I can't." There are two major forms of beriberi: dry and wet.

Dry beriberi affects the nervous system, with symptoms such as loss of muscle function, numbness, and/or tingling. Wet beriberi affects the cardiovascular system resulting in pitting oedema, along with enlargement of the heart.[1]

Another group that is at risk for thiamin deficiency is alcoholics. There are three reasons why alcoholics are prone to becoming deficient.[36]

1. Alcohol displaces foods that are good sources of thiamin
2. Liver damage decreases TPP formation
3. Alcohol increases thiamin excretion

The thiamin deficiency found in alcoholics is known as Wernicke-Korsakoff Syndrome. Symptoms of this condition include paralysis or involuntary eye movement, impaired muscle coordination, memory loss and confusion.[36]

Thiamin toxicity has never been reported from oral intake. Thus, there is little concern about thiamin toxicity.[22]

9.5 Riboflavin

If you've ever taken a 'mega-B' vitamin supplement, you'll be familiar with the vitamin riboflavin. The bright yellow urine which probably surprised you at the time is due to this B vitamin. Indeed, flavin means yellow in Latin, and riboflavin is bright yellow. Riboflavin is water-soluble and so excess that isn't required or assimilated into tissue will be excreted in urine.

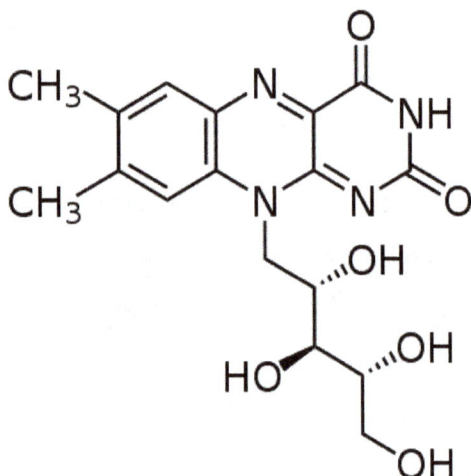

Figure 302. Structure of riboflavin

Riboflavin is important to produce two cofactors: flavin adenine dinucleotide (FAD) & flavin mononucleotide (FMN).

FAD has been introduced before, but structurally you can see where riboflavin is within the compound below.

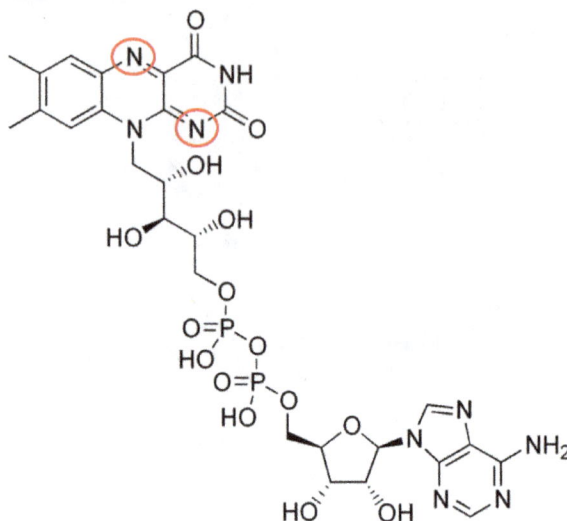

Figure 303. Structure of FAD

The two circled nitrogen are the sites that accept hydrogen to become $FADH_2$ as illustrated below.

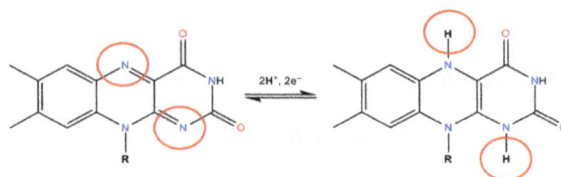

Figure 304. Addition of two hydrogens to the rings of FAD to form $FADH_2$

The structure of FMN as shown below, is like FAD, except that it only contains one phosphate group (as compared to two) and doesn't have the ring structures off the phosphate groups that are found in FAD.

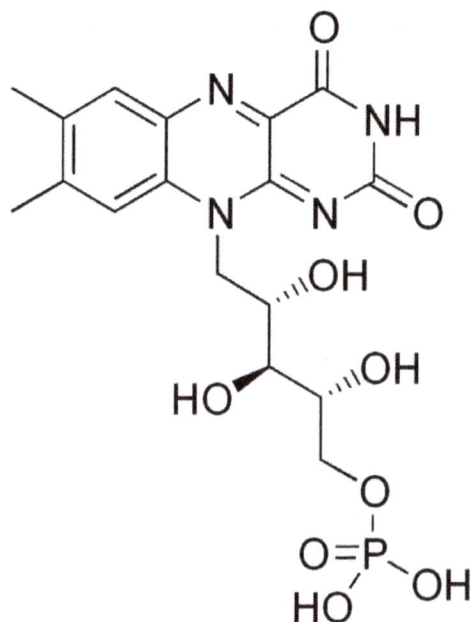

Figure 305. The structure of FMN

Riboflavin is photosensitive, meaning that it can be destroyed by light. When milk was predominantly distributed in glass bottles the riboflavin content could be seriously degraded and this is one of the reasons that milk is now often sold in opaque containers and cartons.

Riboflavin found in foods is free, protein-bound, or in FAD or FMN. Only free riboflavin is absorbed so it must be cleaved, or converted before absorption.[36] Riboflavin is highly absorbed through an unresolved process, though it is believed a carrier is involved.[73] As mentioned earlier, riboflavin is excreted in the urine.

9.5.1 Riboflavin Functions

Riboflavin is required to produce FAD and FMN. Below are some of the functions of FAD and FMN[36]:

1. Citric Acid Cycle
2. Electron Transport Chain
3. Fatty Acid Oxidation
4. Niacin Synthesis
5. Vitamin B₆ Activation
6. Neurotransmitter Catabolism
7. Antioxidant Enzymes

1. Citric Acid Cycle—FAD is reduced to $FADH_2$ in the citric acid cycle when succinate is converted to fumarate by succinic dehydrogenase as circled below.

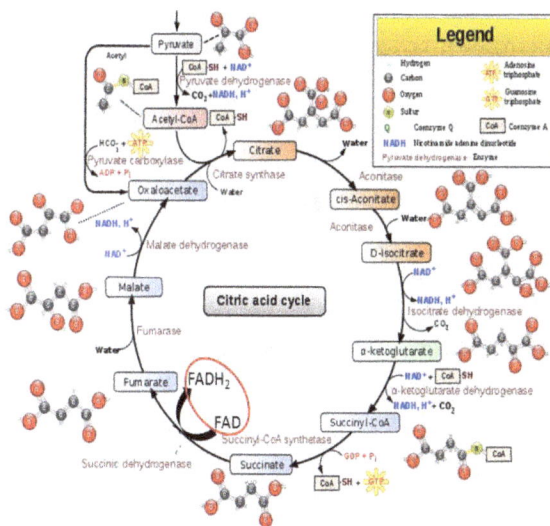

Figure 306. The citric acid cycle requires FAD

2. Electron Transport Chain—Under aerobic conditions, the electron transport chain is where the $FADH_2$ is used to produce ATP. Complex I of the electron transport chain includes an FMN molecule. The electron transport chain is shown below.

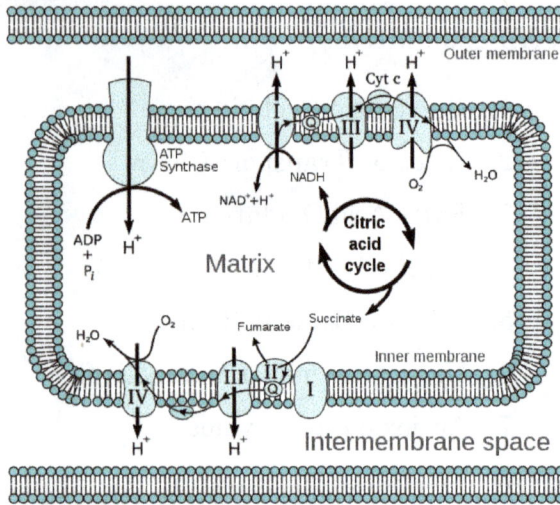

Figure 307. Complex I in the electron transport chain contains FMN

3. Fatty Acid oxidation—During fatty acid oxidation FAD is converted to $FADH_2$ as shown below.

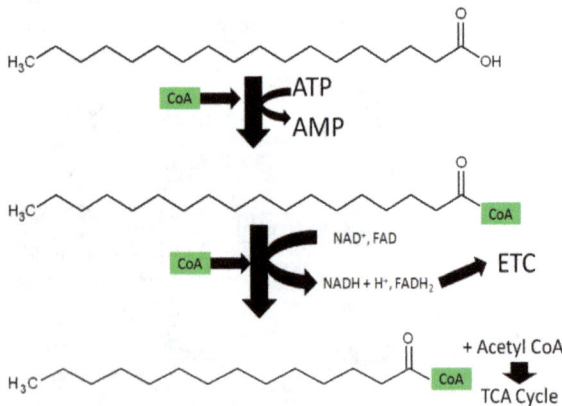

Figure 308. Fatty acid oxidation requires FAD

4. Niacin synthesis—As you will hear more about in the niacin section, niacin can be synthesized from tryptophan as shown below. An intermediate in this synthesis is kynurenine, and one of the multiple steps between kynurenine to niacin requires FAD.

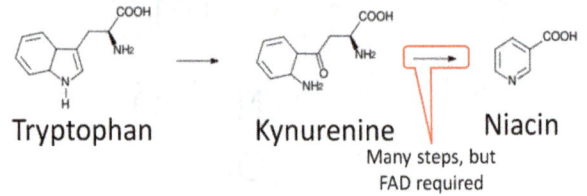

Figure 309. Niacin synthesis from tryptophan requires FAD

5. Vitamin B₆ Activation—The enzyme that creates the active form of vitamin B_6 (pyridoxal phosphate) requires FMN.

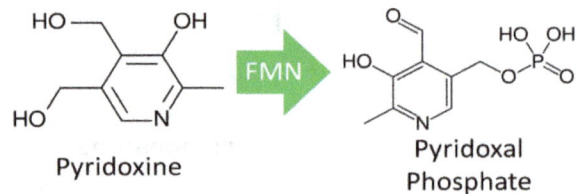

Figure 310. Figure 9.415 Vitamin B6 activation requires FMN

6. Neurotransmitter Catabolism—The enzyme monoamine oxidase (MAO) requires FAD. This enzyme shown below is important in the catabolism of neurotransmitters such as dopamine (shown below) and serotonin.

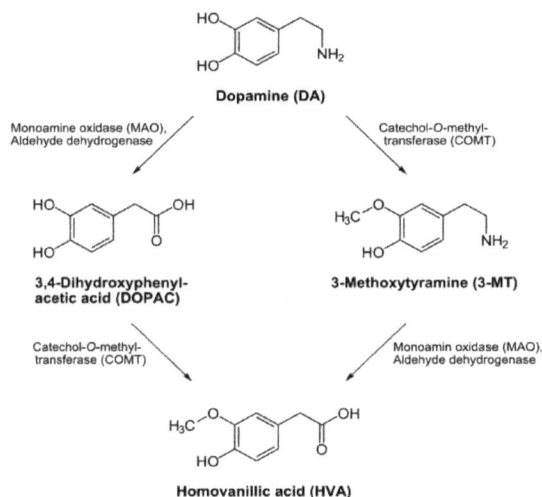

Figure 311. Catabolism of dopamine involves monoamine oxidase, an enzyme that requires FAD[li]

7. Antioxidant Enzymes—The antioxidant enzymes glutathione reductase and thioredoxin reductase both require FAD as a cofactor. Thioredoxin reductase is a selenoenzyme. The function of glutathione reductase is shown in the following link. Glutathione reductase can reduce glutathione that can then be used by the selenoenzyme glutathione peroxidase to convert hydrogen peroxide to water.

In addition to the functions listed above, FAD is also used in folate activation, choline catabolism, and purine metabolism.[36]

There has been no toxicity of riboflavin reported.

9.6 Niacin

There are two forms of niacin: nicotinic acid and nicotinamide (aka niacinamide), that have a carboxylic acid group or amide group, respectively. The structure of nicotinic acid and nicotinamide are shown below.

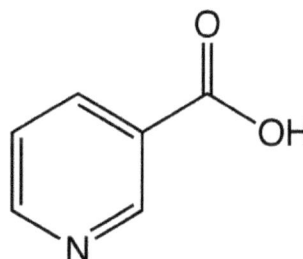

Figure 312. Structure of nicotinic acid

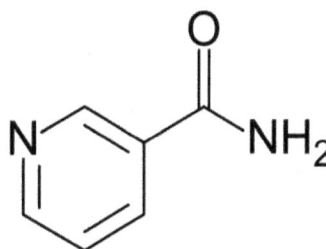

Figure 313. Structure of nicotinamide

Niacin is important to produce two cofactors: nicotinamide adenine dinucleotide (NAD) and nicotinamide adenine dinucleotide phosphate (NADP$^+$). The structure of NAD is shown below; you can clearly see the nicotinamide at the top right of the molecule.

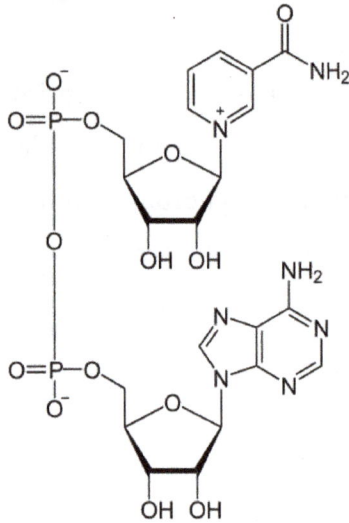

Figure 314. Structure of NAD

NAD is reduced to form NADH, as shown below.

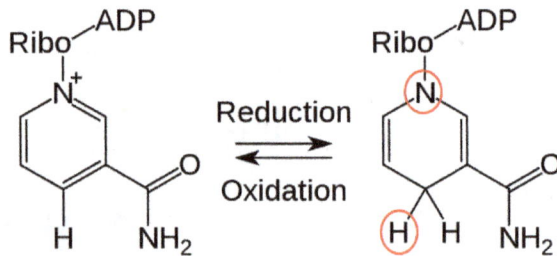

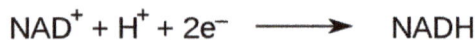

$$NAD^+ + H^+ + 2e^- \longrightarrow NADH$$

Figure 315. Reduction of NAD to NADH

The structure of NADP$^+$ is the same as NAD, except it has an extra phosphate group off the bottom of the structure, as shown below.

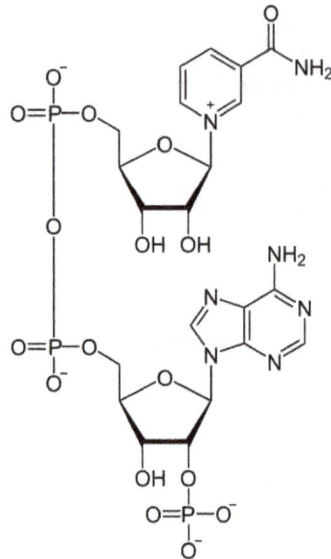

Figure 316. Structure of NADP$^+$

Like NAD, NADP$^+$ can be reduced to NADPH.

Niacin is unique in that it can be synthesized from the amino acid tryptophan as shown below. An intermediate in this synthesis is kynurenine. Many reactions occur between this compound and niacin, and riboflavin and vitamin B$_6$ are required for two of these reactions.

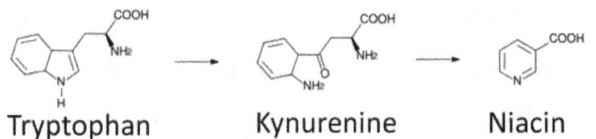

Tryptophan   Kynurenine   Niacin

Figure 317. Tryptophan can be used to synthesize niacin

To account for niacin synthesis from tryptophan, niacin equivalents (NE) were created by the DRI committee to account for niacin in foods as well as their tryptophan content. It takes approximately 60 mg of tryptophan to make 1 mg of niacin. Thus, the conversions to niacin equivalents are:

- 1 mg Niacin = 1 NE
- 60 mg Tryptophan = 1 NE

The tryptophan levels of most foods is not known, but a good estimate is that tryptophan is 1% of amino acids in protein.[16] Using peanut butter as an example[8]:

The peanut butter contains 13.403 mg of niacin and 25.09 g of protein

Step 1: Calculate the amount of tryptophan:

25.09 g X 0.01 (the numerical value of 1%) = 0.2509g of tryptophan

Step 2: Convert Grams to Milligrams

0.2509 g X 1000 mg / g = 250.9 mg of tryptophan

Step 3: Calculate NE from tryptophan

250.9 mg of tryptophan / (60 mg of tryptophan / 1 NE) = 4.182 NE

Step 4: Add NEs together

13.403 NE (from niacin) + 4.182 (from tryptophan) = 17.585 NE

Most niacin we consume is in the form of nicotinamide and nicotinic acid,[36] and in general is well absorbed using an unresolved carrier.[73] However, in corn, wheat, and certain other cereal products niacin bioavailability is low. In these foods, some niacin (~70% in corn) is tightly bound, making it unavailable for absorption. Treating the grains with a base (an alkaline compound such as baking soda) frees the niacin and allows it to be absorbed. This is one of the reasons why traditional processing techniques of grains and legumes and other foods often involved 'activating' and soaking these foods in water with an alkali added. After absorption nicotinamide is the primary circulating form.[16, 36]

9.6.1 Niacin Functions

Approximately 200 enzymes require NAD or NADP+. We will go through some selected functions of NAD and NADP+. The following figures and legends show and describe the functions of NAD and NADP+.

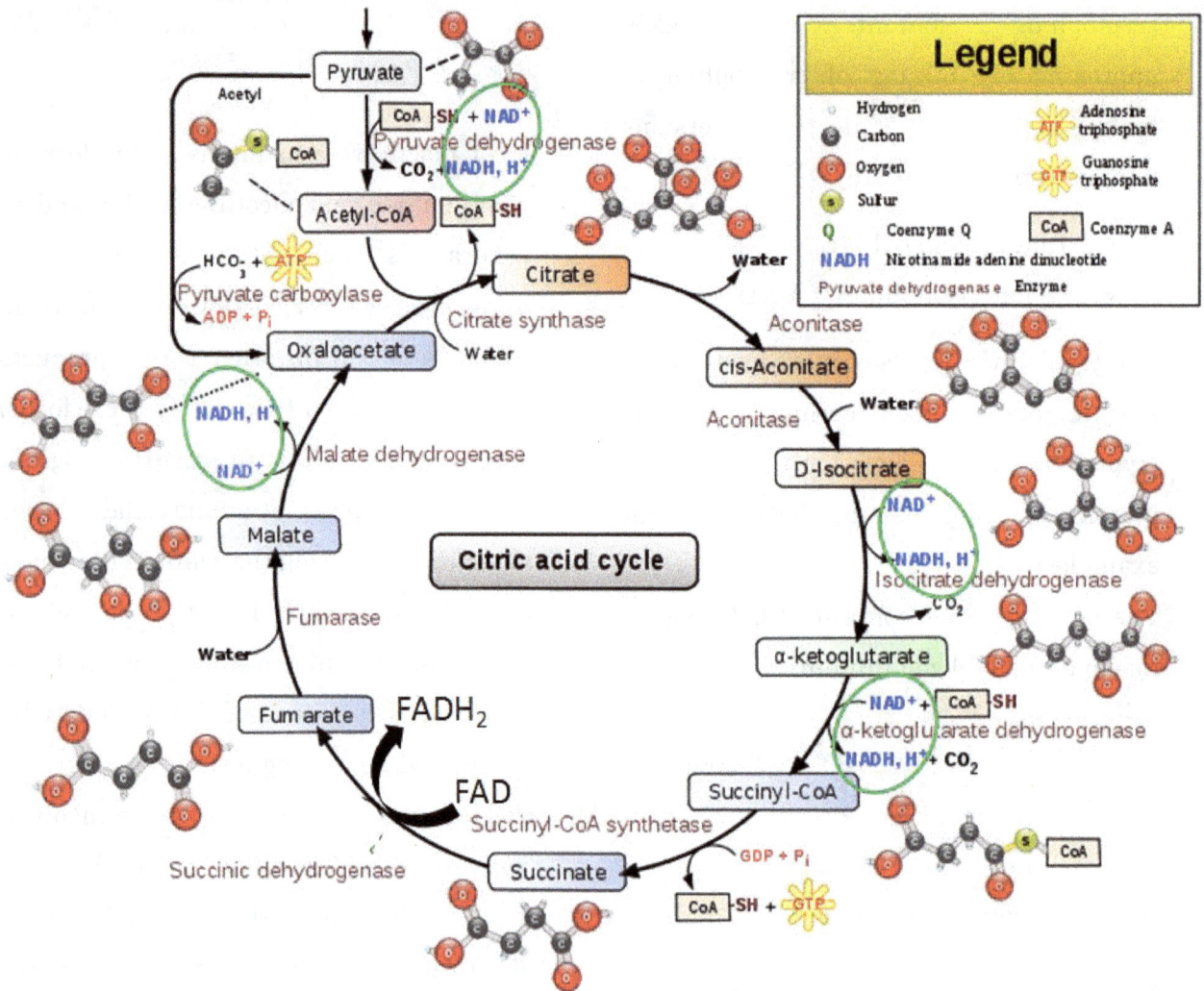

Figure 318. NAD is required for the transition reaction and at three different points in the citric acid cycle

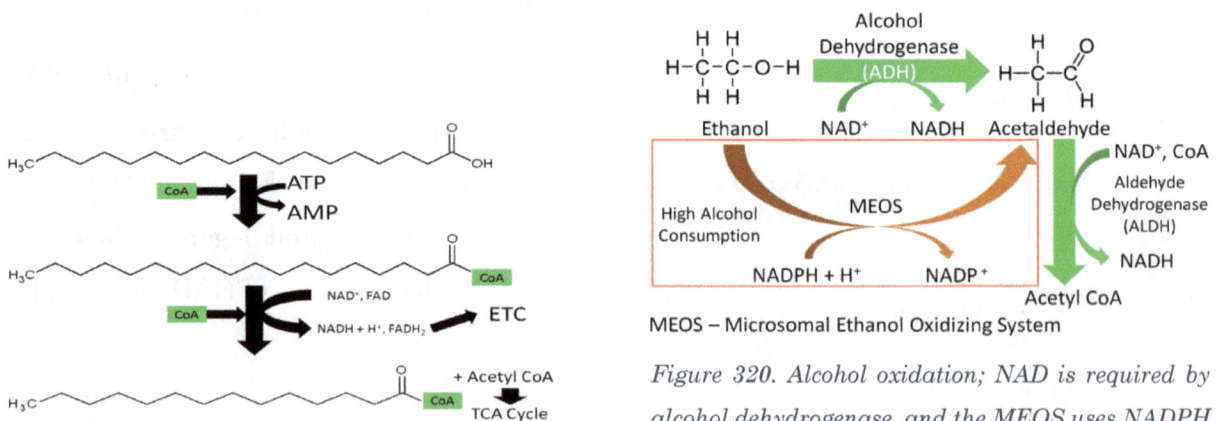

Figure 319. NAD is required for fatty acid oxidation

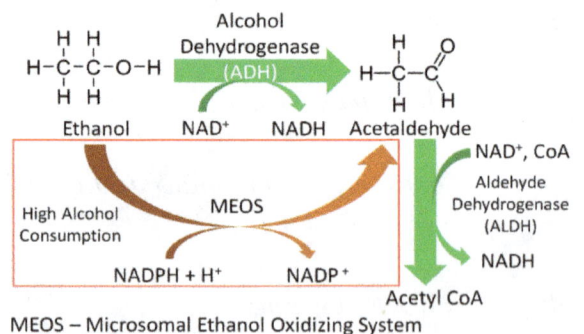

MEOS – Microsomal Ethanol Oxidizing System

Figure 320. Alcohol oxidation; NAD is required by alcohol dehydrogenase, and the MEOS uses NADPH

HMG CoA reductase, the rate-limiting enzyme in cholesterol synthesis, uses NADPH.[36]

9.6.2 Niacin Deficiency & Toxicity

Pellagra is a niacin deficiency. This is no longer a common deficiency in developed countries but was in the U.S. in the early 1900s. This was because corn was a staple crop. As we have discussed, the bioavailability of niacin from corn is poor unless treated with a base (alkaline compound) to release the bound niacin.

The symptoms of pellagra are the three D's:

- Dementia
- Dermatitis
- Diarrhoea

Some refer to four Ds in which the fourth D is death if the condition is not managed. Dietary niacin toxicity is extremely rare. However, nicotinic acid (not nicotinamide) can improve people's lipid profiles when consumed at levels far above the RDA. For instance, the RDA & upper limit (UL) is 14 or 16 (women & men) and 35 mg (both), respectively. Many people are taking 1-2 grams (up to 6 g/day) to get the benefits in their plasma lipid profiles as shown in the table below.[16, 36]

Table 41. Effects of nicotinic acid (>1.5 g/day) on plasma lipid profile

Measure	Change
VLDL	↓ 25-40%
LDL	↓ 6-22%
HDL	↑ 18-35%
Total Cholesterol	↓ 21-44%
Triglycerides	↓ 21-44%

There are special supplements for this purpose that include a slower release nicotinic acid that helps prevent toxicity symptoms (nicotinamide is not toxic).

The most well-known of the toxicity symptoms is "niacin flush", which is a dilation of capillaries accompanied by tingling that can become painful. This symptom is noted to occur at lower levels than the other toxicity symptoms.[18] Other symptoms include gastrointestinal distress and liver damage.

A nicotinic acid receptor (HM74A or GPR109A) has been identified that is believed to mediate the beneficial effects of nicotinic acid on people's lipid profiles and the toxic side-effects.[74]

9.7 Pantothenic Acid

Pantothenic acid has two roles in the body:

1. It is part of coenzyme A (CoA)
2. It is part of acyl carrier protein

1. Coenzyme A

The structure of pantothenic acid is shown alone below and circled within coenzyme A.

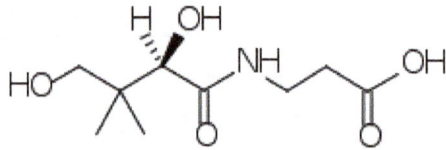

Figure 321. The structure of pantothenic acid

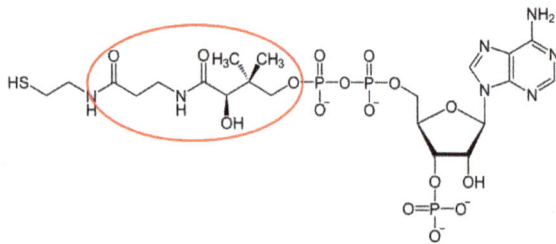

Figure 322. The structure of coenzyme A (CoA) with the pantothenic acid circled

The functions of CoA are shown and described below.[3]

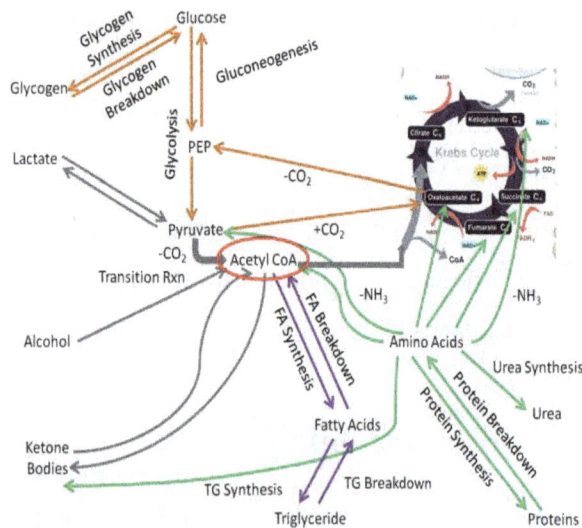

Figure 323. Acetyl-CoA is a pivotal point in metabolism, and contains CoA

2. Acyl Carrier Protein

Acyl carrier protein, is also important in fatty acid synthesis.[36]

Most pantothenic acid in food is found as CoA, which is cleaved prior to absorption. It is then taken up into the enterocyte through the sodium-dependent multivitamin transporter (SMVT) as shown below. Approximately 50% of pantothenic acid is absorbed; it is excreted primarily in urine.[36]

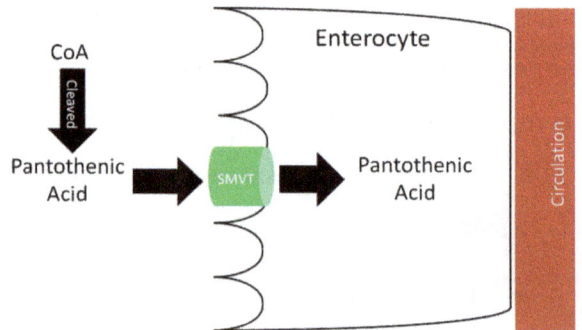

Figure 324. The absorption of pantothenic acid

Deficiency of pantothenic acid is very rare. Pantothenic acid supplementation did relieve the symptoms (burning feet and numbness of toes) of "burning feet syndrome" in prisoners in World War II.[35] It is believed pantothenic acid deficiency was the cause of this syndrome. Other symptoms noted are vomiting, fatigue, weakness, restlessness, and irritability.[36] No toxicity has been reported.

9.8 Vitamin B₆

Vitamin B₆ is composed of three compounds: pyridoxine, pyridoxal, and pyridoxamine. Pyridoxine contains a methylhydroxyl group (-CH₃OH), pyridoxal an aldehyde (-CHO), and pyridoxamine an aminomethyl group (-CH₃NH₂) as shown below.

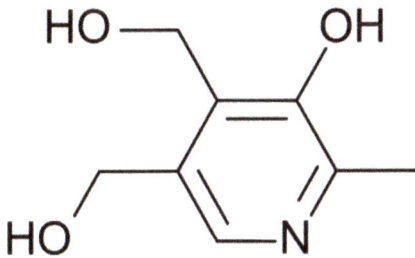

Figure 325. Structure of pyridoxine

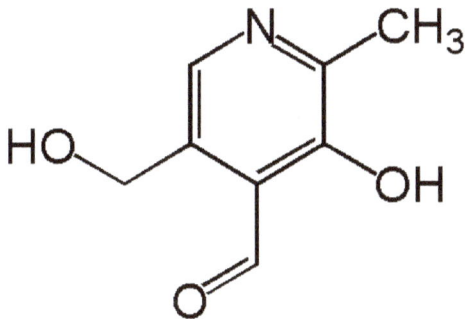

Figure 326. Structure of pyridoxal

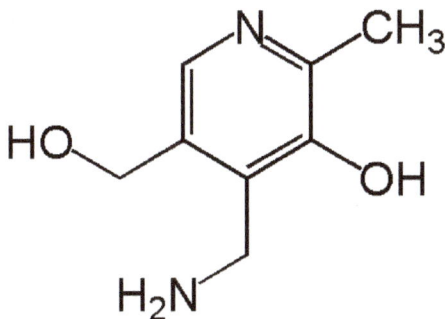

Figure 327. Structure of pyridoxamine

All three forms can be activated by being phosphorylated. The phosphorylated forms can be interconverted to the active, or the cofactor form of vitamin B₆, pyridoxal phosphate (PLP). Thus, any of the three forms is likely to be beneficial, with little real difference noted between them. The active form has a phosphate group added in place of a hydroxyl group. The enzyme that catalyses this reaction requires FMN (riboflavin cofactor) as shown below.

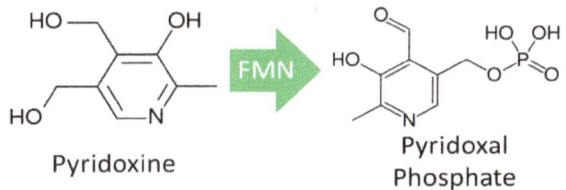

Figure 328. Vitamin B6 activation

In animal products vitamin B₆ is found in its cofactor forms, PLP and pyridoxamine phosphate (PMP). The latter cofactor is less common than PLP. In plants vitamin B₆ is primarily found as pyridoxine, with up to 75% being pyridoxine glucoside, which is believed to be the plant storage form.[35] Pyridoxine glucoside has a glucose added to pyridoxine as shown below.

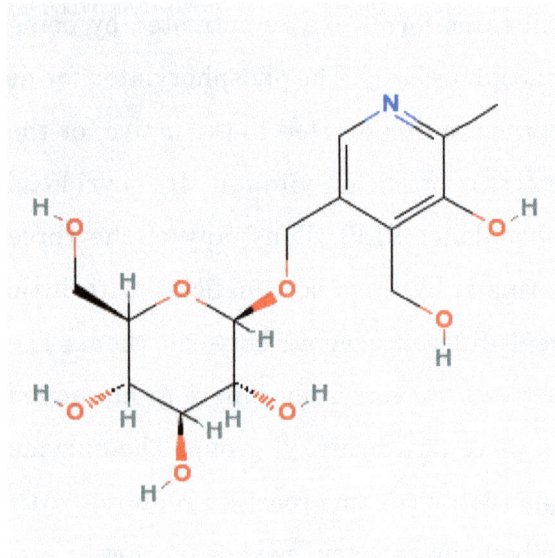

Figure 329. Structure of pyridoxine glucoside

Vitamin B_6 is well absorbed from foods (~75%) through passive diffusion. PLP and PMP are dephosphorylated before uptake into the enterocyte. Some of the pyridoxamine glucoside is cleaved to form free pyridoxine, but some pyridoxine glucoside is absorbed intact. Pyridoxine glucoside absorption is lower (~50%) than pyridoxine alone. The primary circulating forms of vitamin B_6 are pyridoxal and PLP. Vitamin B_6 is primarily excreted in the urine, and like many other B vitamins, vitamin B_6 is destroyed during cooking or heating.[35]

9.8.1 Vitamin B_6 Functions

PLP is a cofactor for over 100 different enzymes, most of which are involved in amino acid metabolism. In fact, without PLP all amino acids would be essential

because we would not be able to synthesize nonessential amino acids. Below are some of the functions of PLP and PMP[36]:

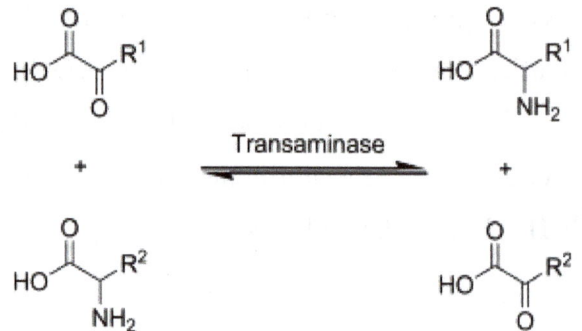

Figure 330. Transaminases require PLP or PMP

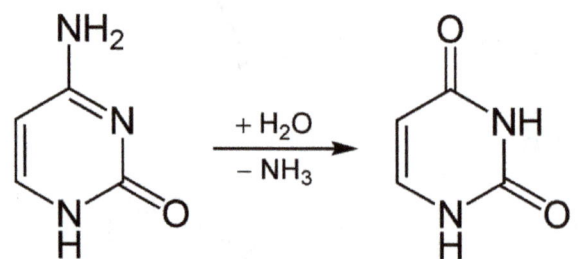

Figure 331. Some deaminases require PLP

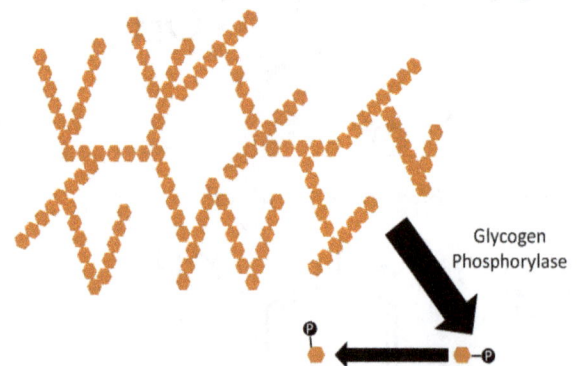

Figure 332. Glycogen phosphorylase requires PLP

PLP is required for decarboxylase enzymes that are involved in the synthesis of the neurotransmitters GABA, serotonin, histamine, and dopamine. As an example,

DOPA decarboxylase uses PLP to convert L-DOPA to dopamine as shown below.[36]

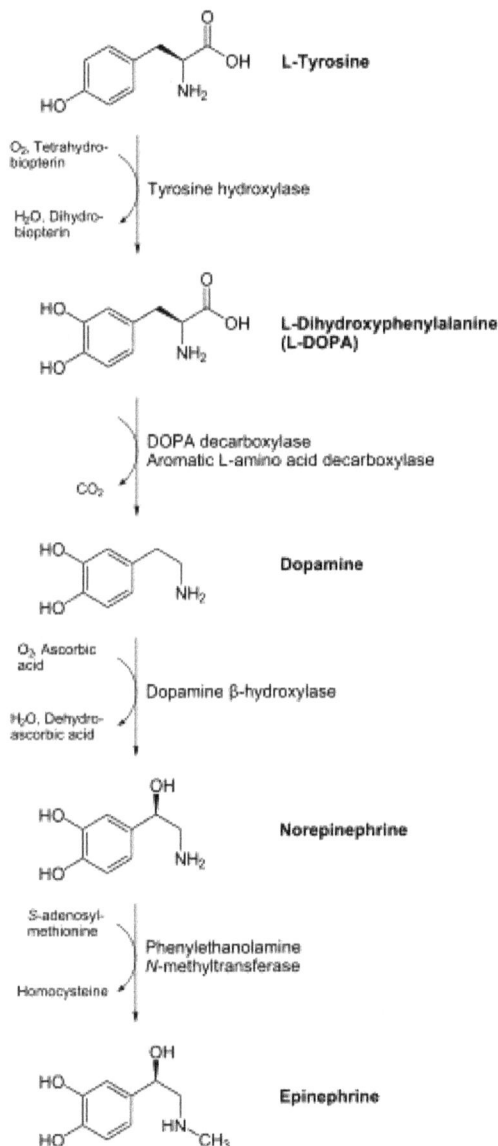

Figure 333. DOPA decarboxylase uses PLP to synthesize dopamine[lii]

PLP is also required by gamma-aminolevulinic acid synthetase that is involved in haeme synthesis. Haeme will be discussed in more detail in the iron section.

PLP is also used in one of the multiple reactions that occurs between kynurenine and niacin in its synthesis from tryptophan.

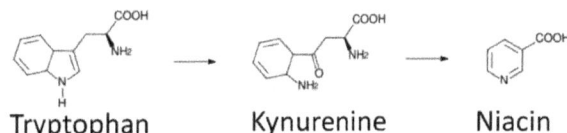

Figure 334. PLP is required for niacin synthesis from tryptophan

In addition, PLP is also involved in:

- Carnitine Synthesis
- 1-Carbon Metabolism

9.8.2 Vitamin B6 Deficiency & Toxicity

Vitamin B6 deficiency is rare, but symptoms include:

- Skin or scalp ailments (seborrheic dermatitis)
- Microcytic hypochromic anaemia (small cells, low colour)
- Convulsions
- Depression
- Confusion

Given what we know about the functions of vitamin B6, these symptoms make sense! The microcytic hypochromic anaemia is a result of decreased haeme synthesis. The neurological symptoms are due to the decreased production of neurotransmitters.[22]

Vitamin B_6 unlike many of the B vitamins can produce toxicity. High doses of vitamin B_6 taken for an extended period of time can lead to neurological damage.[22] It is therefore important that supplementation of high levels of vitamin B_6 is done under the direction of a qualified, registered practitioner (such as a registered nutritionist or clinical nutritionist, or dietician).

Morning sickness that occurs early in pregnancy is another condition where vitamin B_6 supplementation is utilized. The evidence is not clear on whether it is beneficial, but *The American College of Obstetricians and Gynaecologists* makes the following recommendation:

"Treatment of nausea and vomiting of pregnancy with vitamin B_6 or vitamin B_6 plus doxylamine is safe and effective and should be considered first-line pharmacotherapy".

Another condition that vitamin B_6 is commonly supplemented for is premenstrual syndrome (PMS). A systematic literature review found that it is inconclusive whether vitamin B_6 supplementation is beneficial in managing PMS.[75]

9.9 Biotin

The two primary dietary forms of biotin are free biotin and biocytin (aka biotinyllysine).[36] The structure of biotin is shown below.

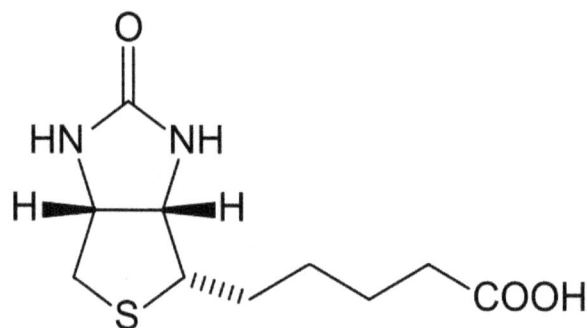

Figure 335. Structure of biotin

Biocytin is biotin bound to lysine as seen in its structure below.

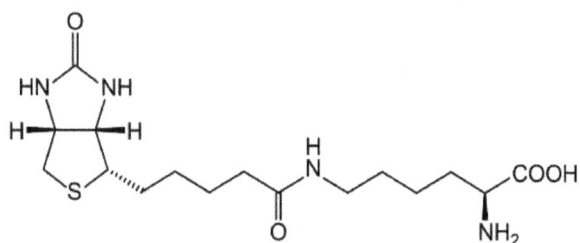

Figure 336. Structure of biocytin

Free biotin is believed to be highly absorbed. Before uptake, biocytin is acted on by the enzyme biotinidase, forming free biotin and lysine. Free biotin is then taken up into the enterocyte through the sodium-dependent multivitamin transporter (SMVT).

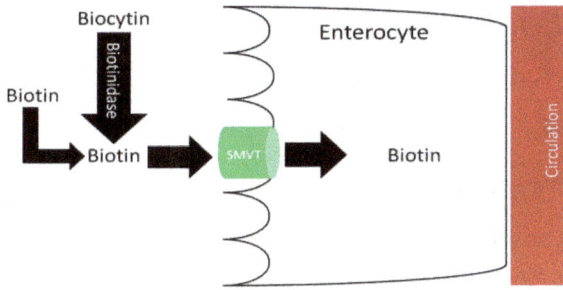

Figure 337. Free biotin is taken up into the enterocyte by the SMVT

Most biotin is excreted in the urine.

9.9.1 Biotin Functions

Biotin is an important cofactor for carboxylase enzymes. These enzymes add carboxylic acid groups (-COOH) to whatever compound they act on. In fatty acid synthesis, biotin is required by the enzyme that forms malonyl CoA from acetyl-CoA.[36]

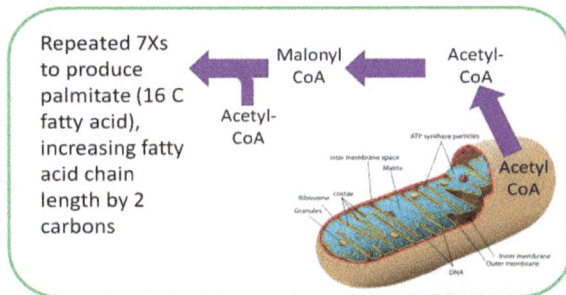

Figure 338. The conversion of acetyl CoA to malonyl CoA in fatty acid synthesis requires biotin

Another biotin-requiring carboxylase converts pyruvate to oxaloacetate in gluconeogenesis.[36]

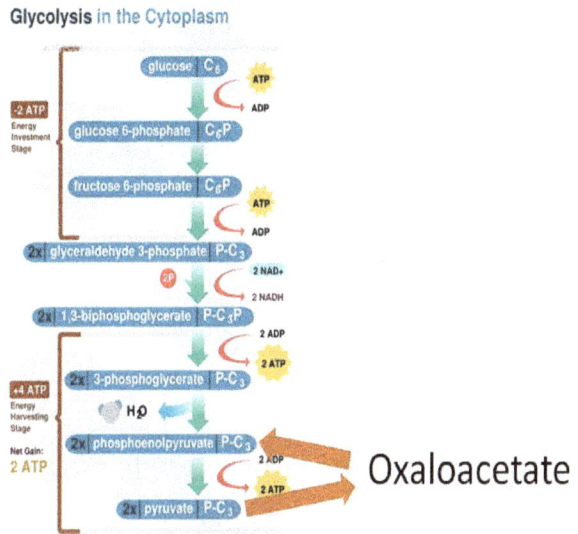

Figure 339. Biotin is required for conversion of pyruvate to oxaloacetate in the oxaloacetate workaround of gluconeogenesis (like glycolysis in reverse with oxaloacetate workaround)

In addition to these two functions, biotin is also important for histone biotinylation and the breakdown of isoleucine, leucine, methionine, and threonine.[36]

Histone biotinylation is an epigenetic modification that is described in the next section.

9.9.2 Epigenetics

What is epigenetics?

Epigenetics means "above the genome." The nucleotide sequence of the human genome is known, and there is surprisingly little difference between individuals. However, two main epigenetic modifications play a significant role in determining what genes are expressed:

- DNA methylation

197

- Histone modification

DNA methylation is the addition of a methyl group to a DNA base, which decreases gene transcription. Conversely, demethylation increases gene transcription.

DNA does not exist simply as long strands of double helix, instead it is packaged and shaped so that it can fit in the nucleus of our cells. The first part of this packaging is that DNA is wrapped around proteins called histones as shown below.

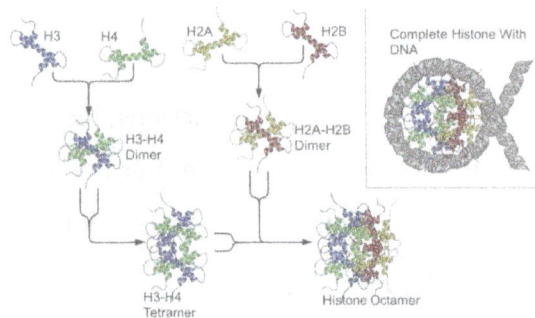

Figure 340. DNA is wrapped around histones[liii]

Histone modification occurs when there are additions or subtractions to the histones themselves. The most common is acetylation (addition of an acetyl group) or deacetylation of histones.

Histone acetylation causes the DNA structure to open so that transcription can occur. Histone deacetylation causes the DNA to become more tightly packed, preventing transcription from occurring.

How does this relate to biotin?

Histones can be biotinylated, or have biotin added to the histone. Through biotinylation, biotin is believed to alter cell growth, gene expression, and DNA repair.[36]

9.9.3 Biotin Deficiency & Toxicity

Biotin deficiency is very rare. Symptoms of biotin deficiency include[16]:

- Skin rash
- Hair loss
- Neurological Impairments

There are a couple of ways that a person could develop a deficiency in biotin. First, a very small number of people are born with a mutation in biotinidase that results in them not being able to cleave biocytin for absorption.[16] Another way is through the excessive consumption of raw eggs. Drinking raw eggs is not something that most people do. However, some have done it as part of various health regimes, bodybuilding and athletic diets (like Sylvester Stallone's movie character Rocky, who consumed them as part of his boxing training regimen). Because of this film a biotin deficiency is sometimes now called "Rocky Balboa Syndrome".

[liii] CC-BY-SA 3.0 Richard Wheeler https://en.wikipedia.org/wiki/File:Nucleosome_structure.png

Specifically, egg whites are the problem for biotin. Raw egg whites contain a protein called avidin which binds to biotin and prevents its absorption. However, it is unlikely that low doses, and occasional raw egg and egg white consumption will cause a biotin deficiency. It has been estimated that more than two dozen egg whites would need to be consumed daily over many months to cause a deficiency.[18] Cooking denatures avidin, preventing it from binding biotin, meaning that cooked eggs are not a concern.

No toxicity of biotin has been reported.

10 One-Carbon Metabolism Micronutrients

Three B vitamins are involved in what is known as 1-carbon metabolism. This is the movement of 1 carbon units, generally methyl groups (CH_3). It is like the movement of the amino group that occurs in transamination. Folate, vitamin B_{12}, and vitamin B_6 are the B vitamins involved in 1-carbon metabolism.

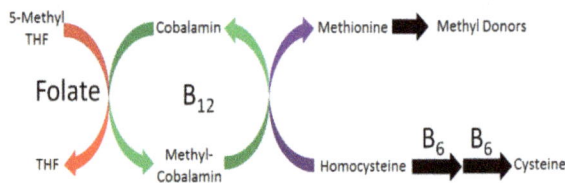

Figure 341. One-carbon metabolism

Vitamin B_6 has been covered already in the previous chapter, so this section is going to focus on folate and vitamin B_{12}. We will examine this figure in pieces, so that hopefully by the time this chapter is completed, you will understand the role of all these vitamins in 1-carbon metabolism.

10.1 Folate & Folic Acid

Folate is a B vitamin that exists in either its reduced (folate), or oxidized form (folic acid). Although often these terms are used interchangeably. Another differentiator between these two terms is that folic acid refers to the synthetic form, while folate refers to the natural form. Folic acid (synthetic or oxidised form) is found in certain foods because they have been fortified with it, not because they produce it. The structure of folic acid is shown below.

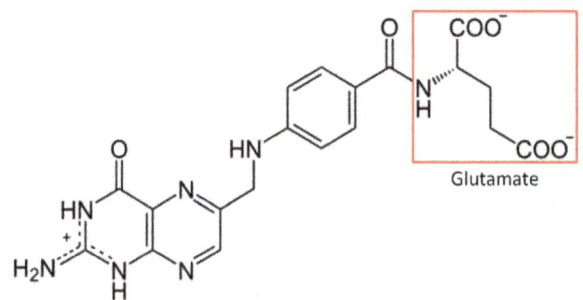

Figure 342. Structure of Folic Acid

Another key difference between folate and folic acid is the number of glutamates in their tails. Notice that glutamate is boxed in the structure of folic acid above. Folic acid always exists as a monoglutamate (especially as the common supplemental form pteroyl monoglutamate), meaning it only contains 1 glutamate. On the other hand, about 90% of the folate found in foods are polyglutamates, meaning there is more than 1 glutamate in their tail. Folic acid is more stable than folate, which can be destroyed by heat, oxidation, and light.[16] Table 10.11 summarizes the key differences between folate and folic acid.

Table 42. Comparison of folate to folic acid

Folate	Folic Acid
Reduced Form	Oxidized Form
Natural	Synthetic
Polyglutamate	Monoglutamate
	More Stable
	May be harmful long-term

The bioavailability of folate was believed to be much lower than folic acid.[76] To account for these differences, the DRI committee created dietary folate equivalents (DFEs) to set the RDAs.[77] DFEs are defined as follows:

1 DFE = 1 ug food folate = 0.6 ug food folic acid = 0.5 ug folic acid on an empty stomach

DFE = ug food folate + (ug folic acid X 1.7)

The factor 1.7 came from research suggesting that folic acid from food was 85% bioavailable, compared to 50% for folate (85%/50% = 1.7). This was established in 1998 by the DRI committee, and it is likely that these conversions & the requirements will change based on the newer evidence suggesting folate's bioavailability from food is actually much higher (80% of folic acid) than previously believed.[76] With this data, the new conversion factor for folic acid would be 1.25 (100%/80%). This conversion factor means that food folate levels are probably contributing more towards our dietary needs than are often currently estimated.

Before folate (polyglutamates) can be taken up into the enterocyte, the extra glutamates must be cleaved prior to uptake into the enterocyte by the reduced folate transporter (RFT, aka reduced folate carrier). Folic acid, because it is a monoglutamate, requires no cleavage for uptake before it is taken up through the RFT. Once inside the enterocyte, the monoglutamate form is methylated and transported into circulation through an unresolved carrier.[35] This series of events is depicted in the figure below.

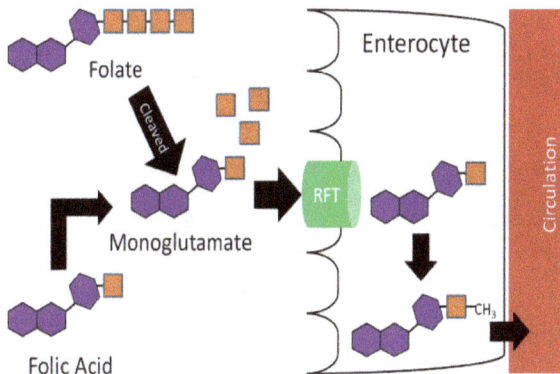

Figure 343. The uptake and absorption of folate and folic acid (orange boxes represent glutamate)

Thus, the methylated monoglutamate form is the circulating form. This is transported to the liver where it is converted back to the polyglutamate form for storage. Folate is excreted in both the urine and faeces.[35]

10.1.1 Folate Functions

The major function of folate is that it participates in 1-carbon metabolism. As described earlier, this is the transfer of 1-carbon units from 1 compound to another. The cofactor form of folate is tetrahydrofolate (THF). As is shown in the figure below, for THF to be formed, a methyl group is transferred to cobalamin (vitamin B_{12}) from 5-methyl THF (THF plus a methyl group), forming methyl-cobalamin. You can see this on the left side of the figure below.

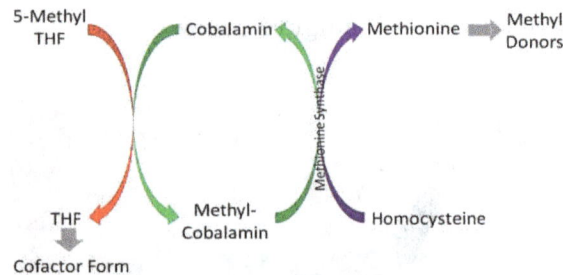

Figure 344. One-carbon metabolism

There are 2 major cofactor functions of THF[36]:

1. DNA Synthesis
THF is required for the synthesis of DNA bases (purines & pyrimidines)[36]. As shown in the link below, N^{10}-formyl-THF (a form of THF) is needed in 2 reactions (3 and 9) in purine synthesis.

2. Amino Acid Metabolism

THF is a cofactor for enzymes that metabolize histidine, serine, glycine, and methionine[36]. The following link shows that THF is a cofactor for serine hydroxymethyltransferase, the enzyme that converts serine to glycine.

10.1.2 Folate Deficiency & Toxicity

Folate deficiency is relatively low in New Zealand (around 2%) although national data on the blood folate status in lacking. The hallmark symptom of folate deficiency is megaloblastic (aka macrocytic) anaemia. Megaloblastic anaemia, as the name suggests, is characterised by large, nucleated (remember that most red blood cells do not have a nucleus), immature red blood cells. This occurs because folate is needed for DNA synthesis; without it red blood cells are not able to divide properly.[16] As a result, fewer and poorer functioning red blood cells are produced that cannot carry oxygen as efficiently as normal red blood cells.[18]

A maternal folate deficiency can lead to neural tube defects in infants. The exact cause of neural tube defects is unknown, but folate supplementation has been shown to markedly decrease the incidence of neural tube defects.[22] The most common of these neural tube defects is spina bifida (1 per 2500 babies born in the United State and 1 per 3000 babies born in NZ), which is a failure of the neural tube to close and the spinal cord and its fluid protrude out the infant's back.[78][4,5,]

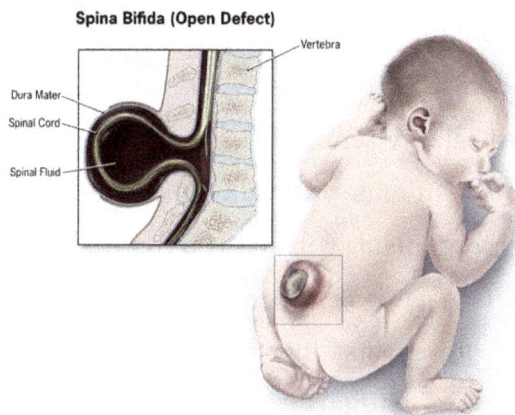

Spina Bifida (Open Defect)

Figure 345. Spina bifida[liv]

The neural tube closes 21-28 days after conception,[16] and with 50% of pregnancies estimated to be unplanned, many women aren't aware they are pregnant during this period.[16, 18] Thus, it is recommended that women of childbearing age consume at least 400mcg of folic acid daily.[1] In addition, in 1998 the United States Food and Drug Administration (FDA) mandated that all refined cereals and grains be fortified with 140mcg folic acid /100 grams of product.[36] Spina bifida incidence rates have been declining in the developed world. For example, rates have been falling in the United States since approximately 1995, before folic acid fortification began.

It is debatable whether folic acid fortification was fully responsible for the decrease in spina bifida rates, but the rates are lower than they were pre-fortification. Folate is not toxic, but it can mask a vitamin B_{12} deficiency and prevent its diagnosis. This is especially pertinent to vegetarians and vegans eating a healthy (i.e. high folate) diet as they may be unaware of a relative vitamin B_{12} deficiency.

10.1.3 Folate or folic acid supplementation?

Folate in any form is not used directly within the body, but is metabolised to a metabolically active co-enzyme, tetrahydrafolate (tetrahydrafolic acid). Pteroylmonoglutamate (synthetic folic acid) in supplements has a greater bioavailability than the natural folates, and while we might initially think that would be beneficial, it can lead to high amounts of unmetabolised folic acid in the blood stream, Increases in blood levels of synthetic folic acid are likely with supplementation and fortification of foods, and when synthetic folates are 'overloaded' into the blood in this fashion they may interfere with the metabolism, cellular transport, and regulatory functions of the

[liv] Public Domain work https://commons.wikimedia.org/wiki/File:Spina-bifida.jpg

natural folates that occur in the body, by competing with them by binding with enzymes, carrier proteins, and binding proteins.[79] The folate receptor has a higher affinity for synthetic folic acid than for methyl-THF (the main natural form of folate that occurs in the blood.)

This may result in:

- Reduced levels of active folates for use as co-enzymes in brain function
- Down-regulation of folate receptors
- Change in gene expression of folate dependent enzymes

There is also considered to be a risk of liver capacity saturation with high dose folic acid supplementation, leading to higher levels of unmetabolised folic acid entering the general circulatory system. This would compound the potential negative effects mentioned above and may have direct effects on other functions such as immunity,[18] and although high folate diets are considered to reduce risk of cancer, high intakes of supplemental folic acid may actually increase carcinogenesis[79] and in fact many cancer drugs are anti-folates due to their ability to inhibit the growth of rapidly dividing cell types found in tumours.

10.2 Vitamin B_{12}

Vitamin B_{12} is unique among vitamins in that it contains an element (cobalt) and is found almost exclusively in animal products. Neither plants nor animals can synthesize vitamin B_{12}. Instead, vitamin B_{12} in animal products is produced by microorganisms within the animal that the products came from. Animals consume the microorganisms in soil or bacteria in ruminant animals that produce vitamin B_{12}.[16] Some plant products, such as fermented soy products (tempeh, miso) and the sea algae supplement, spirulina, are advertised as being good sources of B_{12}. However, fermented soy products are not a reliable vitamin B_{12} source and spirulina contains a 'pseudovitamin' B_{12} that isn't bioavailable.[80]

Vitamin B_{12}'s scientific name is cobalamin, which makes sense when you consider it contains cobalt and many amine groups, as shown in the figure below.

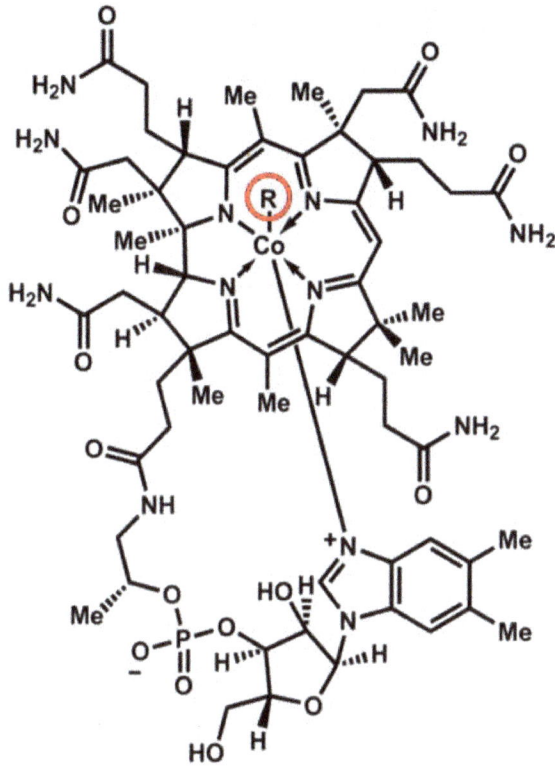

Figure 346. Structure of vitamin B12 (cobalamin)

The other feature that is important in cobalamin is the circled R group. This is what differs between the different cobalamins, whose names and R groups are shown in the following table.

Table 43. Different cobalamin forms

R Group	Name
CN	Cyanocobalamin
OH	Hydroxocobalamin
H_2O	Aquocobalamin
NO_2	Nitritocobalamin
5'-deoxyadenosyl	Adenosylcobalamin*
CH_3	Methylcobalamin*

*Cofactor Forms

The two cofactor forms are adenosylcobalamin and methylcobalamin. We can convert most cobalamins into these two cofactor forms. Most foods contain adenosylcobalamin, hydroxocobalamin, or methylcobalamin.[36] The most common form found in supplements is cyanocobalamin, with some also using methylcobalamin.[6] Both methyl- and adenosyl- forms are considered the 'natural' forms of the vitamin, as these are the forms that occur as active cofactors within the body. These are not always well interconverted within the body. Hydroxocobalamin can be converted to either of the cofactor forms. Cyanocobalamin, the usual form in supplementation is a synthetic form not found in foods in nature. The metabolism of cyanocobalamin leaves behind a cyanide residue that the body must then excrete. This is unlikely to cause problems for most people as the amount of cyanide left is extremely small, however it has been suggested that those with pre-existing kidney problems may have trouble excreting even these small amounts and that a methylcobalamin form is preferred[81] and it has been suggested that cyanocobalamin should be replaced with a non-cyanide form of B_{12} for general safety.[82]

The uptake, absorption, and transport of vitamin B_{12} is a complex process. The following descriptions explain, and figures illustrate this process.

Vitamin B_{12} is normally bound to protein in food. Salivary glands in the mouth produce R protein, which travels with the food into the stomach. In the stomach, acid converts pepsinogen into pepsin, and the protein intrinsic factor is released from the parietal cells.[16, 35]

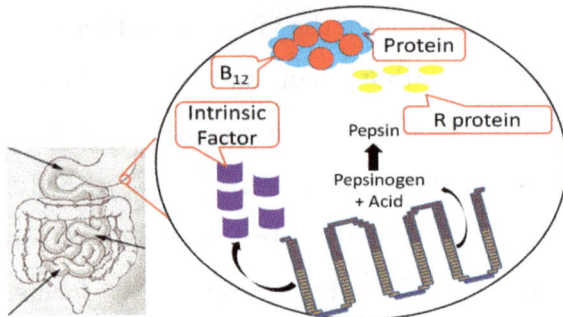

Figure 347. Vitamin B12 in the stomach part 1

As pepsin frees B_{12} from protein, R protein binds to the newly freed vitamin B_{12} (B_{12}+ R protein). Intrinsic factor escapes digestion and, along with B_{12}+ R protein, exits the stomach and enters the duodenum.[16, 35]

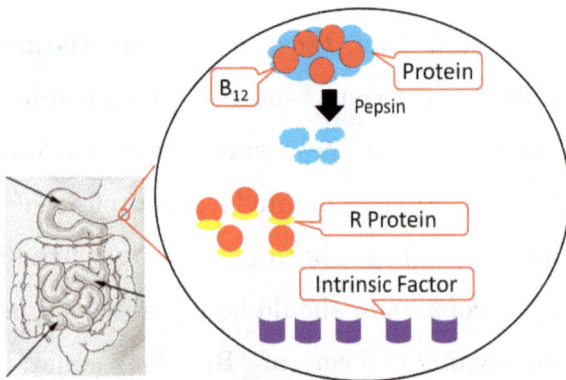

Figure 348. Vitamin B12 in the stomach part 2

In the duodenum, pancreatic proteases break down R protein, and again vitamin B_{12} is freed. Intrinsic factor then binds

vitamin B_{12} (B_{12}+ intrinsic factor); B_{12}+ intrinsic factor continue into the ileum to prepare for absorption.[16, 35]

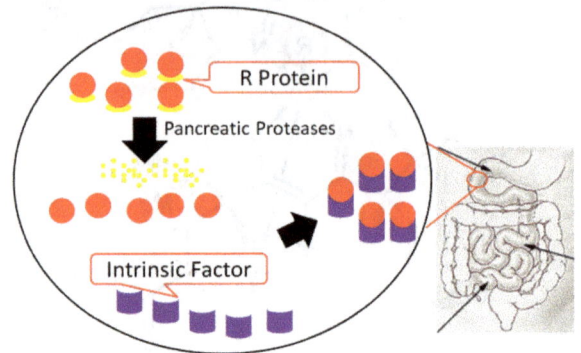

Figure 349. Vitamin B12 in the duodenum

In the ileum, B_{12}+ intrinsic factor is believed to be endocytosed by cubulin (aka intrinsic factor receptor), forming an endosome inside the enterocyte. Intrinsic factor is broken down in the enterocyte freeing vitamin B_{12}. The free vitamin B_{12} is then bound to transcobalamin II (B_{12}+ TC II); B_{12}+ TC II moves into circulation.[35]

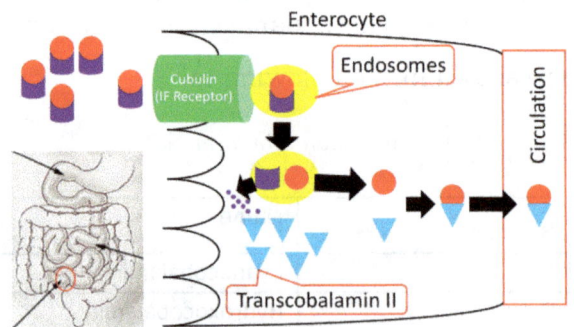

Figure 350. Vitamin B12 absorption

The liver is the primary storage site for vitamin B_{12}. Unlike most other water-soluble vitamins, the liver can maintain significant stores of vitamin B_{12}. Uptake into the liver occurs through the binding of

B_{12}+TC II to the TC II Receptor and the endocytosis of both the compound and the receptor.[35] Vitamin $B_{12}$is once again freed after degradation of TC II. Vitamin B_{12} is primarily stored in the liver as adenosylcobalamin.[35, 36]

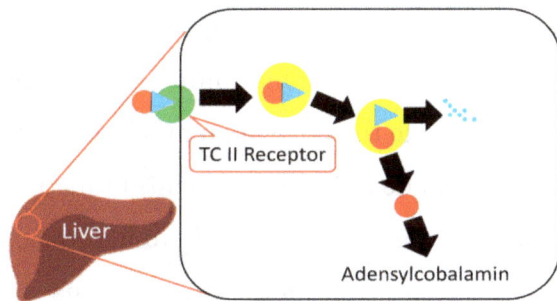

Figure 351. Hepatic uptake and storage of vitamin B12

The overall bioavailability of vitamin B_{12} is believed to be approximately 50%,[80] with the different cobalamin forms having similar bioavailabilities,[6] although some evidence suggests that naturally occurring cobalamins (like methylcobalamin) in food appear to be absorbed at a better rate than synthetic B12 (cyanocobalamin).[83] Sublingual supplements of vitamin B_{12} have been found to be equally efficacious as oral supplements.[6] Excretion occurs mostly through bile, with little loss in urine.[36]

10.2.1 Vitamin B_{12} Functions

Vitamin B_{12} is a cofactor for 2 enzymes:

1. Methionine synthase
2. Methylmalonyl mutase

Methionine Synthase

Methionine synthase is an important enzyme in 1-carbon metabolism that uses methylcobalamin as its cofactor and converts homocysteine to methionine by adding a methyl group. Methionine then is converted to other compounds that serve as methyl donors, as shown below.[16]

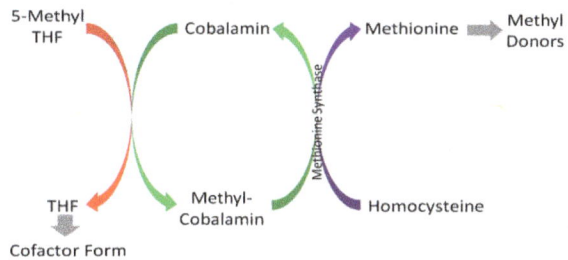

Figure 352. One-carbon metabolism

These methyl donors can donate methyl groups for methylating DNA, an epigenetic modification.[16]

Methymalonyl mutase

This enzyme uses adenosylcobalamin as its cofactor and is important in the breakdown of odd chain fatty acids (5 carbons etc.). As you know, odd chain fatty acids are less common than even chain fatty acids, but this enzyme is required to properly handle these less common fatty acids.[16]

Demyelination

In addition to its role as a cofactor for enzymes, vitamin B12 is also important for preventing degradation of the myelin sheath that surrounds neurons, as shown below.

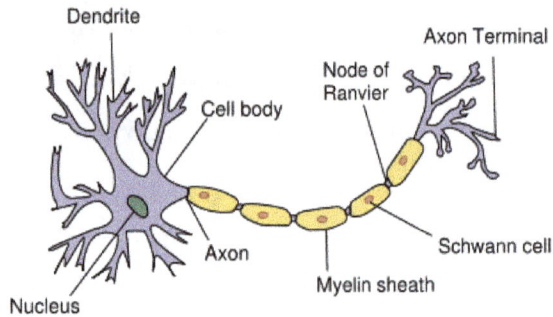

Figure 353. Vitamin B12 is needed to maintain the myelin sheath that surrounds neurons[lv]

The mechanism through which vitamin B12 prevents demyelination is not fully known.[3]

10.2.2 Vitamin B12 Deficiency & Toxicity

There are 2 primary symptoms of vitamin B12 deficiency:

- Megaloblastic (Macrocytic) Anaemia
- Neurological Abnormalities

Megaloblastic (Macrocytic) Anaemia

This is the same type of anaemia that occurs in folate deficiency that is characterized by fewer, enlarged, immature red blood cells. When a product of vitamin B12 deficiency, this occurs because there is not enough cobalamin to

convert 5-methyl THF to THF (illustrated in Figure 10.211). Thus, THF is not available for normal DNA synthesis and the red blood cells do not divide correctly.

Neurological Abnormalities

Vitamin B12 deficiency also results in nerve degeneration and abnormalities that can often precede the development of anaemia. These include a decline in mental function and burning, tingling, and numbness of legs. These symptoms can continue to worsen, and deficiency can be fatal.[16]

The most common cause of vitamin B12 deficiency is pernicious anaemia, a condition of inadequate intrinsic factor production that causes poor vitamin B12 absorption. This condition is common in people over the age of 50 because they have the condition atrophic gastritis.[18] Atrophic gastritis is a chronic inflammatory condition that leads to the loss of glands in the stomach. The loss of glands leads to decreased intrinsic factor production. It is estimated that ~6% of those age 60 and over are vitamin B12 deficient, with 20% having marginal status.[84] In addition to the elderly, vegans are also at risk for vitamin B12 deficiency because they do not consume animal products. However, the deficiency may take years to develop in

---

[lv] Public Domain https://commons.wikimedia.org/wiki/File:Neuron.jpg

adults because of stores and recycling of vitamin B_{12}.[18] Deficiency has the potential to occur much quicker in infants or young children on vegan diets because they do not have stores that adults do.[36]

Folate/Folic Acid masking vitamin B_{12} deficiency

As mentioned above, folate and vitamin B_{12} lead to the same megaloblastic (macrocytic) anaemia. If folate or folic acid is given during vitamin B_{12} deficiency, it can correct this anaemia. This is referred to as masking because it does not rectify the deficiency, but it "cures" this symptom. This is problematic because it does not correct the more serious neurological problems that can result from vitamin B_{12} deficiency. There are some people who are concerned about the fortification of cereals and grains with folic acid because people who are B_{12} deficient might not develop macrocytic anaemia, which makes a vitamin B_{12} deficiency harder to diagnose.[18]

No toxicity of vitamin B_{12} has been reported.

10.3 B Vitamins, Homocysteine & Cardiovascular Disease

Homocysteine is a sulphur containing, nonproteinogenic (not used for making proteins) amino acid whose structure is shown in the figure below.

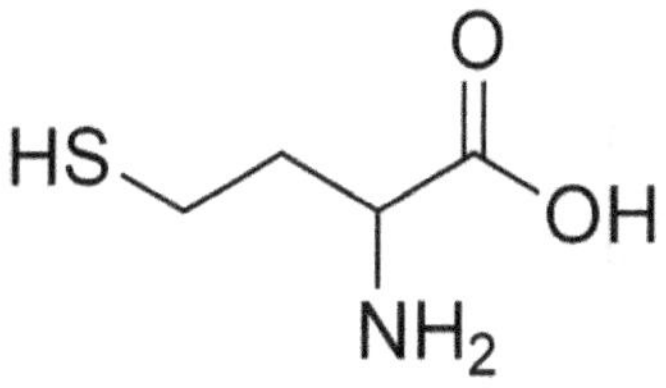

Figure 354. Structure of homocysteine

Elevated circulating homocysteine levels have been found in people with cardiovascular disease. Folate, vitamin B_6, and vitamin B_{12} contribute to the conversion of homocysteine to methionine by providing methyl groups, thereby decreasing homocysteine levels, as illustrated in the figure below. Thus, based on these facts, it was hypothesized that intake of these B vitamins may decrease the risk of cardiovascular disease.

Research has found that intake of these B vitamins does decrease circulating homocysteine levels. However, most studies have not found that this reduction improves cardiovascular disease outcomes. It is debated why B vitamin intake has not resulted in improved outcomes. Some think it is because the studies haven't focused on individuals with elevated homocysteine levels,[85] while others believe that homocysteine is a biomarker or indicator of cardiovascular disease, not a causative or contributing factor to cardiovascular disease development.[86]

11 Blood, Bones & Teeth Micronutrients

This chapter is a collection of vitamins and minerals that are involved in the structure or function of blood, bones and teeth.

11.1 Vitamin D

Vitamin D is unique among the vitamins in that it is considered both a vitamin and a hormone (or pro-hormone). It is considered at least hormone-like for two reasons: (1) we can synthesize it, and (2) it has hormone-like functions. The amount synthesized, however, is often not enough to meet our needs especially with modern considerations of reduced sun exposure (for example working long hours indoors), increased sunblock and SPF cosmetic use (which reduces vitamin D production), and seasonal and latitudinal variations in sun exposure. Thus, we may need to consume this vitamin under certain circumstances, meaning that vitamin D is a conditionally essential micronutrient.

There are two major dietary forms of vitamin D: the form produced by plants and yeast is vitamin D_2 (ergocalciferol), and the form made by animals is vitamin D_3 (cholecalciferol). The structures of these two forms are shown below. Notice that the only difference is the presence of a double bond in D_2 that is not in D_3.

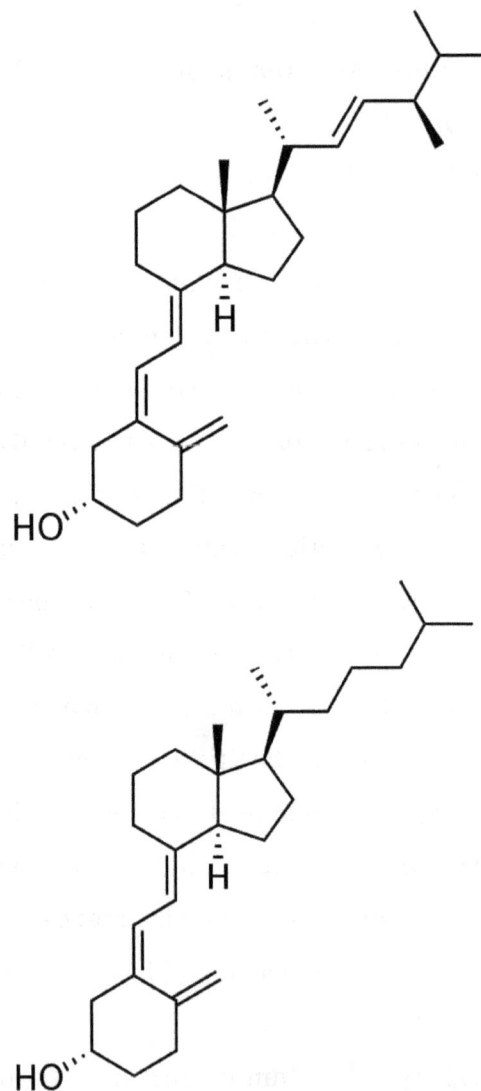

Figure 355. Structure of vitamin D2 (ergocalciferol) and vitamin D3 (cholecalciferol)

We synthesize vitamin D_3 from cholesterol, as shown below. In the skin, cholesterol is converted to 7-dehydrocholesterol. In the presence of UV-B light, 7-

dehydrocholesterol is converted to vitamin D_3. Synthesized vitamin D will combine with vitamin D-binding protein (DBP) to be transported to the liver. Dietary vitamin D_2 and D_3 is transported to the liver via chylomicrons and then taken up in chylomicron remnants. Once in the liver, the enzyme 25-hydroxylase (25-OHase) adds a hydroxyl (-OH) group at the 25th carbon, forming 25-hydroxy vitamin D (25(OH)D, calcidiol).[36] This is the circulating form of vitamin D, thus 25(OH)D blood levels are measured to assess a person's vitamin D status. The active form of vitamin D is formed with the addition of another hydroxyl group by the enzyme 1alpha-hydroxylase (1alpha-OHase) in the kidney, forming 1,25 hydroxy vitamin D $(1,25(OH)_2D)$. The synthesis and activation of vitamin D is shown in the figures below.

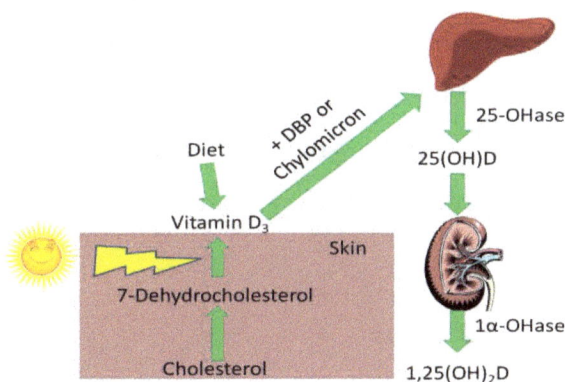

Figure 357. Synthesis of 25(OH)D (calcidiol) from vitamin D3 by 25-hydroxylase

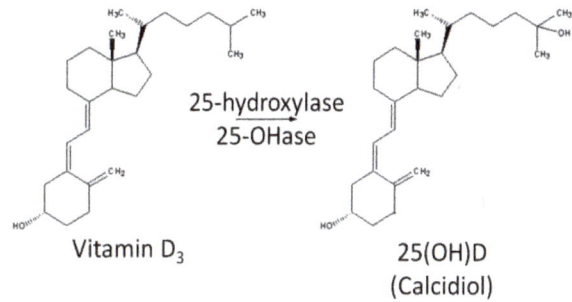

Figure 358. Synthesis of 1,25(OH)2D (calcitriol) from 25(OH)D by 1alpha-hydroxylase

However, there are several other tissues that have been found to have 1alpha-hydroxylase activity. Therefore, tissues can activate circulating 25(OH)D to $1,25(OH)_2D$ for their own use.

Vitamin D_2 and D_3 were once thought to be equivalent forms of vitamin D, but more recent research found that D_3 is "87% more potent in raising and maintaining serum 25(OH)D concentration and produces a 2 to 3 fold greater storage of vitamin D" than D_2[87] and a Cochrane Database review suggests that only supplemental vitamin D3 improves mortality outcomes.

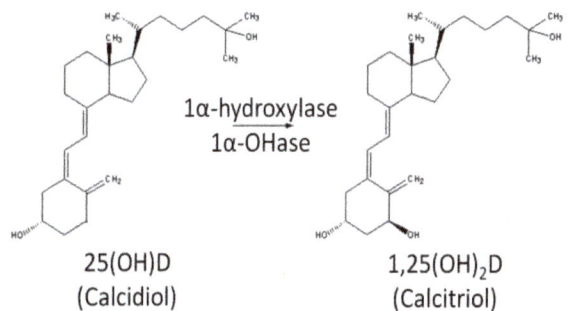

Figure 356. Vitamin D synthesis and activation

11.1.1 Environmental Factors That Impact Vitamin D_3 Synthesis

There are several environmental factors that affect vitamin D_3 synthesis:

- Latitude
- Season
- Time of Day
- Skin Colour
- Body mass index (BMI)
- Age
- Clothing
- Sunscreen

11.1.1.1 Latitude

The latitude at which someone lives affects that person's ability to synthesize vitamin D_3. There is an inverse relationship between distance from the equator and UV light exposure. Thus, with increased distance from the equator (increased latitude), there is decreased UV light exposure and vitamin D_3 synthesis.

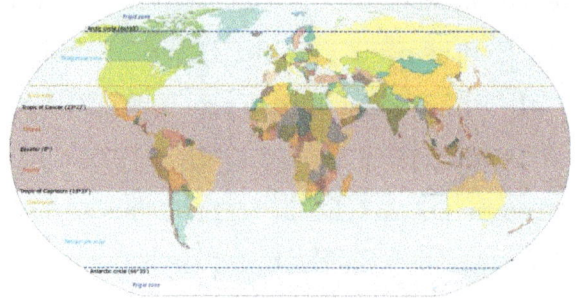

Figure 359. World map showing selected latitudes and tropic zones[lvi]

Seasons

Seasons also make a difference in vitamin D_3 synthesis. For example, research has demonstrated that in major cities in North America, vitamin D synthesis varies markedly in various locations, at various times of the year. Boston (42° N), vitamin D synthesis only occurs from March-October, because during late fall and winter not enough UV-B reaches the earth's surface to synthesize vitamin D_3. However, in Los Angeles (34° N), vitamin D_3 synthesis occurs year round.[2] The difference is the angle of the sun relative to latitude and how many UV-B photons are absorbed before they reach the earth's surface.[35]

11.1.1.2 Time

Time of day is also a crucial factor in affecting vitamin D_3 synthesis. Vitamin D_3 synthesis increases in the morning before peaking at noon, then declines the rest of the day.[3]

11.1.1.3 Skin pigmentation

Another factor that plays a vital role in vitamin D_3 synthesis is skin pigmentation.

As shown in the figure below, skin pigmentation tends to be darker around the equator to help protect inhabitants from the harmful effects of sun exposure.

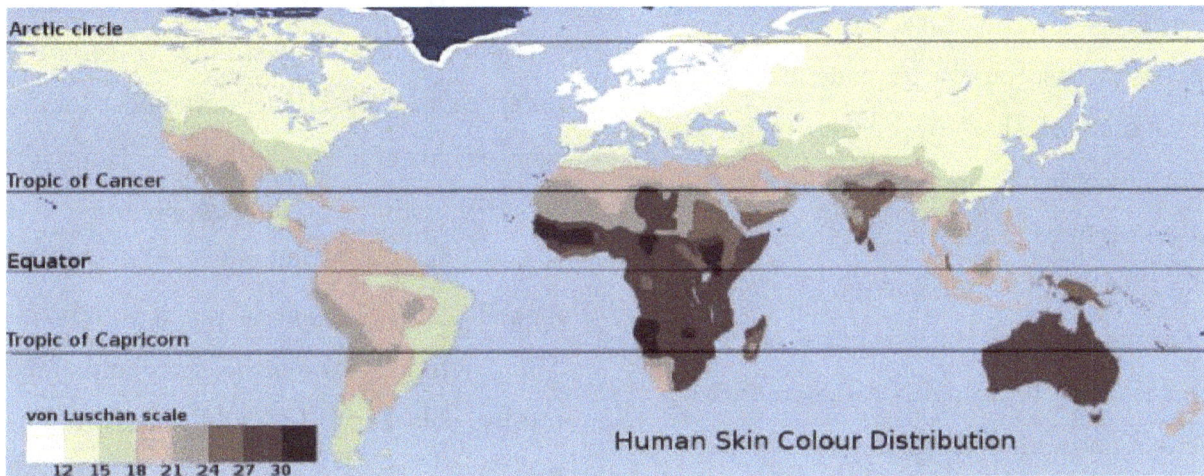

Figure 360. Skin colour distribution. Darker skinned people typically need more sun exposure to produce adequate Vitamin D[lvii]

Skin colour is the result of increased production of the pigment melanin. Populations that have lived closer to the equator over a very long time have developed a much higher production of this pigment. However, as you can see form the image above this is not completely uniform. This is due to migration patterns over relatively shorter periods of time. The 'beach-hopper' migration out of Africa which spread throughout the southern Asian coast down through the Indonesian, Melanesian and Polynesian areas helped to spread darker-skinned peoples to areas

with lower latitudes. Another consideration with migration patterns like these, and regional variations alike is that sun exposure is also affected by other factors such as proximity to the sea (which reflects UVB rays and therefore amplifies exposure), mountainous areas that are relatively clear-skied, which have high UVB exposure (such as in the Andes as compared to the Amazon rainforest), and local climate which can serve to provide more cloud cover.

Very dark skin colour can provide a sun protection factor (SPF).[88] These

---

[lvii] https://en.wikipedia.org/wiki/File:Map_of_skin_hue_equi3.png

individuals will require approximately 5-10 times greater sunlight exposure than a light-skinned person to synthesize the same amount of vitamin D_3.[22, 88]

11.1.1.4 Body Mass Index

Serum 1,25-dihydroxy vitamin D is inversely associated with body mass index It is thought that the bigger we become (with increased adiposity), the less vitamin D we produce in the skin *and* absorb from the diet and supplements. Weight-loss improves vitamin D levels in the body, and this is likely to be highly correlated with a reduction in insulin resistance.

11.1.1.5 Age

Age also plays a factor in vitamin D_3 synthesis. Aging results in decreased 7-dehydrocholesterol concentrations in the skin, resulting in an approximately 75% reduction in the vitamin D_3 synthesis capability by age 70.[22]

11.1.1.6 Clothing

Clothing is another factor that influences vitamin D_3 synthesis. More clothing means that less sun reaches your skin, and thus less vitamin D_3 synthesis.

11.1.1.7 Sunscreen, "Sensible Sun Exposure", and Tanning

There is quite a spirited debate on sunscreen, sun exposure, skin cancer, and vitamin D synthesis. On one side are the vitamin D researchers, on the other side are dermatologists. Vitamin D research found that SPF 8 sunscreen almost totally blocked vitamin D_3 synthesis.[22] However, the SPF value equals 1/(# photons that reaches your skin) meaning that SPF 30 means 1/30 UV photons reach your skin. Thus, vitamin D_3 synthesis shouldn't be totally blocked. In addition, studies indicate that consumers apply 1/2 or less of the amount required to get the listed SPF protection.[89] Researchers recommend sun exposure on the face, arms, and hands for 10-15 minutes 2-3 times per week between 10AM-3PM.[15, 88] However, dermatologists do not like "sensible sun exposure" because this is also the peak time for harmful sun exposure. Dermatologists say that "sensible sun exposure" appeals to those who are looking for reasons to support tanning and are at highest risk (primarily young, fair-skinned females) of sun damage. They argue that vitamin D can be provided through supplementation.[89]

What about tanning beds? Not all tanning beds provide UV-B rays that are needed for vitamin D_3 synthesis. In fact, some advertise that they only use UV-A rays that are safer, even though this is not the case.[18] Virtually every health organization advises against using tanning beds, because the risks are far greater than the potential benefits.[18, 90]

11.1.2 Dietary or Supplemental Vitamin D

Because of the potential dangers of over-sun exposure for the synthesis of vitamin D, especially for those that have become unaccustomed to sun (and thus more likely to burn), consuming vitamin D from the diet or supplements is an alternative.

Vitamin D is rare naturally in foods, with useful sources of vitamin D being fatty fish (salmon, tuna, etc.) and their oils (such as cod liver oil). The amount in fatty fish varies greatly with wild-caught fish such as herring and salmon being the highest. One study showed that farmed salmon contained almost 75% less vitamin D than wild-caught salmon.[91] It is not known whether this disparity exists between other types of farmed and wild-caught fish varieties.

Table 44. High Vitamin D content foods (unfortified)

Fish	Vitamin D (iu/100g)
Herring	1628
Sockeye Salmon	763
Pink Salmon	624
Steelhead Trout	604
Halibut	600
Catfish	500
Sardines	480

Conversions for international units (iu) to micrograms (µg) are:

- 1 µg of D_3 = 40 IU
- 1 µg of 25-OH-D = 200 IU[92]

Many commonly consumed foods do not contain vitamin D, and so in the US and Canada many brands of milk have been fortified with vitamin D_2 or D_3 (100 IU/8 oz) since the 1930s.[22] This is becoming more common in New Zealand and Australia with several brands of fortified milks entering the market. However, the levels stated on labels may be considerably lower than that which can be measured. Part of this problem stems from a lack of a standardized method for measuring vitamin D in the past. Without standardized analysis, there inevitably was a wide range of variation from lab to lab in the reported amount of vitamin D. Some fortified milks are also reduced fat varieties which can impede the absorption of vitamin D, a fat-soluble vitamin. It has been demonstrated that fat in a meal increases absorption of vitamin D.

Another issue with relying on dairy products to provide vitamin D is the widespread problem of lactose intolerance. Lactose intolerant individuals don't have lactase, the enzyme needed to break down lactose. Common symptoms of this condition include:

- Abdominal Pain
- Abdominal Bloating
- Gas
- Diarrhoea
- Nausea[6]

Lactose intolerance is a widespread problem worldwide, as shown in the map below.

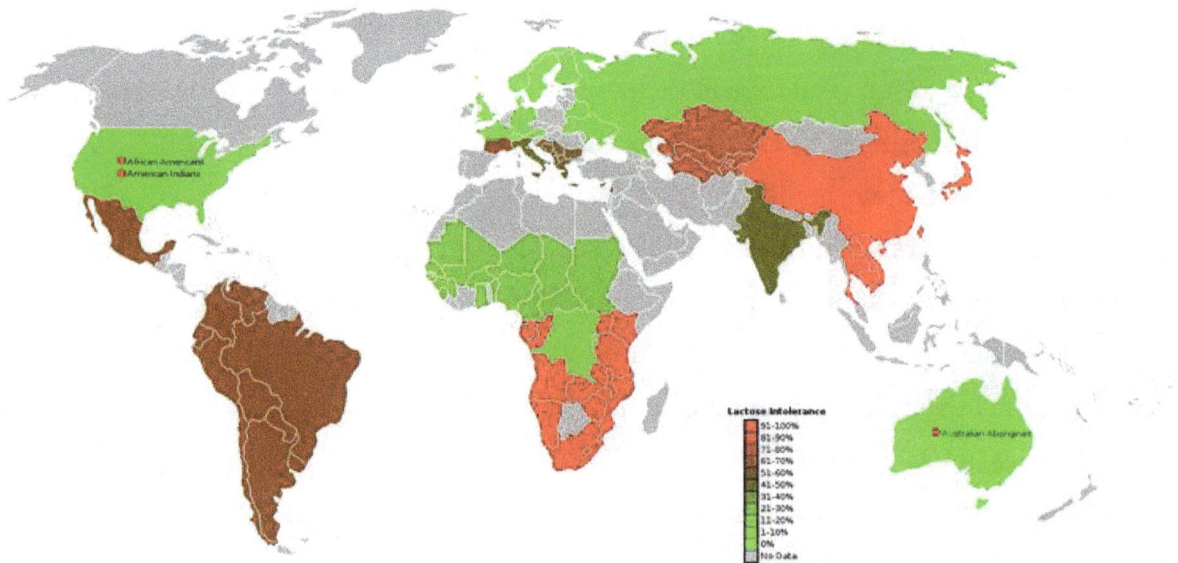

Figure 361. Lactose intolerance worldwide[lviii]

The following table shows the percent of people who are lactose intolerant by race:

Table 45. Lactose intolerance rates

Race or ethnicity	% Lactose Intolerant
Southeast Asian	98%
Native Americans	62-100%[93]
Asian Americans	90%
Alaskan Eskimo	80%

African-American Adults	79%
Mexicans (rural communities)	74%
North American Jews	69%
Greek Cypriots	66%
Cretans	56%
Mexican American Males	55%
Indian Adults	50%
African-American Children	45%
Indian Children	20%
Descendants of N. Europeans	5%

lviii https://en.wikipedia.org/wiki/File:LacIntol-World2.png

Thus, you can see that many people are lactose intolerant. Coincidentally, many of these people have darker pigmented skin, meaning that they have an increased risk of vitamin D deficiency/insufficiency because they require greater sun exposure to synthesize adequate amounts of vitamin D_3.

Other foods that are sometimes fortified are breakfast cereals and orange juice. Even though orange juice doesn't contain fat, and vitamin D is fat-soluble, vitamin D is quite bioavailable in orange juice, however fortification of what are typically high-sugar and high glycaemic load (GL) foods could be considered counter to overall nutrition and may provide a 'health halo' for these foods.

Vitamin D in supplements is found as vitamin D_2 or D_3. However, based on the recent evidence suggesting that D_2 isn't as potent as D_3, many are being reformulated to contain D_3.[11]

11.1.3 Response to Low Blood Calcium

One of the major functions of vitamin D is to assist in maintaining blood calcium concentrations. The other major regulators of blood calcium levels are two hormones: parathyroid hormone (PTH) and calcitonin, which are released from the parathyroid glands and thyroid glands, respectively. Bone serves as the calcium

depot, or reservoir, if there is a sufficient concentration in the body. In bone, calcium is found in hydroxyapatite crystals on a collagen matrix.

The chemical formula of hydroxyapatite is:
$$Ca_{10}(PO_4)_6(OH)_2$$

Calcium and phosphorus are either jointly deposited (deposition) or jointly liberated (resorption) from bone hydroxyapatite to maintain/achieve blood calcium concentrations. Osteoblasts are bone cells that are responsible for bone formation or depositing hydroxyapatite. Osteoclasts are the bone cells that are responsible for breaking down or resorption of bone. A straightforward way to remember the function of these cells is:

- Osteoblasts "build" bone
- Osteoclasts "chew" bone

Bone resorption is the process of liberating calcium and phosphorus from hydroxyapatite.

Bone deposition is the process of depositing calcium and phosphorus in bone as hydroxyapatite.

11.1.3.1 Response to Low Blood Calcium

The parathyroid senses low blood calcium concentrations and releases PTH. These steps are designed to maintain consistent blood calcium levels, but also affects phosphate (phosphorus) levels. PTH has 3 effects:

1. Increases bone resorption

2. Decreases calcium and increases phosphorus urinary excretion

3. Increases 1,25(OH)$_2$D activation in the kidney[18, 36]

The first effect of PTH is increased bone resorption. Hydroxyapatite must be broken down to release both calcium and phosphate. This effect is illustrated below.

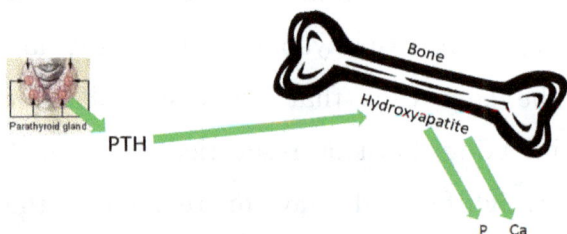

Figure 362. PTH effect 1: increased bone resorption[lix]

The second effect of PTH is decreased calcium excretion in urine. This is a result of increased calcium reabsorption by the kidney before it is excreted in urine. Kidney phosphate reabsorption is decreased, meaning the net effect is less calcium, but more phosphate urinary excretion, as shown in the figure below.

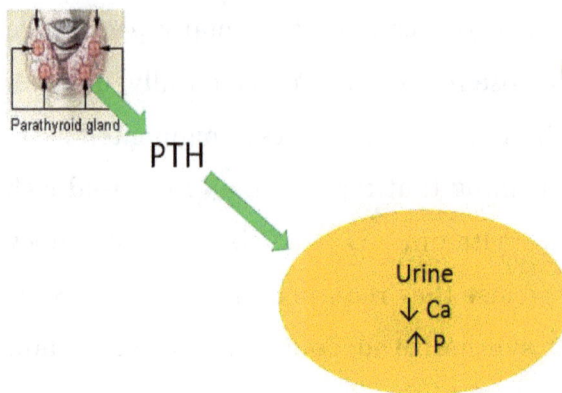

Figure 363. PTH effect 2: decreased calcium, increased phosphorus excretion

The 3rd effect of PTH is that it increases 1,25(OH)$_2$D activation in the kidney, by increasing 1alpha-hydroxylase levels. The 1,25(OH)$_2$D then increases calcium and phosphorus absorption in the small intestine to help raise blood calcium levels, as shown below. This mechanism will be discussed in more detail in the vitamin D receptor subsection.

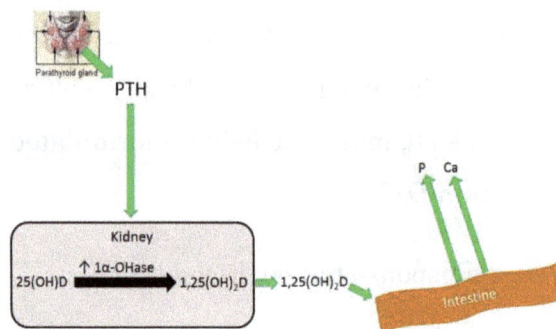

Figure 364. PTH effect 3: increased 1,25(OH)2D activation

Overall PTH causes more calcium and phosphate to be leached from bone, and absorbed from the intestine, into the blood.

[lix] http://en.wikipedia.org/wiki/File:Illu_thyroid_parathyroid.jpg

Coupled with decreased calcium and increased phosphate urinary excretion, means that blood calcium levels rise without a marked rise in phosphate levels, as depicted in the figure below.

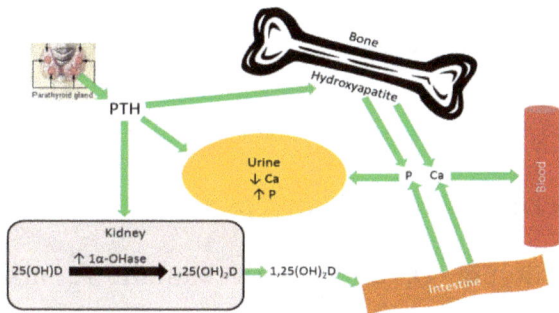

Figure 365. Increased calcium and phosphorus absorption

Figure 11.134 1,25(OH)$_2$D

11.1.4 Response to High Blood Calcium

In adults, it is rare for blood calcium levels to get too high. However, in infants and young children whose bodies, and thus bones, are not as large, the hormone calcitonin helps to prevent blood calcium levels from getting too high.

High blood calcium levels are sensed by the thyroid, which releases calcitonin. This response is designed to maintain/achieve normal blood calcium levels, but also affects phosphate (phosphorus) levels. Calcitonin has 3 effects[18, 36]:

1. Decreases bone resorption, increases bone deposition

2. Increases calcium and phosphorus excretion in urine

3. Decreases 1,25(OH)$_2$D activation in the kidney

The first effect of calcitonin is to inhibit bone resorption, thus promoting the deposition of calcium and phosphorus into bone as hydroxyapatite.

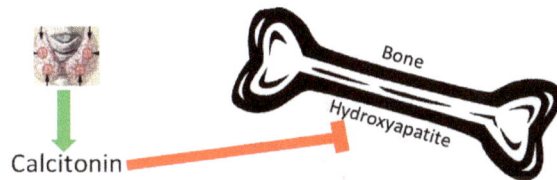

Figure 366. Calcitonin effect 1: increased bone deposition

The second effect of calcitonin is to increase calcium and phosphorus excretion in urine.

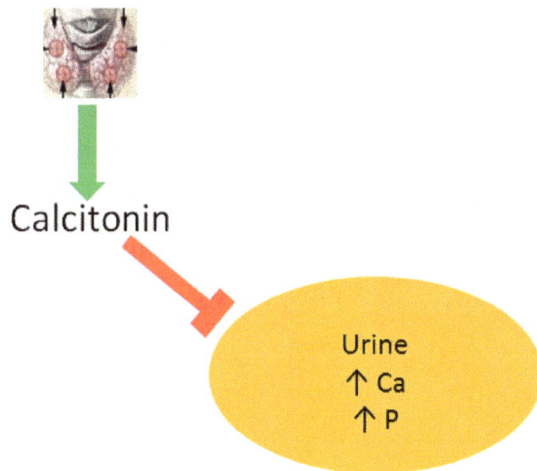

Figure 367. Calcitonin effect 2: increased calcium and phosphorus excretion

The third effect of calcitonin is to decrease 1alpha-hydroxylase levels, which decreases the activation of 1,25(OH)$_2$D. As a result, the absorption of calcium and phosphorus from the small intestine is decreased, as shown below.

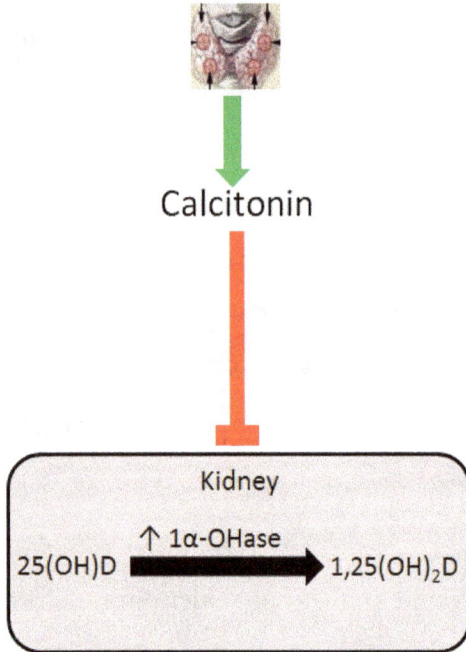

Figure 368. Calcitonin effect 3: decreased 1,25(OH)2D activation

Overall, calcitonin inhibits the 3 actions that PTH uses to increase blood calcium levels. Thus, more calcium and phosphate are deposited into bones and excreted into urine, as shown below. This causes blood calcium levels to decrease.

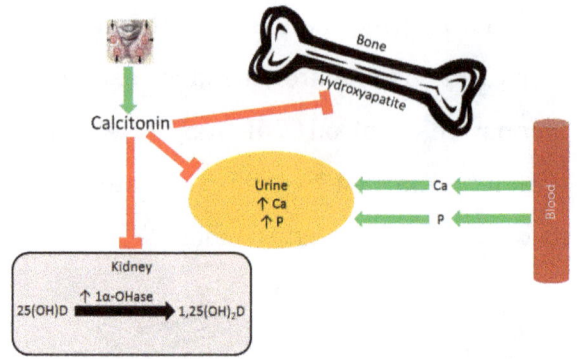

Figure 369. Response to high blood calcium

11.1.5 Vitamin D Receptor

Vitamin D, along with vitamin A, are unique among the vitamins because they have nuclear receptors. Many steroid hormones have nuclear receptors. The following figure illustrates the action of a nuclear hormone receptor.

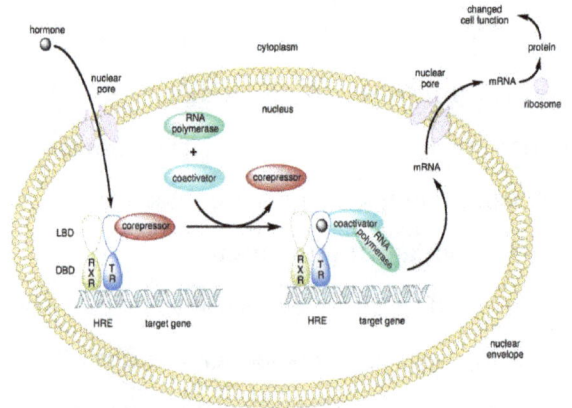

Figure 370. Nuclear hormone receptors action[lx]

In the figure above the hormone (in this case thyroid hormone) is the receptor's ligand (something that binds to the receptor), enters the nucleus and binds to the thyroid hormone receptor (TR). The TR

[lx] https://en.wikipedia.org/wiki/File:Type_ii_nuclear_receptor_action.png

has paired (formed a dimer) with the retinoid X receptor (RXR) on the hormone response element (HRE) in the promoter of target genes. The HRE for thyroid hormone is the thyroid hormone response element. Target genes are those whose transcription is altered by the hormone binding to its receptor on the response element. The mRNA produced then leaves the nucleus where it is translated into protein.

Vitamin A and D have nuclear receptors that act in the same fashion as nuclear hormone receptors.

$1,25(OH)_2D$ is the active form of vitamin D because it is the form that binds to the vitamin D receptor (VDR). There is a vitamin D response element (VDRE) in the promoter of specific vitamin D target genes. In the figure below, 25(OH)D, the major circulating form of vitamin D, is usually transported through the blood to the kidney by vitamin D binding protein (DBP). Again, the kidney converts 25(OH)D to $1,25(OH)_2D$ by use of the enzyme 1alpha-hydroxylase. $1,25(OH)_2D$ moves from the kidney or the tissue itself into the nucleus where it binds to the vitamin D receptor (VDR), that is dimerized to the RXR on the vitamin D response element of the target gene. Consequently, this then increases transcription of mRNA. The mRNA then

moves into the cytoplasm to synthesize specific proteins. This process is shown in the figure below.

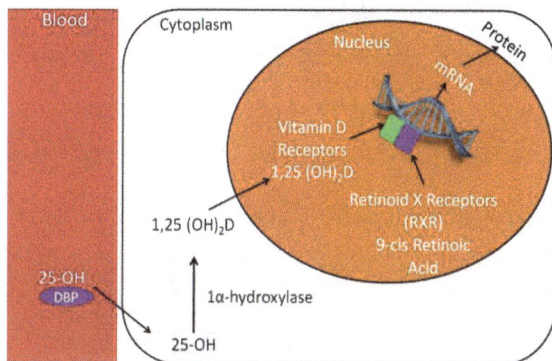

Figure 371. Vitamin D receptor and a generic target gene

It's through this action that $1,25(OH)_2D$ can increase calcium absorption. In this case, the target gene is the calcium-binding protein calbindin. Thus, increased $1,25(OH)_2D$ leads to increased calbindin mRNA that increases calbindin protein levels. Calbindin will be discussed in more detail in the calcium section.

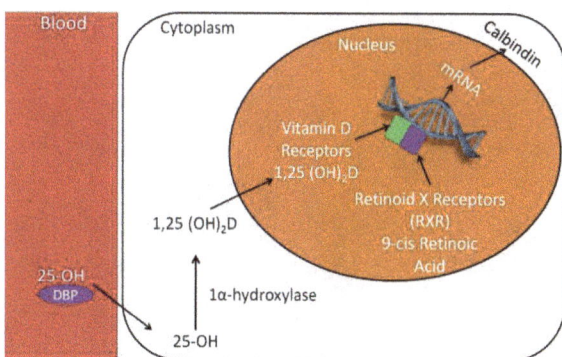

Figure 372. Vitamin D receptor and calbindin

221

11.1.6 Vitamin D Deficiency, Toxicity & Insufficiency

Rickets is a vitamin D deficiency in infants and children. A lack of vitamin D leads to decreased bone mineralization, causing the bones to become weak. The bones then bow under pressure, leading to the characteristic bowed legs, as seen below.

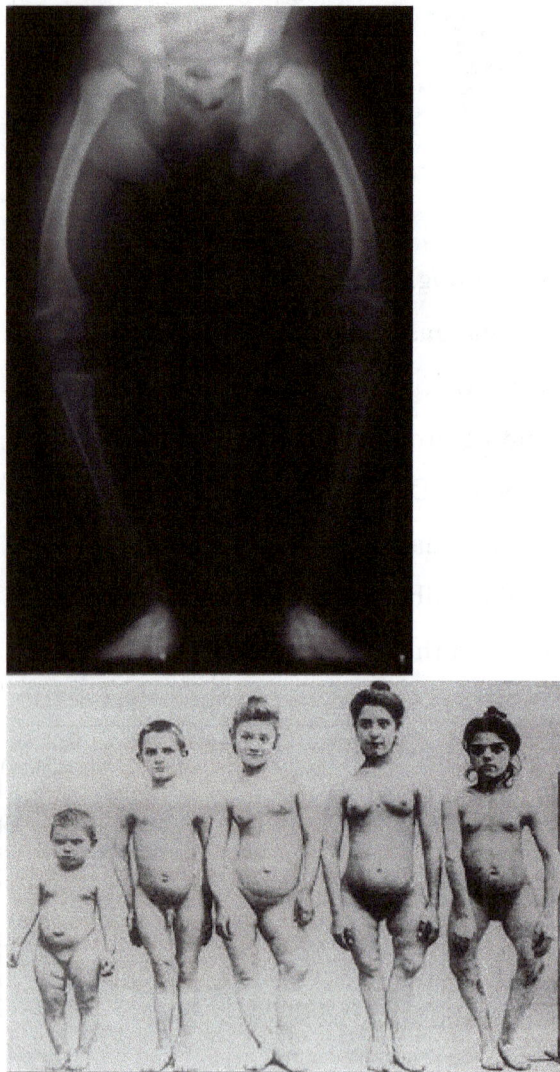

Figure 373. Children suffering from rickets[lxi]

Another characteristic symptom of rickets is rachitic rosary, or beaded ribs. The beading occurs at the areas where cartilage meets bone on the rib cage. Osteomalacia is a vitamin D deficiency in adults and results in poor bone mineralization. The bone becomes soft, resulting in bone pain and an increased risk of fractures.[18]

While rickets and osteomalacia are rare in the United States, it is believed that vitamin D insufficiency might be much more widespread. Insufficiency means that the level of intake or body status is suboptimal (neither deficient nor optimal). The figure below illustrates this concept.

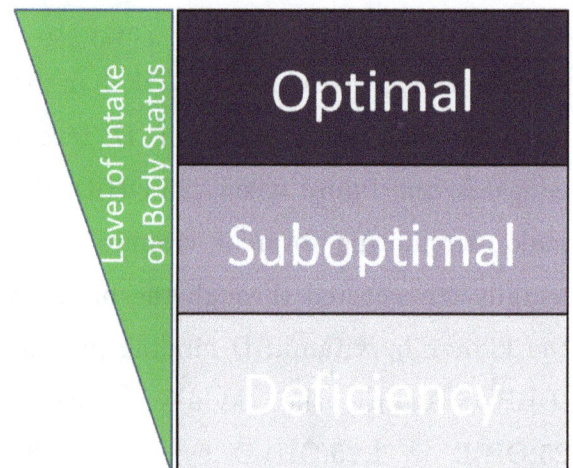

Figure 374. Illustration of insufficient or suboptimal levels

Suboptimal/insufficient means intake or status is higher than deficient, but lower than optimal. Thus, higher intake levels will provide additional benefits. The

---

lxi https://en.wikipedia.org/wiki/File:Rickets_USNLM.gif

functions of vitamin D are growing by the day due to increased research discoveries. These functions now include benefits beyond bone health, further supporting the importance of vitamin D. In late 2010, an RDA for vitamin D was established (was an Adequate Intake before), to make it, along with calcium, the first micronutrients to have their DRIs revised[4]. The RDA for vitamin D is three-times higher than the previous AI. Many believe these are more reasonable levels, while others think that the new RDA is still not high enough.

Vitamin D from supplements can become toxic but toxicity is generally considered unlikely. You cannot develop vitamin D toxicity from sun exposure, because the sunlight degrades a precursor of vitamin D_3 in the skin.[35] Vitamin D toxicity results in hypercalcaemia or high blood calcium levels. These become problematic because it can lead to the calcification of soft tissues.

11.2 Calcium

Calcium is a macromineral and the most abundant mineral in the body. The reason for calcium's abundance is its distribution in the skeleton, which contains 99% of the calcium in the body.

11.2.1 Calcium Absorption

Calcium is taken up into the enterocyte through Transient Receptor Potential V6 (TRPV6), a calcium channel found on the brush border. Calbindin is the calcium binding protein that facilitates both uptake through the channel and transport across the enterocyte. Ca^{2+}-Mg^{2+} ATPase functions to pump calcium out of the enterocyte and into circulation and to pump magnesium into the enterocyte, as shown below.[36]

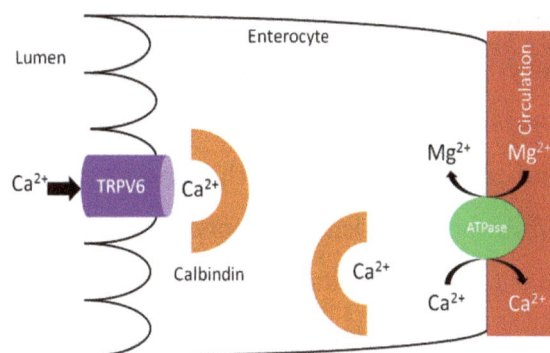

Figure 375. Calcium uptake and absorption

As we have previously discussed, increased $1,25(OH)_2D$ synthesis in the kidney causes increased binding to the vitamin D receptor, which increases calbindin synthesis that ultimately increases calcium uptake and absorption.

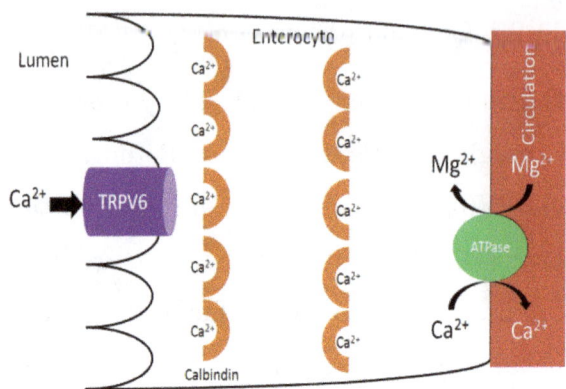

Figure 376. Increased calbindin increases calcium absorption

There are a couple of calcium-binding compounds that inhibit its absorption. Therefore, even though some foods are a good source of calcium, the calcium is not very bioavailable. Oxalate, found in high levels in spinach, rhubarb, sweet potatoes, and dried beans, is the most potent inhibitor of calcium absorption.[35] Recall that calcium oxalate is one of the compounds that makes up kidney stones. Based on this understanding, it should not be a surprise that formation of this compound inhibits calcium absorption.

Another inhibitor of calcium absorption is phytate. Phytate is found in whole grains and legumes.[3]

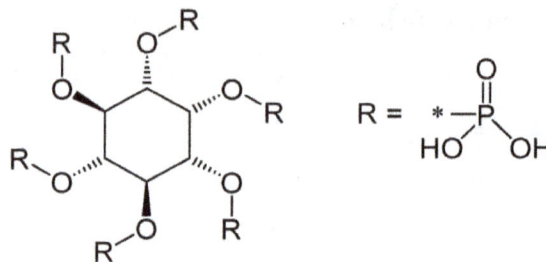

Figure 377. Structure of phytate

11.2.2 Calcium Bioavailability

Calcium bioavailability varies greatly from food to food, as shown in the table below. This table gives the serving size, calcium content of that food, and percent absorbed. The calcium content is multiplied by the absorption percentage to calculate the estimated calcium absorbed. Finally, it shows the servings of each food needed to equal the estimated calcium absorbed from one serving of milk.

Table 46. Bioavailability of calcium from different foods sources

Food	Serving Size (g)	Calcium content (mg)	Absorption (%)	Estimated Calcium Absorbed	Servings needed to equal 240 mL milk
Milk	240	300	32.1	96.3	1.0
Almonds, dry roasted	28	80	21.2	17.0	5.7
Beans, Pinto	86	44.7	26.7	11.9	8.1
Beans, Red	172	40.5	24.4	9.9	9.7
Beans, White	110	113	21.8	24.7	3.9
Bok Choy	85	79	53.8	42.5	2.3

Broccoli	71	35	61.3	21.5	4.5
Brussel Sprouts	78	19	63.8	12.1	8.0
Cabbage, Chinese	85	79	53.8	42.5	2.3
Cabbage, Green	75	25	64.9	16.2	5.9
Cauliflower	62	17	68.6	11.7	8.2
Cheddar Cheese	42	303	32.1	97.2	1.0
Chinese mustard greens	85	212	40.2	85.3	1.1
Chinese spinach	85	347	8.36	29	3.3
Fruit Punch (CCM)	240	300	52	156	0.62
Kale	85	61	49.3	30.1	3.2
Kohlrabi	82	20	67.0	13.4	7.2
Mustard Greens	72	64	57.8	37.0	2.6
Orange juice (CCM)	240	300	36.3	109	0.88
Radish	50	14	74.4	10.4	9.2
Rhubarb	120	174	8.54	10.1	9.5
Rutabaga	85	36	61.4	22.1	4.4
Sesame seeds, no hulls	28	37	20.8	7.7	12.2
Soy milk (tricalcium phosphate)	240	300	24.0	72.0	1.3
Soy milk (calcium carbonate)	240	300	21.1	66.3	1.0
Spinach	85	115	5.1	5.9	16.3
Sweet Potatoes	164	44	22.2	9.8	9.8
Tofu with Ca	126	258	31.0	80.0	1.2
Turnip Greens	72	99	51.6	51.1	1.9
Watercress	17	20	67.0	13.4	7.2
Yogurt	240	300	32.1	96.3	1.0

Notice that the foods high in oxalate like spinach, rhubarb, sweet potatoes, and dried beans are poorly absorbed. But there are still a number of calcium sources outside of milk.

The most common forms of calcium found in supplements are calcium carbonate and calcium citrate. As you can see in the figure below, they differ in the amount of elemental calcium they contain. This shows how much of the molecular weight of the compound is calcium.[4]

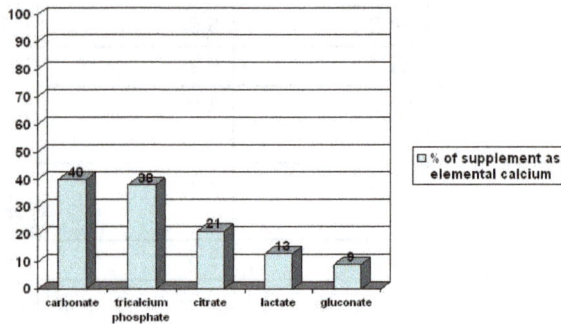

Figure 378. Percent of calcium supplements that is elemental calcium

The higher the percent elemental calcium, the greater the amount of calcium you will receive per given weight of that compound versus a compound that has a lower elemental calcium percentage. Both carbonate and citrate forms are well absorbed, but individuals with low stomach acid absorb citrate better. Also, carbonate is best absorbed when taken with food, while for citrate it is equally well absorbed when taken alone.[4]

Older research suggested that calcium citrate malate was more bioavailable than other calcium sources. However, more recent clinical research found no difference in the bioavailability of calcium from calcium citrate malate in orange juice, skim milk, or calcium carbonate supplements.[94] There is some evidence to suggest that even though bioavailability is the same among these different forms,

they might not be equally effective in improving bone measures.[95]

11.2.3 Calcium Functions

Calcium in hydroxyapatite is a major component of bones and teeth but there are also several non-bone functions of calcium. Calcium is an intracellular signalling molecule. Because of this, intracellular calcium is tightly controlled, primarily stored within organelles.

11.2.3.1 Neurotransmitter release

Neurotransmitter release is stimulated by the opening of voltage-gated Ca^{2+} channels. This stimulates the synaptic vesicle to fuse with the axon membrane and release the neurotransmitter into the synapse, as shown below.[15]

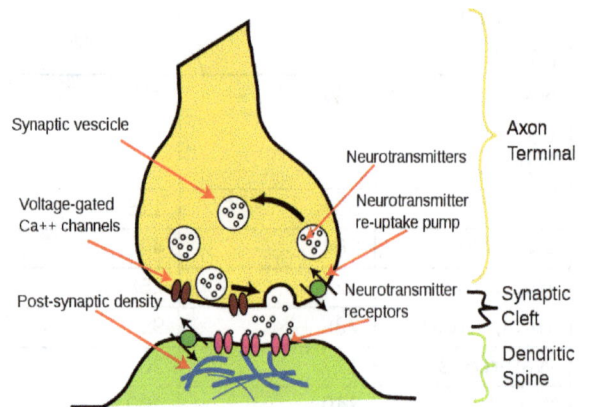

Figure 379. Calcium regulates neurotransmitter release

11.2.3.2 Muscle contraction

Calcium is released in muscle cells, where it binds to the protein troponin, changes its shape, and removes the tropomyosin blockade of actin active sites so that contraction can occur.[3]

11.2.3.3 Hormone release

Calcium acts as an intracellular messenger for the release of hormones, such as insulin. In the beta cells of the pancreas, the opening of voltage-gated calcium channels stimulates the insulin granules to fuse with the beta cell membrane to release insulin.

11.2.3.4 Blood Clotting

As will be discussed more in the vitamin K section, calcium binding to activated Gla proteins is important in the blood clotting cascade.[36]

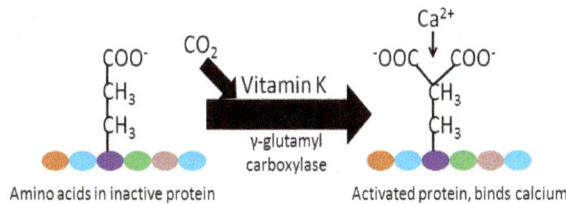

Figure 380. Calcium bind to Gla proteins

11.2.3.5 Enzyme regulation

The binding of calcium to calcium-binding proteins also regulates the action of a number of enzymes.[36]

11.2.4 Calcium Deficiency & Toxicity

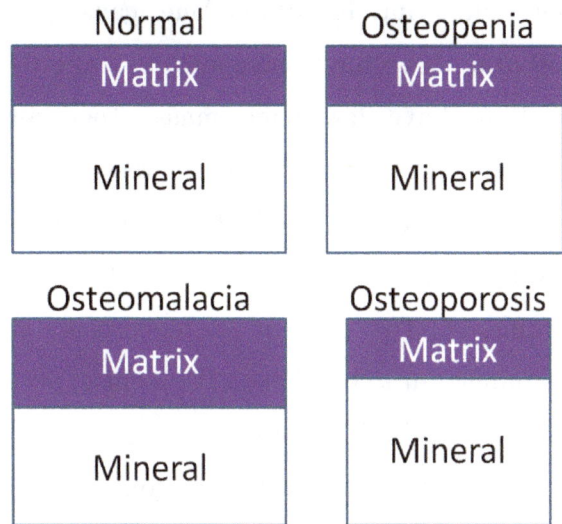

Figure 381. Bone states; the width of each figure represents the bone mass. The height of the matrix and mineral boxes represents the relative proportion for matrix to mineral in the bone. [Adapted from reference 3]

Osteomalacia—Bone mass is normal, but the matrix to mineral ratio is increased, meaning there is less mineral in bone.

Osteopenia—Bone mass is decreased, but the matrix to mineral ratio is not altered from normal bone. This condition is intermediate in between normal and osteoporosis.

Osteoporosis—Bone mass is further decreased from osteopenia, but the matrix to mineral ratio is not altered from normal bone.[3]

227

The National Osteoporosis Foundation estimates that 10 million Americans aged 50 and above have osteoporosis, while 34 million have low bone mass. Together these 44 million Americans represent 55% of people aged 50 and above. Of the 10 million with osteoporosis, 80% are women.[4] To prevent osteoporosis it is important to build peak bone mass, 90% of which is built in females by age 18 and age 20 in males but can continue to increase until age 30. After that time, bone mass starts to decrease. For women after menopause, bone mass decreases dramatically because of the decrease in oestrogen production, as shown in the link below.[5]

A measure of bone status is bone mineral density. As the name indicates, bone mineral density is a measure of the amount of mineral in bone. Dual energy X-ray absorptiometry (DEXA) accurately measures bone mineral density using a small amount of radiation.

A person lies down on the table and the arm of the machine moves slowly over them.

From the scan, a bone mineral density t-score is generated. As shown below, normal bone mineral density has a t-score of greater than -1, osteopaenia is from -1 to -2.5, and osteoporosis is a t-score of less than -2.5.

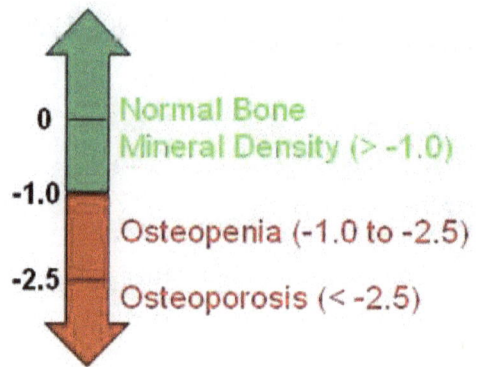

Figure 382. DEXA bone mineral density t-scores

There are other methods of measuring bone mineral density, such as peripheral DEXA and ultrasound. These typically are done on the wrist or heel, but are not as accurate because that one area might not reflect the bone mineral density in other parts of the body.[15]

Calcium toxicity is rare, occurring in those with hyperparathyroidism or high calcium supplementation levels. Like vitamin D, toxicity can lead to calcification of soft tissues.[15] In addition, a very high intake of calcium can lead to kidney stone formation.

11.3 Phosphorus

We have already talked about how blood phosphate levels are regulated in the body by PTH, calcitonin, and $1,25(OH)_2D$. Animal products are rich sources of phosphate. Plant products contain phosphorus, but some is in the form of phytic acid (phytate). In grains, over 80%

of the phosphorus is phytate. This structure is shown below.[36]

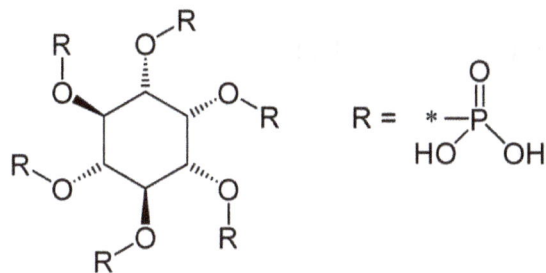

Figure 383. Structure of phytic acid

The bioavailability of phosphorus from phytate is poor because we lack the enzyme phytase. Nevertheless, ~50-70% of phosphorus is estimated to be absorbed from our diet.[36] Another source of phosphorus for many is phosphoric acid that is used to acidify soft drinks. Epidemiological studies have found that soft drink consumption is associated with decreased bone mineral densities, particularly in females. It has been hypothesized that phosphoric acid plays some role in this effect, but there is limited evidence to support this belief. Most phosphorus is excreted in the urine.

Phosphorus deficiency is rare but can hinder bone and teeth development. Other symptoms include anorexia, weakness and bone pain.[15] Toxicity is also rare, but it causes low blood calcium concentrations and tetany.[36]

11.3.1 Phosphorus Functions

Phosphorus has a number of functions in the body.[36] As discussed earlier, it is a component of hydroxyapatite in bones and teeth.

11.3.1.1 Phosphorylation

Phosphates are used to activate and deactivate several proteins. In addition, compounds are also frequently phosphorylated, like the monosaccharides shown below.

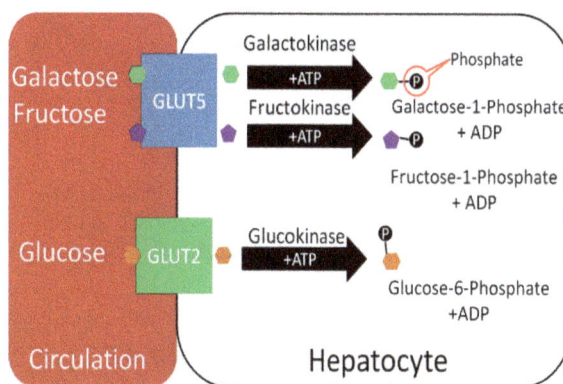

Figure 384. Uptake of monosaccharides into the hepatocyte

11.3.1.2 Phospholipids

Phosphates are a component of phospholipids, as shown below.

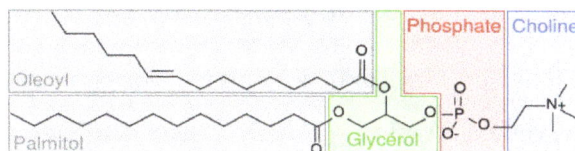

Figure 385. Structure of phosphatidylcholine (lecithin)

229

11.3.1.3 DNA/RNA

DNA/RNA have a phosphate backbone as shown below.

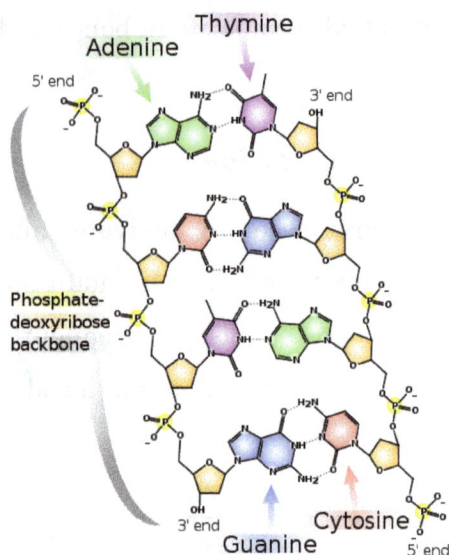

Figure 386. Structure of DNA[lxii]

11.3.1.4 ATP

The major energy currency, ATP, stores energy in its phosphate bonds.

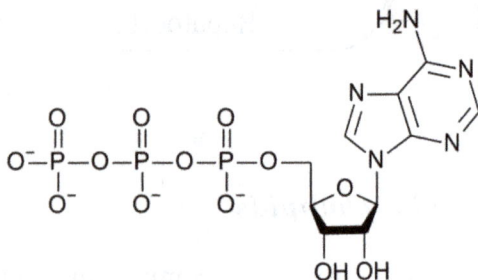

Figure 387. Structure of ATP

11.3.1.5 Secondary Messengers

The intracellular secondary messengers cyclic AMP (cAMP) and inositol triphosphate (IP$_3$) both contain phosphate.

11.4 Fluoride

Fluoride is a nonessential mineral. It is not required by the body and it is not widely found in the food supply. Most of the fluoride we consume comes from fluoridated water. Other non-dietary sources are fluoridated toothpaste and dental rinses.[15] Absorption of fluoride is near 100% for both dietary and non-dietary forms and it is rapidly excreted in the urine.[36]

Fluoride alters the mineralization of bones and teeth. It does this by replacing hydroxyl (OH) ions in hydroxyapatite ($Ca_{10}(PO_4)_6(OH)_{2)}$, forming fluorohydroxyapatite.

Fluorohydroxyapatite is more resistant to acid degradation than hydroxyapatite, leading to fewer cavities.[36]

Since it is a nonessential mineral, there is no fluoride deficiency. However, fluoride can be quite toxic. Acute toxicity symptoms from large intakes of fluoride include[15]:

- Nausea
- Vomiting
- Diarrhoea
- Convulsions

Chronic toxicity results in an irreversible condition known as fluorosis,

---

characterized by the mottling and pitting of teeth as shown below.

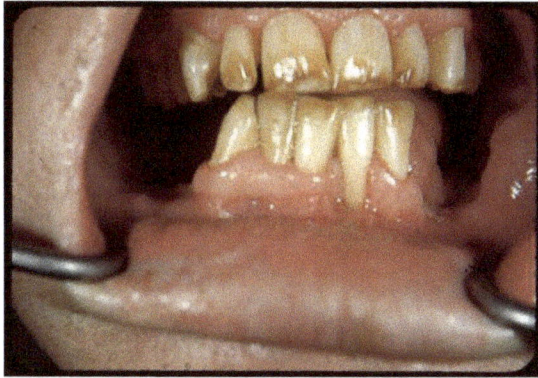

Figure 388. Severe fluorosis[lxiii]

As you can see from the figure below, fluorosis is more prevalent in the United States than most people would probably believe.[96]

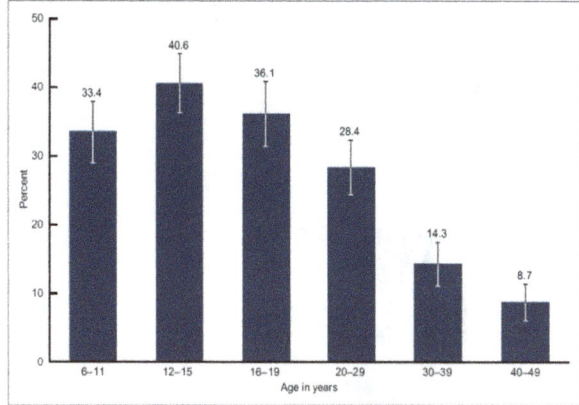

Figure 2. Prevalence of dental fluorosis among persons aged 6–49, by age group: United States, 1999–2004

NOTES: Dental fluorosis is defined as having very mild, mild, moderate, or severe forms and is based on Dean's Fluorosis Index. Error bars represent 95% confidence intervals.
SOURCE: CDC/NCHS, National Health and Nutrition Examination Survey, 1999–2004.

Figure 389. Fluorosis prevalence by age in the United States

A comparison of the prevalence of fluorosis in US children, ages 12-15, indicates an increase from the late 1980s to the early 2000s.[96]

Figure 3. Change in dental fluorosis prevalence among children aged 12–15 participating in two national surveys: United States, 1986–1987 and 1999–2004

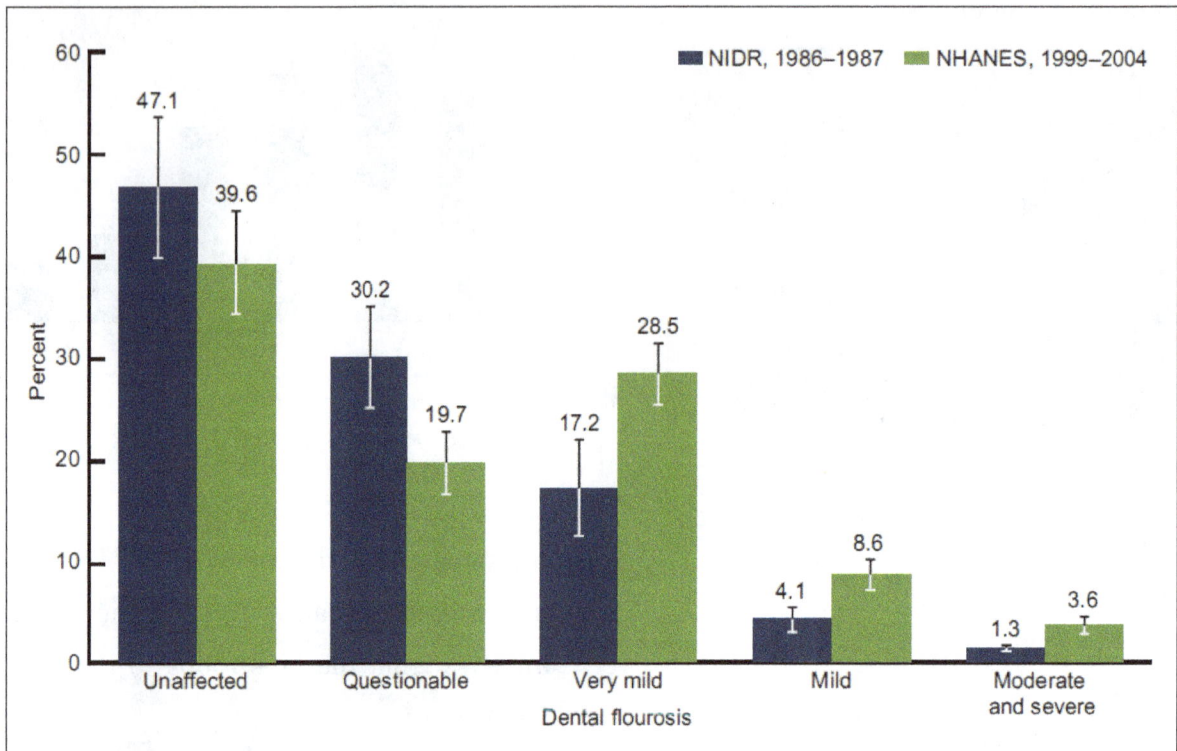

NOTES: Dental fluorosis is defined as having very mild, mild, moderate, or severe forms and is based on Dean's Fluorosis Index. Percentages do not sum to 100 due to rounding. Error bars represent 95% confidence intervals.
SOURCES: CDC/NCHS, National Health and Nutrition Examination Survey, 1999–2004 and National Institute of Dental Research, National Survey of Oral Health in U.S. School Children, 1986–1987.

Figure 390. Change in dental fluorosis in 12-15-year-old US children

There has been an ongoing debate in many countries about the role of fluoridation in health, and while the impact of fluoridation on dental health is clear, the necessity of having fluoridated water has been brought into question. With the prevalence of fluoride containing toothpastes and improved dental hygiene practices the ingestion of fluoride in water may be unnecessary.[97]

11.5 Vitamin K

There are three forms of vitamin K. Phylloquinone (K1), the plant form of vitamin K, is the primary dietary form of vitamin K. Its structure is shown below.

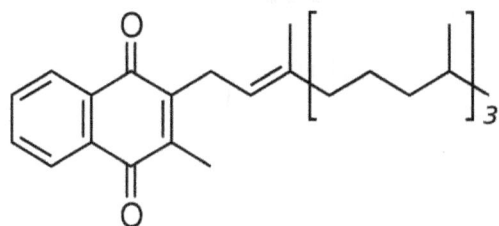

Figure 391. Structure of phylloquinone (K1), the 3 outside of the brackets indicates the structural unit inside the brackets is repeated 3 times

Green leafy vegetables, broccoli, Brussels sprouts, and asparagus are foods that are good sources of phylloquinone.[90] Another form of vitamin K, menaquinone (K2), is synthesized by bacteria in the colon. Menaquinone comprises ~10% of absorbed vitamin K every day and can also be found in lesser amounts in animal products. Its structure is shown below.[15]

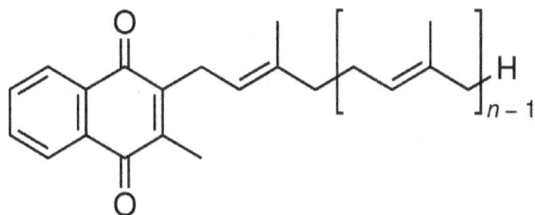

Figure 392. Structure of menaquinone (K2). Menaquinones have side chains of varying length

In the structure above, if it was menaquinone-8, there would be 7 (8-1) repeating units of the structure inside the brackets above.

The synthetic form of vitamin K is menadione, whose structure is shown below.

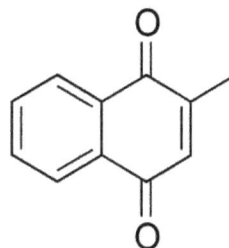

Figure 393. Structure of menadione

A tail, like the one found in menaquinone, must be added to menadione for it to be biologically active.

Vitamin K is absorbed like other fat-soluble substances. Approximately 80% of phylloquinone and menaquinone are incorporated into chylomicrons and stored primarily in the liver.[36, 90]

Once metabolized, vitamin K is primarily excreted via bile in the faeces, with a lesser amount excreted in urine.[36]

11.5.1 Vitamin K Functions

Vitamin K is a cofactor for carboxylation reactions that add a CO_2 to the amino acid glutamic acid (glutamate) in certain proteins. The structure of glutamic acid is shown below.

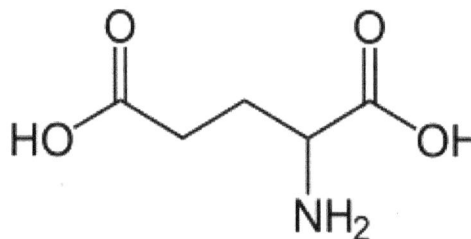

Figure 394. Structure of glutamic acid

The enzyme, gamma-glutamyl carboxylase, using a vitamin K cofactor, converts glutamic acid to gamma-carboxyglutamic acid (Gla). Gla proteins are those that contains glutamic acid(s) that have been converted to gamma-carboxyglutamic acid(s). The formation of Gla proteins allows the 2-positive charge of calcium to bind between the 2 negative charges on the carboxylic acid groups (COO^-) in the Gla. The binding of calcium activates these proteins.[36]

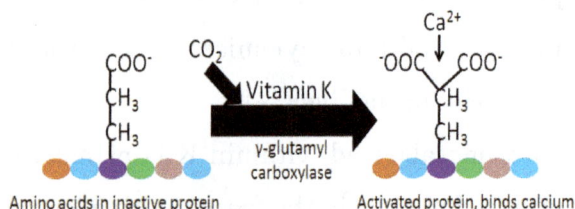

Figure 395. Gamma-glutamyl carboxylase for Gla proteins

Gla proteins are important is in blood clotting. Within the blood clotting cascade, there several Gla proteins, as shown in the figure below.

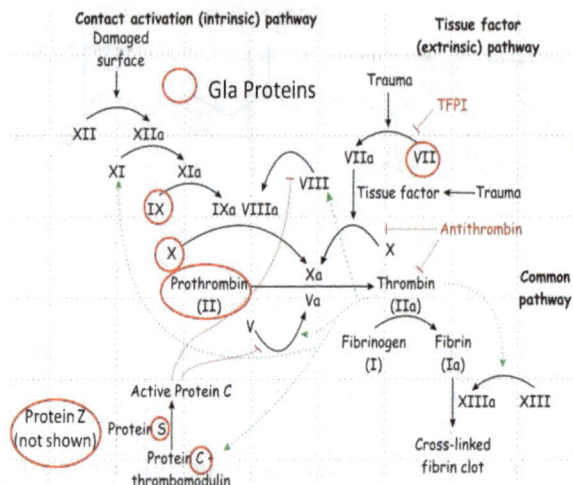

Figure 396. Blood clotting cascade with Gla proteins circled

After being used as a cofactor by gamma-glutamyl carboxylase to produce a Gla protein, vitamin K becomes vitamin K epoxide. Vitamin K epoxide needs to be converted back to vitamin K to serve as a cofactor again. Warfarin (Coumadin) and dicoumarol are blood thinning drugs that inhibit this regeneration of vitamin K. This reduces the amount of Gla in the blood clotting proteins and thus, reduces the clotting response. The structure of warfarin and dicoumarol are shown below.[5]

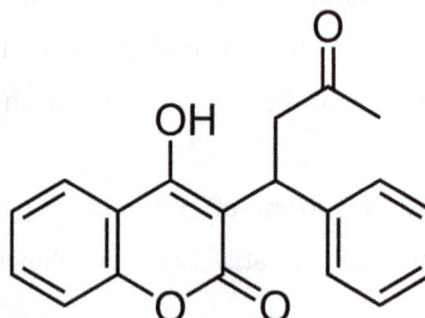

Figure 397. Structure of warfarin

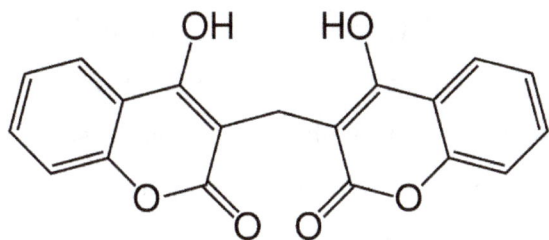

Figure 398. Structure of dicoumarol

Vitamin K is also important for bone health. There are three Gla proteins found in bone: osteocalcin, matrix Gla protein (MGP), and protein S.[35] Osteocalcin is a major bone protein, constituting 15-20% of all non-collagen proteins in bone. However, overall the function of these three proteins in bone is not known.[15, 36] Research suggests that higher vitamin K status or intake decreases bone loss.

11.5.2 Vitamin K Deficiency & Toxicity

Prolonged antibiotic treatment (which kills bacteria in the gastrointestinal tract) and lipid absorption problems can also lead to vitamin K deficiency.[90] Vitamin K deficient individuals have an increased risk of bleeding or haemorrhage. Remember that high levels of vitamin E intake can also interfere with vitamin K's blood clotting function. It is believed that a vitamin E metabolite, with similar structure to the vitamin K quinones, antagonizes the action of vitamin K.[15]

Phylloquinone and menaquinone have no reported toxicities. However, menadione can cause liver damage[36] and is not recommended as a supplemental form of vitamin K.

11.6 Vitamin A

There are 3 forms of vitamin A (retinol, retinal, and retinoic acid) that collectively are known as retinoids. Retinol is the alcohol (OH) form, retinal is the aldehyde (COH) form, and retinoic acid is the carboxylic acid (COOH) form, as shown in the figure below (areas of difference are indicated by red in the figure below).

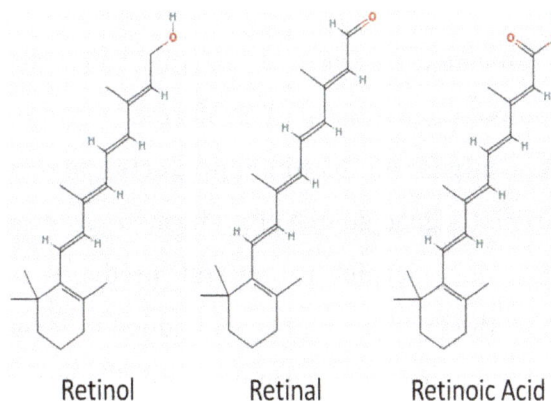

Retinol   Retinal   Retinoic Acid

Figure 399. Structure of the retinoids

Among these different retinoids, retinol and retinal are fairly interchangeable. Either form is readily converted to the other. However, only retinal is used to form retinoic acid, and this is a one-way reaction. Thus, once retinoic acid is formed it can't be converted back to retinal, as shown in the figure below.

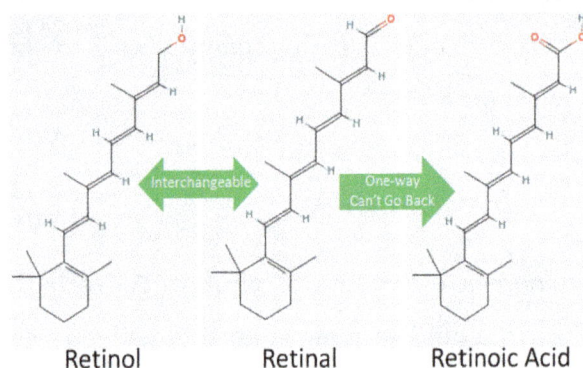

Figure 400. Metabolism of retinoids

There are 2 primary dietary sources of vitamin A:

- Retinyl/retinol esters (Animal Products)
- Provitamin A Carotenoids (Plants)

Preformed vitamin A means that the compound is a retinoid. Preformed vitamin A is only found in animal products (carrots are not a good source of preformed vitamin A!) Most retinol in animal products is esterified or has a fatty acid added to form retinyl esters (aka retinol esters). The most common retinyl ester is retinyl palmitate (retinol + the fatty acid palmitate) whose structure is shown below.

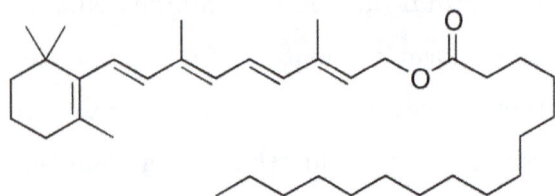

Figure 401. Retinyl palmitate

Provitamin A is a compound that can be converted to vitamin A in the body, but currently isn't in vitamin A form. The next section will talk about carotenoids, some of which are provitamin A compounds. International units are also used for vitamin A, such that: 1 IU = 3.33 ug retinol

11.6.1 Carotenoids

There are many hundreds of carotenoids consumed in foods. Some of the most common are:

- Beta-carotene
- Alpha-carotene
- Beta-cryptoxanthin
- Lutein
- Zeaxanthin
- Lycopene

Many carotenoids are pigments, meaning they are coloured. The table below gives the colour of some of these carotenoids, as well as some food sources.

Table 47. Carotenoids' colour and food sources

Carotenoid	Colour	Food Sources
Beta-carotene	Orange	Carrots, Sweet Potatoes, Leafy Greens
Lycopene	Red	Tomatoes, Watermelon, Pink Grapefruit
Lutein/Zeaxanthin	Yellow	Kale, Corn, Egg Yolks, Spinach

Carotenoids can be further classified as provitamin A or non-provitamin A. Provitamin A carotenoids are those that can be cleaved to form retinal, while the non-provitamin A carotenoids cannot. The structure and classification of the six major carotenoids is shown below.

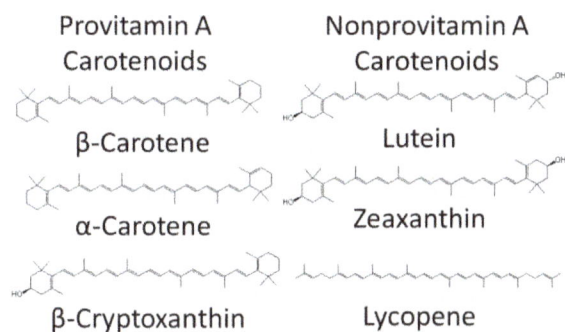

Figure 402. Structure and classification of the 6 major carotenoids

After provitamin A carotenoids are taken up into the enterocyte, some are cleaved to form retinal. In the case of symmetrical beta-carotene, it is cleaved in the centre to form 2 retinal molecules as shown below.

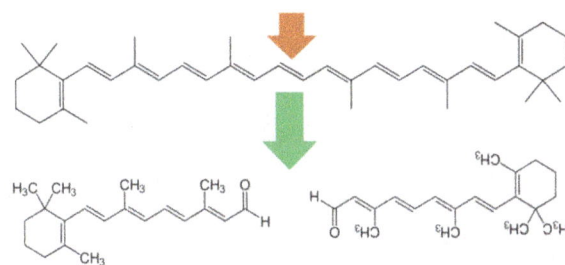

Figure 403. Cleavage of beta-carotene 2 to retinal molecules

Alpha-carotene and beta-cryptoxanthin are asymmetrical, thus they can be used to form only one retinal.

To help account for the fact that retinol can be made from carotenoids, the DRI committee made retinol activity equivalents (RAE) that consider the bioavailability and bioconversion of the provitamin A carotenoids.

1 ug RAE

= 1 ug of retinol

= 2 ug of supplemental beta-carotene

= 12 ug of dietary beta-carotene

= 24 ug of alpha-carotene or beta-cryptoxanthin[98]

11.6.2 Vitamin A Uptake, Absorption, Transport & Storage

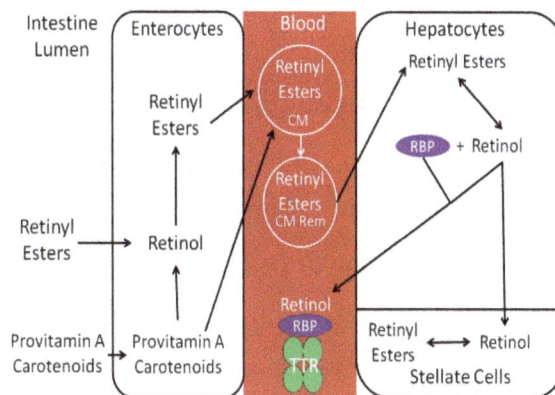

Figure 404. Vitamin A uptake, absorption, transport, and storage. [22]

Esters are removed by esterases so that free retinol can be taken up into the enterocyte. Preformed vitamin A is highly bioavailable (70-90%) if consumed with some fat.[36] Carotenoids have a much lower bioavailability, which varies based on the carotenoid and matrix it is in when consumed. Conversion rates of beta-carotene to usable vitamin A differ by a factor of nine-fold.[99] In whole food such as spirulina or types of rice, beta-carotene may be required in amounts around four times higher than taking pre-formed vitamin A.

Higher body-fat levels may also negatively affect beta-carotene conversion.[99]

Once provitamin A carotenoids are taken up into the enterocytes, they are: (1) cleaved to retinal and then converted to retinol or (2) absorbed intact and incorporated into chylomicrons.

Retinol in the enterocyte is esterified, forming retinyl esters. The retinyl esters are packaged into chylomicrons (CM) and enter the lymph system. Once the chylomicrons reach circulation, triglycerides are cleaved off to form chylomicron remnants (CM Rem). These are taken up by hepatocytes, where the retinyl esters are de-esterified to form retinol.

The liver is the major storage site of vitamin A. For storage, the retinol will be transported from the hepatocytes to the stellate cells and converted back to retinyl esters, the storage form of vitamin A. If vitamin A is needed to be released into circulation, retinol will combine with retinol binding protein (RBP). Retinol + RBP are then bound to a large transport protein, transthyretin (TTR). It is believed that retinol + RBP would be filtered out by the kidney and excreted in urine if it was not bound to TTR.[22]

After it is further metabolized, 60% of vitamin A is excreted in the urine, 40% in faeces.[36]

11.6.3 Vitamin A Nuclear Receptors

As shown in the figure below, all-trans retinol is brought to the cell by RBP and TTR. All-trans retinol is converted to all-trans-retinal, and then to all-trans-retinoic acid. RAR and RXR are paired, or dimerized, on retinoic acid response element (RARE) in the promoter region of target genes. The binding of all-trans retinoic acid causes the transcription and ultimately the translation of target proteins.

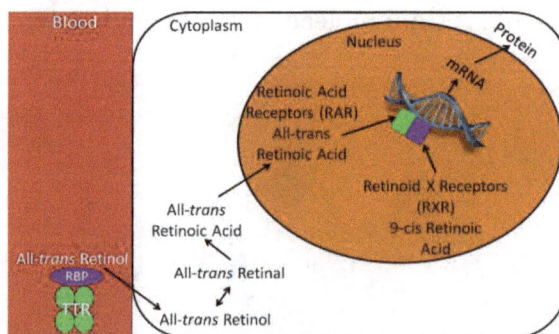

Figure 405. All-trans retinoic acid and retinoid X receptors

All-trans retinoic acid is the active form of vitamin A because it is the ligand for

RARs, and thus causes increased production of target proteins.

11.6.4 Vitamin A Functions

Vitamin A has several crucial functions in the body.

11.6.4.1 Vision

The retina is the inner back lining of the eye that takes visual images and turns them into nerve signals that are sent to the brain to form the images that we "see". Inside the retina are the photoreceptor cells, rods and cones. Cones are responsible for colour vision, while rods are important for seeing black and white. Within the rods, 11-cis retinal combines with the protein, opsin, to form rhodopsin. When light strikes rhodopsin, the compound splits into opsin and all-trans retinal. This sends a signal to your brain for us to "see". This process is illustrated in the figure below.[15]

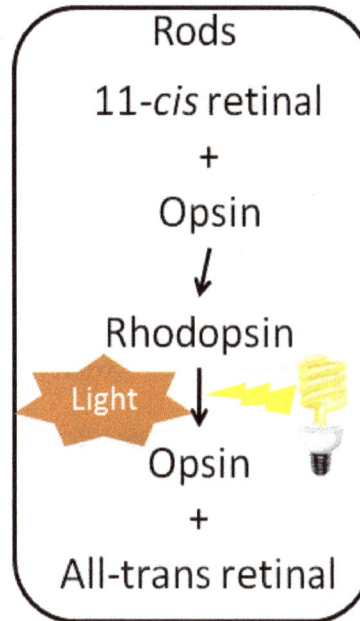

Figure 406. Vitamin A in the rod

Most all-trans retinal is converted back to 11-cis retinal through a series of steps so it can continue to be used to form rhodopsin. However, this recycling is not 100% efficient. Vitamin A stores, or continued intake, is required to provide the 11-cis retinal needed to continue to form rhodopsin. Normally, our eyes adapt to darkness by increasing the amount of rhodopsin available so we can see under reduced light conditions.[15] If a person does not have enough rhodopsin he/she will become night blind, meaning their eyes do not adjust, or adjust very slowly, so that he/she can see under limited light conditions.

239

11.6.4.2 Cell Differentiation

Vitamin A, retinoic acid, is important for cell differentiation, or the ability of stem cells to develop into specialized cells.

Other functions that vitamin A is important for include:

- Growth and development
- Reproduction
- Immune function

11.6.5 Vitamin A Deficiency & Toxicity

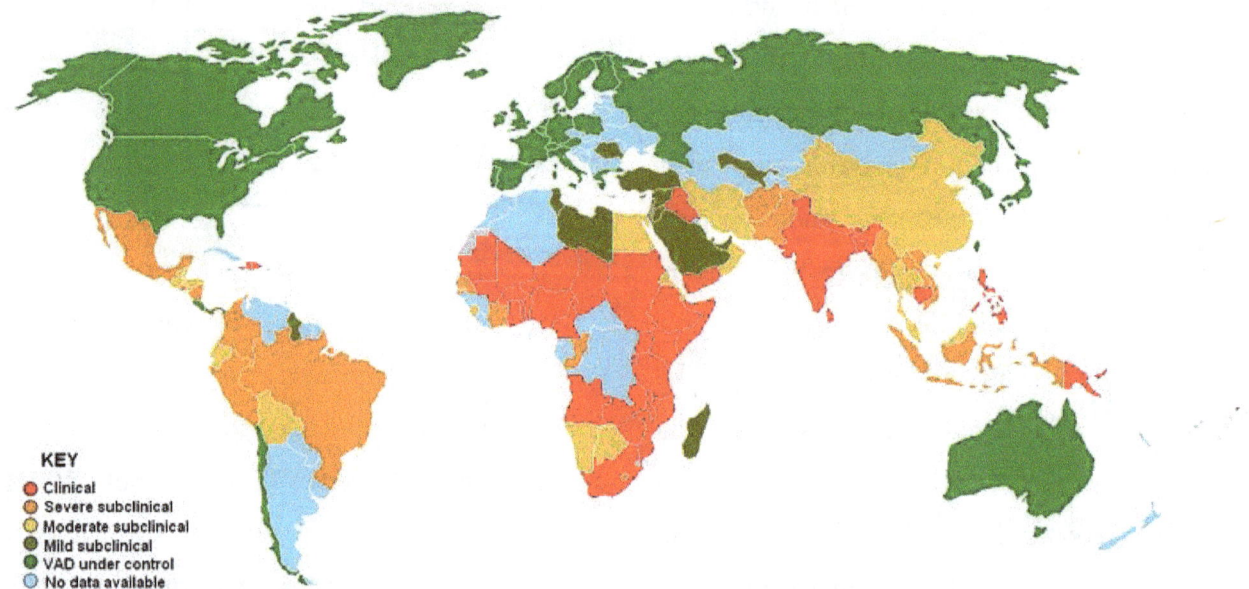

Figure 407. Prevalence of vitamin A deficiency worldwide[lxiv]

Often the earliest symptom of vitamin A deficiency is night blindness, due to the insufficient production of rhodopsin. There are further changes to the eye that occur during vitamin A deficiency, collectively referred to as xerophthalmia. Ultimately the person can become blind and vitamin A deficiency is the leading cause of blindness in some parts of the world.[90]

Another symptom of vitamin A deficiency is hyperkeratosis. In this condition, cells overproduce the protein keratin, causing the skin to become rough and irritated.

Vitamin A can be very toxic and can cause serious symptoms, such as blurred vision, liver abnormalities, skin disorders, and joint pain.[15, 90] In addition, research has suggested that people who consume high levels of vitamin A are more prone to bone

---

[lxiv] Public Domain work https://en.wikipedia.org/wiki/File:Vitamin_A_deficiency.PNG

fractures.[90] Toxic levels of vitamin A are also teratogenic, which means they could cause birth defects.

This is important to keep in mind because a vitamin A derivative isotretinoin is the active ingredient in a common oral acne medication, Accutane and Roaccutane. Due to the number of adverse events reported from its consumption, Accutane was recalled from the US market in 2009.[4] Retin-A is a topical product of all-trans retinoic acid. Women of childbearing age need to exercise caution when using these products due to the risk of birth defects, should they become pregnant.[15] People should not consume huge doses of vitamin A expecting to get the same effects seen from these medications.[18]

It is important to note that you cannot develop vitamin A toxicity from consuming too much beta-carotene or other provitamin A carotenoids. Instead, a nontoxic condition known as carotenodermia occurs when copious amounts of beta-carotene are consumed, where the accumulation of the carotenoid in the fat below the skin causes the skin to look orange.

11.7 Iron

There are two major dietary forms of iron: haeme and non-haeme. Haeme iron is only found in foods of animal origin, within haemoglobin and myoglobin. The structure of haeme iron is shown below.

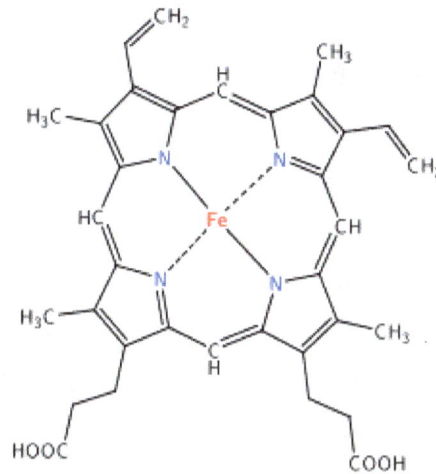

Figure 408. Structure of haeme iron

Approximately 40% of iron in meat, fish, and poultry is haeme-iron, and the other 60% is non-haeme iron.[18]

Non-haeme iron is the mineral alone, in either its oxidized or reduced form. The two forms of iron are:

- Ferric (Fe^{3+}, oxidized)
- Ferrous (Fe^{2+}, reduced)

It is estimated that 25% of haeme iron and 17% of non-haeme iron are absorbed.[18]

Approximately 85-90% of the iron we consume is non-haeme iron.[18,3]

In addition to getting iron from food sources, if food is cooked in cast iron cookware, a small amount of iron can be transferred to the food. Reductions in use of cast iron cookware has likely influenced iron status in many countries.

11.7.1.1 Supplements

Most iron supplements use ferrous (Fe^{2+}) iron, because this form is better absorbed, as discussed in the next section.

Vitamin C does not increase absorption of ferrous supplements because they are already in reduced form, as discussed in the following subsection.[18] Iron chelates are marketed as being better absorbed than other forms of iron supplements, but this hasn't been proven.[36] It is recommended that supplements are not to be taken with meals, because they are better absorbed when not consumed with food.[18]

11.7.2 Iron Uptake & Absorption

There are two transporters for iron, one for haeme iron and one for non-haeme iron. The non-haeme transporter is the divalent mineral transporter 1 (DMT1), which transports Fe^{2+} into the enterocyte. Haeme iron is taken up through haeme carrier protein 1 (HCP-1), and then metabolized to Fe^{2+}. Fe^{2+} may be used by enzymes and other proteins or stored in the enterocyte bound to ferritin, the iron storage protein. To reach circulation, Fe^{2+} is transported through ferroportina.[35, 36] This process is summarized in the figure below.

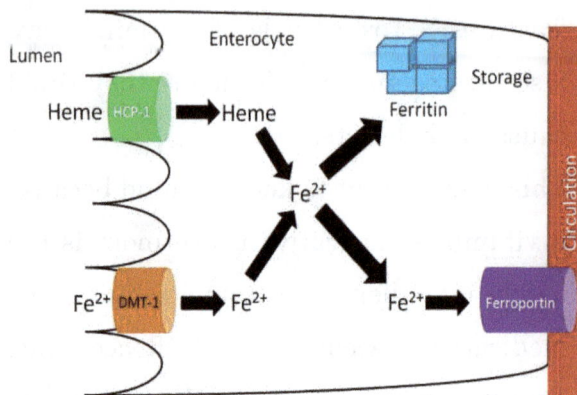

Figure 409. Iron uptake into the enterocyte

Since only the reduced form of non-haeme iron (Fe^{2+}) is taken up, Fe^{3+} must be reduced. There is a reductase enzyme on the brush border, duodenal cytochrome b (Dcytb), that catalyses the reduction of Fe^{3+} to Fe^{2+}, as shown below. Vitamin C enhances non-haeme iron absorption because it is required by Dcytb for this reaction. Thus, if dietary non-haeme iron is consumed with vitamin C, more non-haeme iron will be reduced Fe^{2+} and taken up into the enterocyte through DMT-1.

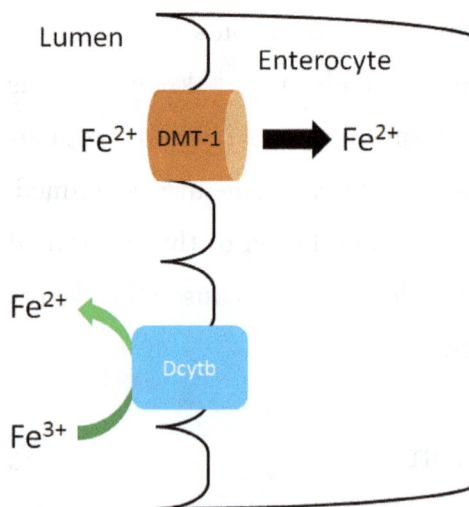

Figure 410. Reduction of non-haeme iron by Dcytb

In addition to vitamin C, there is an unidentified factor in muscle that enhances non-haeme iron absorption if consumed at the same meal.[100] This unidentified factor is referred to as meat protein factor (MPF). The table shows how MPF can increase non-haeme iron absorption.

Table 48. Non-haeme iron absorption from chicken or beef muscle fraction

Mean Fe Absorption (% of Dose)	Egg Albumin	Whole Muscle	Whole Muscle Protein	Haeme-Free Muscle Protein
Chicken	8.41	16.43	26.98	36.81
Beef	11.21	31.52	44.15	38.29

Albumin is a protein, so the egg albumin represents a non-meat protein standard for comparison. You can see that absorption is much higher with whole muscle. When only consuming muscle protein, there is a slight increase from muscle itself, and when they look at haeme-free muscle iron, absorption is still higher than egg albumin.[100]

Inhibitors of non-haeme iron absorption typically chelate, or bind, the iron to prevent absorption. Phytates (phytic acid), which also inhibit calcium absorption, chelate non-haeme iron decreasing its absorption.

Other compounds that inhibit absorption are:

Polyphenols (coffee, tea)[36]

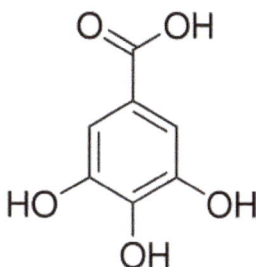

Figure 411. Structure of gallic acid, a polyphenol

Oxalate (spinach, rhubarb, sweet potatoes, and dried beans)[35]

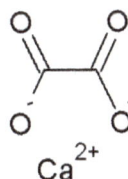

Figure 412. Structure of calcium oxalate

Calcium is also believed to inhibit iron uptake by competing for the DMT.

11.7.3 Iron Transport & Storage

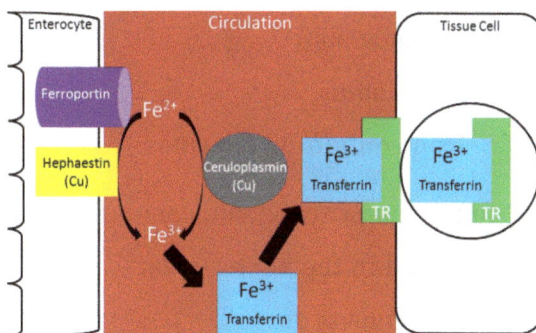

Figure 413. Transport and uptake of iron

Once inside cells, the iron can be used for cellular purposes (cofactor for enzyme etc.) or it can be stored in the iron storage proteins ferritin or hemosiderin. Ferritin is the primary iron storage protein, but at

243

higher concentrations, iron is also stored in hemosiderin.[36]

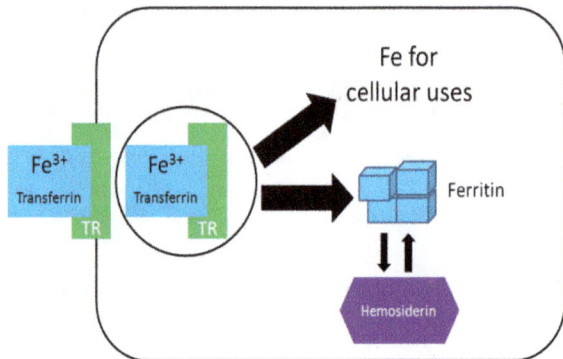

Figure 414. Fates of iron within cells

There are three major compartments of iron in the body[22]:

1. Functional Iron
2. Storage Iron
3. Transport Iron

Functional iron consists of iron performing some function. There are three functional iron sub compartments.

1. Haemoglobin
2. Myoglobin
3. Iron-containing enzymes

The functions of these sub-compartments are discussed in the next section.

Iron Stores consist of:

1. Ferritin
2. Hemosiderin

The liver is the primary storage site in the body, with the spleen and bone marrow being the other major storage sites.

Circulating iron is the iron found in transferrin.[22]

The following table shows how much iron is distributed among the different compartments.[22]

Table 49. Iron Distribution in adults (mg Fe/kg body weight)

	Men	Women
Functional iron		
Haemoglobin	32	28
Myoglobin	5	4
Fe-containing enzymes	1-2	1-2
Storage iron		
Ferritin and hemosiderin	~11	~6
Transport iron		
Transferrin	0.04	0.04

The majority of iron is in the functional iron compartment. The figure below further reinforces this point, showing that most of iron is found in red blood cells (haemoglobin) and tissues (myoglobin).[3]

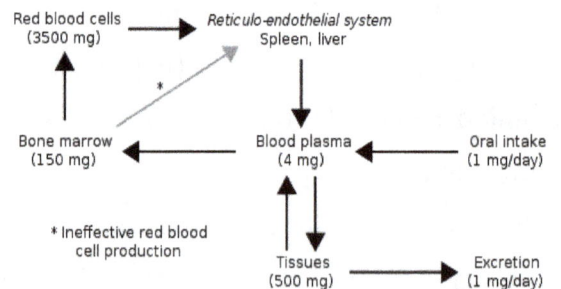

Figure 415. Iron distribution in different compartments

Also, notice how small oral intake and excretion are compared to the amount found in the different compartments in the body. As a result, iron recycling is important, because red blood cells only live for 120 days. Red blood cells are broken down in the liver, spleen, and bone marrow and the iron can be used for the same purposes as described earlier: cellular use, storage, or transported to another tissue on transferrin.[36] Most of this iron will be used for haeme and ultimately red blood cell synthesis. The figure below summarizes the potential uses of iron recycled from red blood cells.

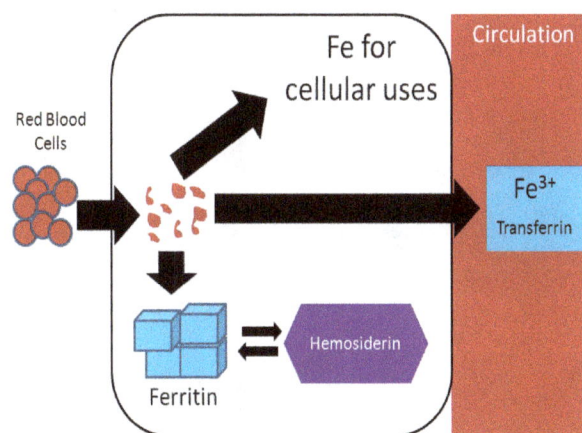

Figure 416. Iron recycling from red blood cells

Iron is unique among minerals in that our body has limited excretion ability. Thus, absorption is controlled by the hormone hepcidin. The liver has an iron sensor so when iron levels get high, this sensor signals for the release of hepcidin. Hepcidin causes degradation of ferroportin. Thus, the iron is not allowed to be transported into circulation.[101]

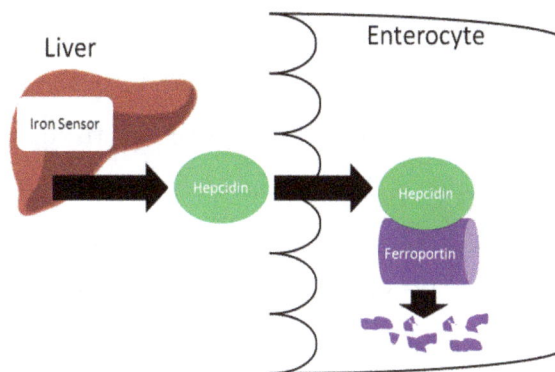

Figure 417. Action of hepcidin

The iron is trapped in the enterocyte, which is eventually sloughed off and excreted in faeces. Thus, iron absorption is decreased through the action of hepcidin.[101]

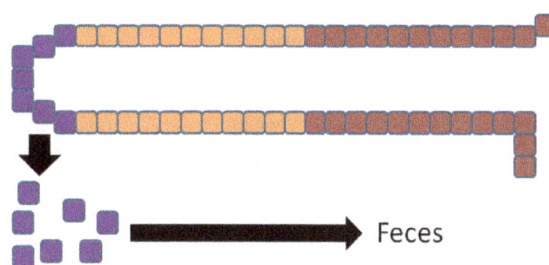

Figure 418. Enterocytes are sloughed off the villus and unless digested and their components reabsorbed, they will be excreted in faeces (feces in US image above)

11.7.4 Iron Functions

As we talked about in the previous subsection, there are three primary functional iron sub-compartments.

1. Haemoglobin
2. Myoglobin
3. Iron-containing enzymes

Haemoglobin contains haeme that is responsible for red blood cells' red colour. Haemoglobin carries oxygen to tissues. Myoglobin is like haemoglobin in that it can bind oxygen. However, instead of being found in blood, it is found in muscle. The colour of meat products is a result of that myoglobin.

There are several enzymes that use iron as a cofactor.

Iron is a cofactor for the antioxidant enzyme catalase that converts hydrogen peroxide to water, as shown below.

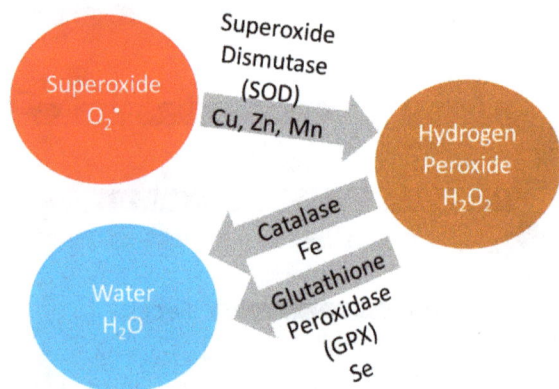

Figure 419. Catalase uses iron as a cofactor

Iron is also a cofactor for proline and lysyl hydroxylases that are important in collagen cross-linking. This is discussed in greater depth in the vitamin C section. The function of these enzymes is shown below.

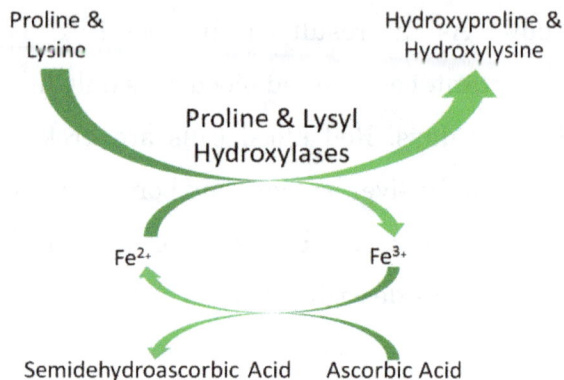

Figure 420. Importance of ascorbic acid to proline and lysyl hydroxylases

Haeme iron is also found in cytochromes, like cytochrome c in the electron transport chain.[36]

11.7.5 Iron Deficiency & Toxicity

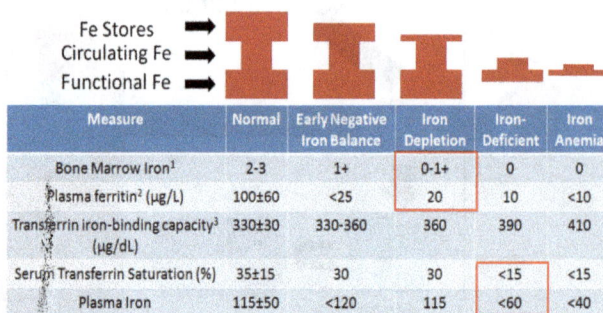

Measure	Normal	Early Negative Iron Balance	Iron Depletion	Iron-Deficient	Iron Anemia
Bone Marrow Iron[1]	2-3	1+	0-1+	0	0
Plasma ferritin[2] (μg/L)	100±60	<25	20	10	<10
Transferrin iron-binding capacity[3] (μg/dL)	330±30	330-360	360	390	410
Serum Transferrin Saturation (%)	35±15	30	30	<15	<15
Plasma Iron	115±50	<120	115	<60	<40

[1] Great measure, but invasive

[2] Small amounts are released from liver, bone, and spleen – proportional to body stores

[3] Also referred to as Total iron-binding capacity

The most common measures of iron status are haemoglobin concentrations and haematocrit (described below) levels. A decreased amount of either measure indicates iron deficiency, but these two measures are among the last to reflect the development of iron deficiency. This is because, as you can see in the figure above, circulating iron (plasma iron) levels aren't altered until you reach iron deficiency. Thus, other measures are likely better choices.[36]

The haematocrit, as illustrated in the figure below, is a measure of the proportion of red blood cells (erythrocytes) as compared to all other components of blood. The components are separated by a centrifuge. The red blood cells remain at the bottom of the tube. They can be quantified by measuring the packed cell volume (PCV) relative to the total whole blood volume.

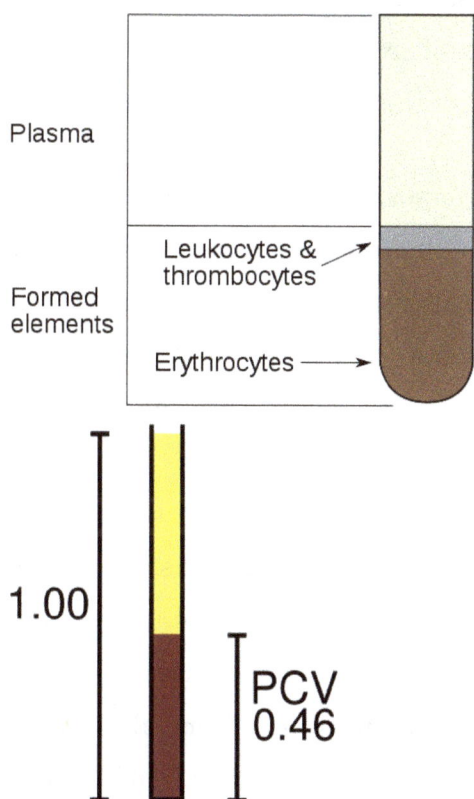

Figure 421. Haematocrit figures[lxv]

One of the best measures of iron status is bone marrow iron, but this is an invasive measure and is therefore not commonly used. Plasma ferritin, the iron storage protein, is also found in lower amounts in the blood (plasma) and is a good indicator of iron stores. Thus, it is a sensitive measure to determine if someone is in negative iron balance or iron depleted. It is not as useful a measure beyond this stage because the iron stores have already been exhausted. Transferrin iron binding capacity (aka total iron binding capacity), as it sounds, is a measure of how much iron transferrin can bind. An increase in transferrin iron binding capacity indicates deficiency (>400 indicates deficiency). But the best measure for deficiency or anaemia is either percent serum transferrin saturation or plasma iron. A lower % saturation means that less of the transferrin are saturated or carrying the maximum amount of iron that they can handle. Plasma iron is easily understood as the amount of iron within the plasma.[36] Iron deficiency is the most common nutritional deficiency worldwide, estimated to affect 1.6 billion people. In the so-called developed nations, it is less common, but an estimated 10% of toddlers and women of childbearing age are deficient. Deficiency often results in a microcytic (small cell), hypochromic (low colour) anaemia, that is a result of decreased haemoglobin production. With decreased haemoglobin, the red blood cells cannot carry as much oxygen and without decreased oxygen energy metabolism slows. A person with this anaemia feels fatigued, weak, apathetic, and can experience headaches.[18] Other side effects include decreased immune function and delayed cognitive development in children.[15]

Those who are at greater risk are[15, 36]:

- Women of childbearing age—because of losses due to menstruation
- Pregnant women—because of increased blood volume
- Vegetarians—because they do not consume haeme iron sources
- Infants—because they have low iron stores that can quickly be depleted

Thus, recommended daily allowances reflect the increased demands for women compared to men.[98]

- Women of reproductive age   18 mg/day

- Pregnancy   27 mg/day
- Men   8 mg/day

To put this in perspective, 100 g of beef contains ~3 mg of iron. Thus, it can be a challenge for some women to meet their iron requirements. The RDA committee in the US also estimates the iron requirements to be 80% and 70% higher for vegans and endurance athletes, respectively. The increased requirement for endurance athletes is based on loss due to "foot strike haemolysis", or the increased rupture of red blood cells due to the striking of the foot on hard surfaces.[90]

Overt iron toxicity is rare in adults but can occur in children who consume too many supplements containing iron. Symptoms of this acute toxicity include nausea, vomiting, and diarrhea.[15] Additionally approximately 3-10 out of 1000 newborns[102] are born with the genetic condition, haemochromatosis. In this condition, there is a mutation in a protein in the enterocyte that prevents the normal decrease of intestinal iron absorption. Without this protein these individuals cannot decrease iron absorption. Since the body cannot excrete iron, it accumulates in tissues, ultimately resulting in organ failure.[36]

Sub-clinical iron overload is considered to be a risk-factor for conditions such as heart disease and cancer,[103] possibly due to pro-oxidant effects but its prevalence is not well described in the literature, with the exception of dietary iron-overload in sub-Saharan Africa due to the high intakes of traditional beers with high iron content.

11.8 Zinc

Animal products account for most of the zinc consumed in western nations. Approximately 70% of the zinc North Americans' consume is from animal products[15] and this amount is similar to Australia and New Zealand [REF]. An estimated 15-40% of consumed zinc is absorbed.[18] Zinc is taken up into the enterocyte through the Zir-and Irt-like protein 4 (ZIP4). Once inside the enterocyte, zinc can:

1. Bind to the zinc storage protein thionein. Once thionein has bound a mineral (or a metal) it is known as metallothionein.
2. Be used for functional purposes.
3. Bind to the cysteine-rich intestinal protein (CRIP) where it is shuttled to a zinc transporter (ZnT), after moving through, zinc primarily

binds to the circulating protein albumin.[36]

These functions are represented in the figure below.

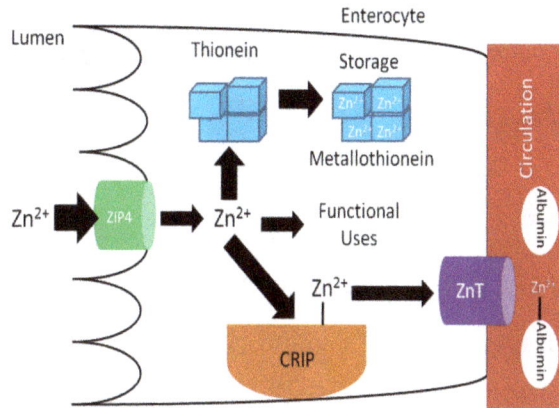

Figure 422. Fates of zinc once it is taken up into the enterocyte

The zinc attached to albumin is transported to the liver through the portal vein. There is not a major storage site of zinc, but there are pools of zinc in the liver, bone, pancreas, and kidney.[36] Zinc is primarily excreted in faeces.

There are some similarities in how zinc and iron are absorbed. Increased zinc consumption results in increased thionein synthesis in the enterocyte. As a result, more zinc is bound to thionein (forming metallothionein) and not used for functional uses or transported into circulation, as represented by the thick and thin arrows in the figure below.

249

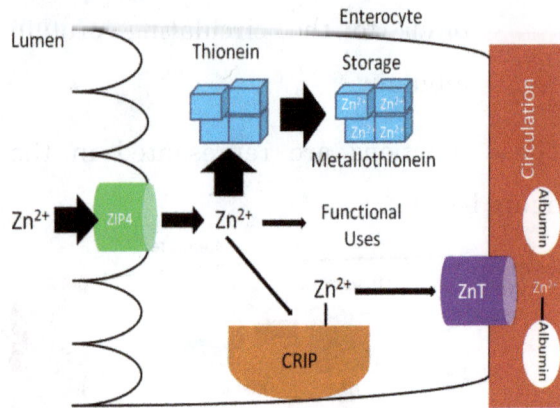

Figure 423. Fate of zinc under high zinc status

The enterocytes are then sloughed off preventing the bound zinc from being absorbed.

There are several inhibitors of zinc absorption, similarly to the other minerals like iron:

- Phytate (phytic acid), which inhibits calcium and iron absorption, also binds to and inhibits zinc absorption.[36]

- Oxalate (spinach, rhubarb, sweet potatoes, and dried beans)[36]

- Non-haeme iron also inhibits zinc absorption.

In supplements, zinc is found in several forms, such as[36, 104]:

- Zinc oxide - 80% zinc

- Zinc chloride - 23% zinc

- Zinc sulphate - 23% zinc

- Zinc gluconate - 14.3% zinc

Zinc oxide is the least bioavailable form, but since it is 80% zinc, it is commonly used in supplements.[104]

11.8.1 Zinc Functions

Zinc is a cofactor for up to 300 enzymes in the body. Enzymes that use zinc as a cofactor are known as metalloenzymes. Some examples include:

Zinc is a cofactor for the antioxidant enzyme superoxide dismutase that converts superoxide to hydrogen peroxide, as shown below.

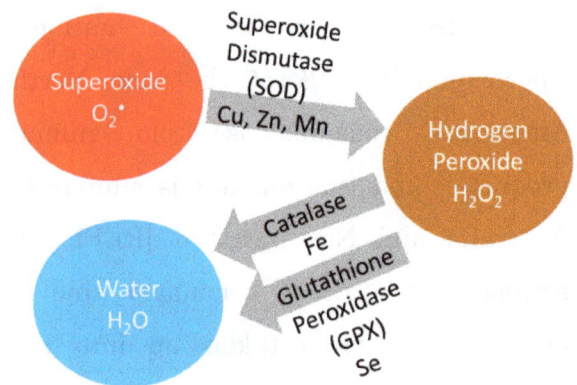

Figure 424. Superoxide dismutase uses zinc as a cofactor

Alcohol dehydrogenase uses four zincs per enzyme. Its role in ethanol metabolism is shown below.[36]

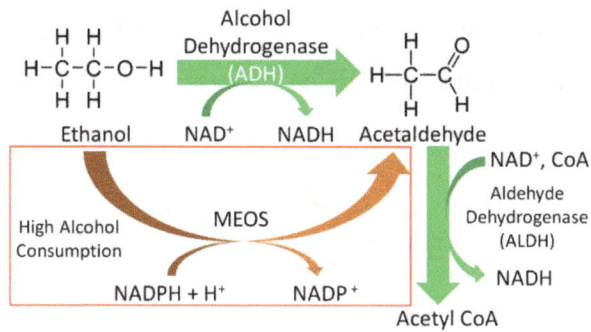

MEOS – Microsomal Ethanol Oxidizing System

Figure 425. Ethanol metabolism

Delta-aminolevulinic acid dehydratase (ALA dehydrogenase), which is involved in haeme synthesis, uses eight zincs enzymes to form porphobilinogen.

The enzyme that cleaves the extra glutamates from folate so that it can be taken up into the enterocyte is a metalloenzyme.[36] The cleavage of folate is shown in the figure below.

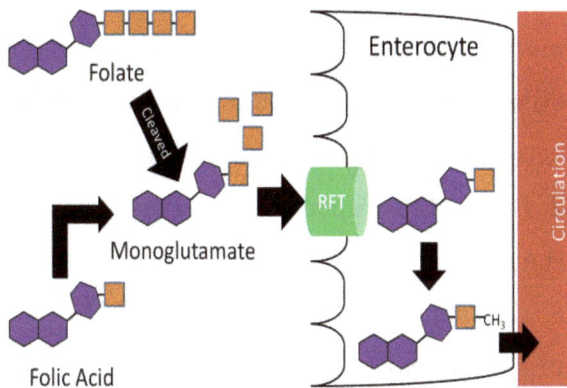

Figure 426. The absorption of folate and folic acid

Other notable metalloenzymes include DNA and RNA polymerase.[36]

Zinc is also important for the formation of zinc fingers in proteins. Zinc fingers help proteins bind to DNA.[36]

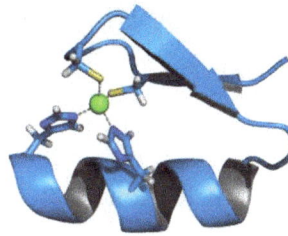

Figure 427. Structure of a zinc finger. Zinc is the green atom bound in the centre[lxvi]

Figure 11.815 Structure of a zinc finger, zinc is the green atom bound in the center[6]

Zinc is also important for growth, immune function, and reproduction.[36]

A recent Cochrane review concluded that when taken within 24 hours of the onset of symptoms, that zinc lozenges or syrup results in a significant decrease in the duration and severity of common cold symptoms.[105] Thus, commonly used zinc lozenges may be an effective way to combat the common cold. However, large intakes of zinc can be problematic for copper and ultimately iron levels in the body, as described in the last copper subsection.

11.8.2 Zinc Deficiency & Toxicity

A frank zinc deficiency is rare in the developed world but evidence suggests that many people, around 25% overall and

45% of men, do not consume enough zinc from diet alone.[106]

At particular risk are children, pregnant women, elderly and the poor.[15] Symptoms of zinc deficiency include[15, 36]:

- Growth retardation
- Delayed sexual maturation
- Dermatitis
- Hair loss
- Impaired immune function Skeletal abnormalities

A cause of zinc deficiency is mutation of ZIP4 that results in the condition acrodermatitis enteropathica. Without ZIP4, zinc cannot be taken up efficiently into the enterocyte. This condition is managed by administering very high levels of zinc, some of which is absorbed through other mechanisms.[36]

Zinc toxicity is not common, but an acute toxicity results in[15]:

- Nausea
- Vomiting
- Intestinal cramps
- Diarrhoea

An acute toxicity can occur with high-dose zinc supplementation, especially in those trying to avoid the effects of a cold, the primary symptoms being nausea and intestinal cramps.

Chronic toxicity can result in copper deficiency, as will be discussed in the last copper subsection.[36]

11.9 Copper

Like iron, copper is found in 2 forms:

1. Cupric (Cu^{2+}), oxidized

2. Cuprous (Cu^{1+}), reduced

Cu^{1+} is the form that is primarily absorbed, thus Cu^{2+} is reduced to Cu^{1+} in the lumen. It is believed that, like iron, enzymatic reduction of Cu^{2+} is stimulated by ascorbate (vitamin C). The exact transporter that takes up the copper into the enterocyte is not known. It may be DMT1 that takes up non-haeme iron. Once inside the enterocyte, Cu^{1+} can[36]:

1. Bind to thionein to form metallothionein. While zinc is a better stimulator of thionein levels, copper is actually a more avid binder to this protein.

2. Be used for functional uses discussed in the next subsection

3. Transported across the cell by an unknown carrier and then exported by ATP7A, an ATPase transporter.

Like zinc, copper is transported through the portal vein to the liver bound to albumin, as shown below. Albumin has a high affinity for Cu^{2+}, so Cu^{1+} is oxidized before transported to albumin through ATP7A, as illustrated below.

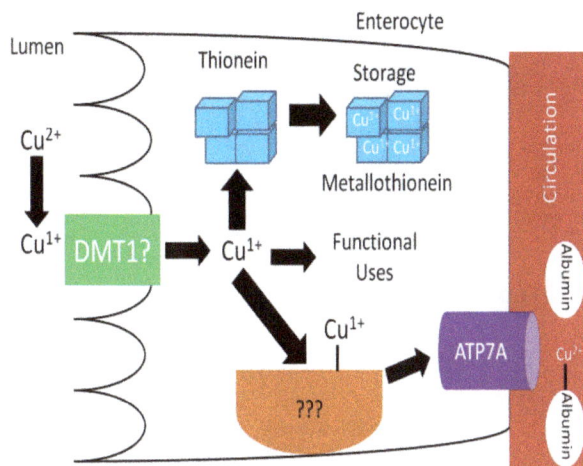

Figure 428. Copper absorption

Like zinc, there is not much storage of copper in the body. The liver is the primary site of storage, where copper is taken up through an unknown transporter. If it is going to be stored, it will bind with thionein to form metallothionein. Copper to be sent out to the body is transferred to the copper transport protein ceruloplasmin, which can bind 6 coppers/protein as shown below.[36]

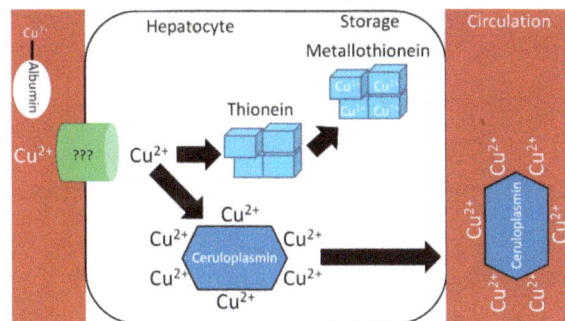

Figure 429. Copper in the hepatocyte

Legumes, whole grains, nuts, shellfish, and seeds are good sources of copper.[18] It is estimated that over 50% of copper consumed is absorbed.[36] Copper is primarily excreted in the faeces.

There are number of different forms of copper used in supplements:

- Copper sulphate (25% copper)
- Cupric chloride (47% copper)
- Cupric acetate (35% copper)
- Copper carbonate (57% copper)
- Cupric oxide (80% copper)

All these forms of copper are bioavailable, except cupric oxide. Assays have shown that it is not absorbed at all. Nevertheless, some supplements still use this form of copper.[36, 107]

11.9.1 Copper Functions

Copper has several functions that are described and shown below.

Two copper-containing proteins, ceruloplasmin and hephaestin, oxidize Fe^{2+} to Fe^{3+}. Fe^{3+} is the form that binds to transferrin, as shown below.[36]

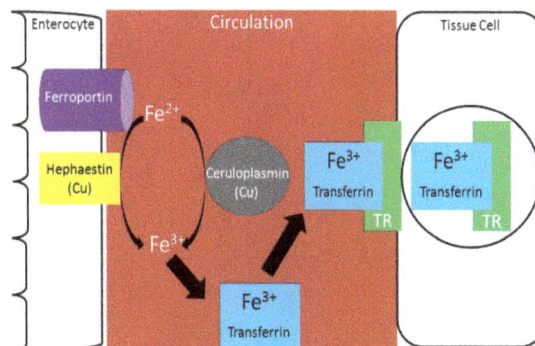

Figure 430. Transport and uptake of iron

253

Because copper is needed for this function, it is important for iron absorption.

Copper is also a cofactor for superoxide dismutase, which converts superoxide to hydrogen peroxide, as shown below.

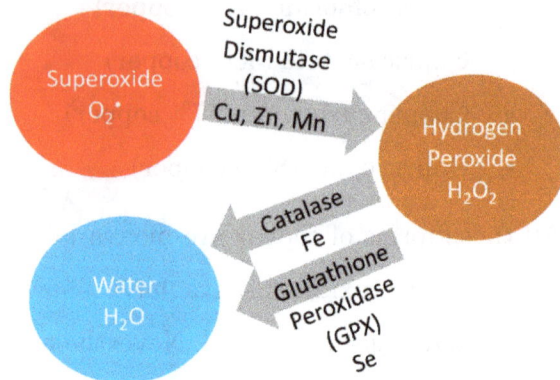

Figure 431. Superoxide dismutase uses zinc as a cofactor

Copper is also needed for hormone synthesis. For example, it is a cofactor for dopamine beta-hydroxylase, which converts dopamine to norepinephrine, as shown below.[36]

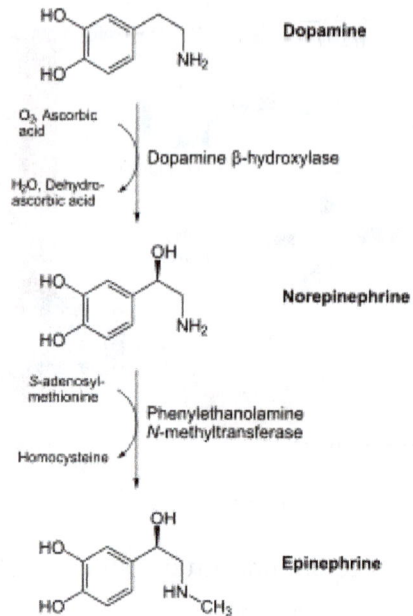

Figure 432. Dopamine beta-hydroxylase requires copper

The pathway below has been discussed in the vitamin C functions subsection. Ascorbic acid reduces Cu^{2+} back to Cu^{1+} so that this enzyme can continue to function, as shown below.[36] This is analogous to how ascorbic acid reduces Fe^{3+} back to Fe^{2+} so proline and lysyl hydroxylases can continue to function.

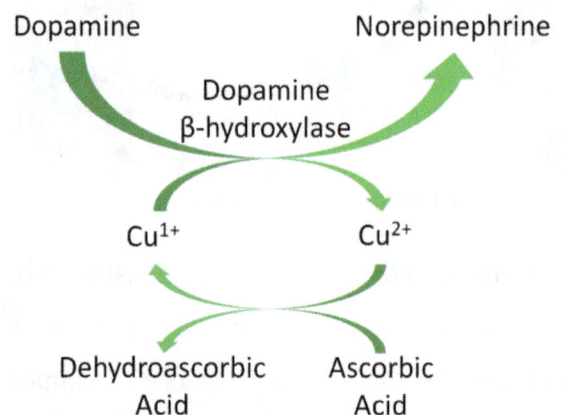

Figure 433. Dopamine beta-hydroxylase

Cytochrome c oxidase (complex IV) in the electron transport chain is a copper-containing enzyme that reduces oxygen to form water.[36]

Lysyl oxidase, an enzyme that is important for cross-linking between structural proteins (collagen and elastin) requires copper as a cofactor.[36]

11.9.2 Copper Deficiency & Toxicity

Copper deficiency is rare in humans, but results in the following symptoms[15, 36]:

- Hypochromic anaemia
- Decreased white blood cell counts leading to decreased immune function
- Bone abnormalities

Copper deficiency can result in a secondary iron deficiency, since Fe^{2+} cannot be oxidized to Fe^{3+} to bind to transferrin. This can cause the hypochromic anaemia that occurs in iron deficiency.

Menke's disease is a genetic disorder that results in copper deficiency. It is believed that individuals with this disease have a mutation in ATP7A that prevents copper from leaving the enterocyte, thus preventing absorption.[36]

Copper toxicity is also rare in humans, but acute toxicity results in the following symptoms[15, 36]:

- Nausea
  Vomiting
- diarrhoea
- Abdominal pain

Chronic symptoms include[15, 36]:

- Brain, liver, and kidney damage
- Neurological damage

Wilson's disease is a genetic disorder where a mutation in ATP7B prevents copper excretion, resulting in copper toxicity. One notable symptom is that individuals with this disease have golden to greenish-brown Kayser-Fleischer rings around the edges of the cornea.[15, 36]

11.9.3 How High Zinc Intake Can Lead to Copper & Iron Deficiencies

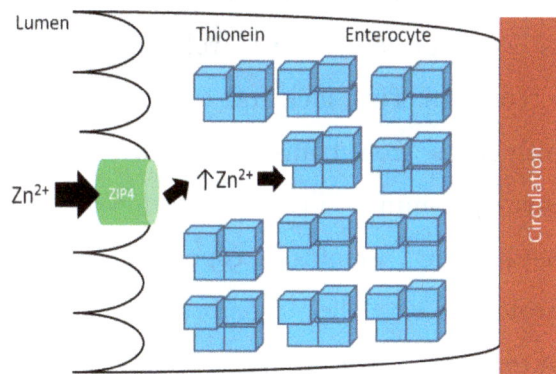

Figure 434. Zinc increases thionein production

The elevated levels of thionein will bind any copper that is taken up into the enterocyte (as metallothionein), "trapping" the copper in the enterocyte and preventing it from being absorbed into circulation, as shown below.

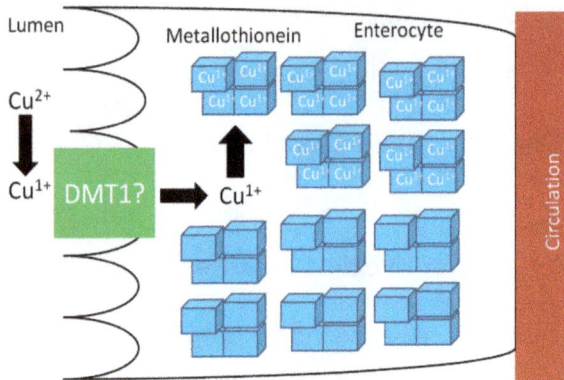

Figure 435. Copper taken up into the enterocyte is bound to thionein forming metallothionein

The enterocytes containing the "trapped" copper move up the crypt and are sloughed off and excreted in faeces. The copper consumed essentially is lost from the body through this process.

Without adequate copper being transported to the liver, no ceruloplasmin is produced and released into circulation. The lack of copper further influences iron transport by decreasing ceruloplasmin in circulation and hephaestin (another copper-containing protein) on the membrane of the enterocyte. These proteins normally convert Fe^{2+} to Fe^{3+} so that iron can bind to transferrin.

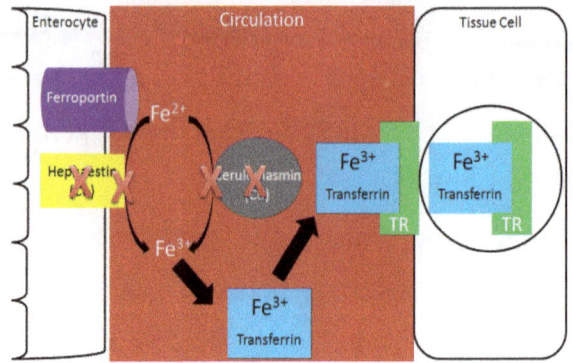

Figure 436. Lack of copper means that hephaestin and ceruloplasmin aren't available to oxidize Fe^{2+} to Fe^{3+}

Without hephaestin and ceruloplasmin, Fe^{3+} is not formed from Fe^{2+}. As a result, Fe^{2+} is "trapped" in the enterocyte because it can't bind to transferrin as shown below.

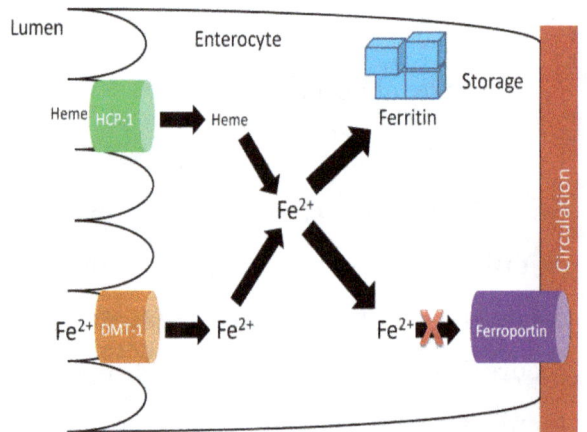

Figure 437. Fe^{2+} is trapped in the enterocyte

The enterocytes containing the "trapped" iron move up the crypt and are also sloughed off and excreted in faeces. The iron consumed essentially is lost from the body through this process.

In summary, high zinc intake increases thionein production, which traps all copper; the lack of copper decreases circulating ceruloplasmin and hephaestin, which causes all iron to be trapped as well. This example illustrates the interconnectedness of zinc, copper, and iron.

12 Electrolyte Micronutrients

In this chapter electrolytes will be explained generally along with further explanation about the electrolyte minerals. Hypertension will be discussed in brief, along with explanations of how the electrolyte minerals affect this condition.

12.1 Electrolytes

Electrolytes are compounds that separate into ions (molecules with a charge) in water. Electrolytes can be separated into two classes:

- Cations: ions that have a positive charge
- Anions: ions that have a negative charge

The following table summarises the major intracellular and extracellular electrolytes by giving their milliequivalents (mEq)/L.[15, 18] Milliequivalents are a measure of charge. Thus, a higher value means that the cation or anion is accounting for more charge.

Table 50. *Major intracellular and extracellular electrolytes*

Cations	Anions	Cations	Anions
Potassium (K^+) 150*	Phosphate (PO^{4-}) 104	Sodium (Na^+) 142	Chloride (Cl^-) 103
Magnesium (Mg^{2+}) 40	Proteins 57		Bicarbonate (HCO^{3-}) 27
	Sulphate (SO_4^{2-}) 20		Proteins 16

*mEq/L

The following figure graphically shows the major intracellular and extracellular cations (green) and anions (red).[18]

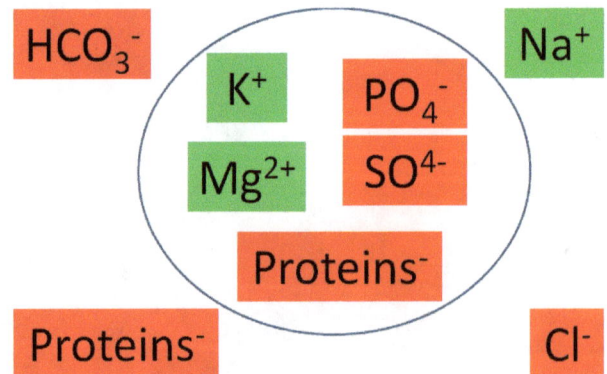

Figure 438. *Major intracellular and extracellular cations (green) and anions (red)*

Electrolytes, along with proteins are critical for preserving appropriate fluid balance in the body. Your body is 60% water by weight. Two-thirds of this water is intracellular, or within cells. One-third of the water is extracellular, or outside of cells. A quarter of the extracellular fluid is plasma, while the other three quarters is interstitial (between cells) fluid. Thus, when considering total body water, 66% is intracellular fluid, 25% is interstitial fluid, and 8% is plasma.[36,4]

Fluid distribution between the different compartments are shown below.[36]

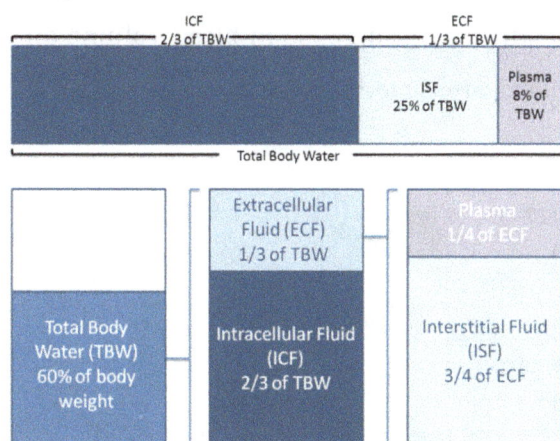

Figure 439. Distribution of fluid in the body[lxvii]

12.2 Sodium

Salt (NaCl) contributes almost all the sodium that people consume. In the United States for example, 75-85% of the salt consumed is from processed foods while only around 10% is that naturally occurring in foods. Of course, a diet that is lower in refined and processed foods will derive less sodium from those sources and more from natural foods, however, the total sodium intake is also going to be a lot lower. Added salt contributes around 10-15% of salt in the diet.[15]

95-100% of consumed sodium is absorbed.[36] Sodium is taken up into the enterocyte through multiple mechanisms before being pumped out of the enterocyte by sodium-potassium (Na^+/K^+) ATPase. Sodium-potassium ATPase is an active carrier transporter that pumps three sodium ions out of the cell and two potassium ions into the cell, as shown below.

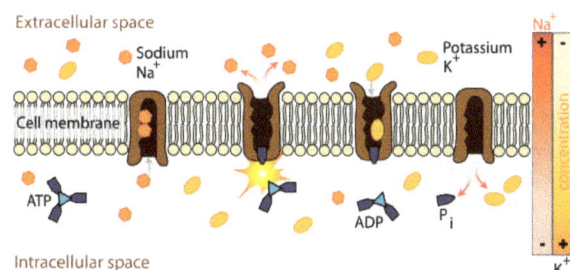

Figure 440. Sodium-potassium ATPase (aka sodium-potassium pump) an active carrier transporter[lxviii]

Sodium is the major cation in extracellular fluid.

Sodium has three main functions[15]:

1. Fluid balance
2. Aids in monosaccharide and amino acid absorption

---

lxvii Adapted by Brian Lindshiled from http://www.netterimages.com/image/21248.htm

lxviii Public Domain by LadyHats https://en.wikipedia.org/wiki/File:Scheme_sodium-potassium_pump-en.svg

3. Muscle contraction and nerve transmission

12.2.1.1 Fluid balance

The body regulates sodium and fluid levels through a series of processes as shown below. A decrease in plasma volume and blood pressure signals the kidney to release the enzyme renin. Renin activates angiotensin that is converted to angiotensin II. Angiotensin II signals the adrenal glands to secrete the hormone aldosterone. Aldosterone increases sodium reabsorption in the kidney, thus decreasing sodium excretion. These actions cause plasma sodium concentrations to increase, which is detected by the hypothalamus. The hypothalamus stimulates the pituitary gland to release antidiuretic hormone (ADH) that causes the kidneys to reabsorb water, decreasing water excretion. The net results is an increase in blood volume and blood pressure.[15]

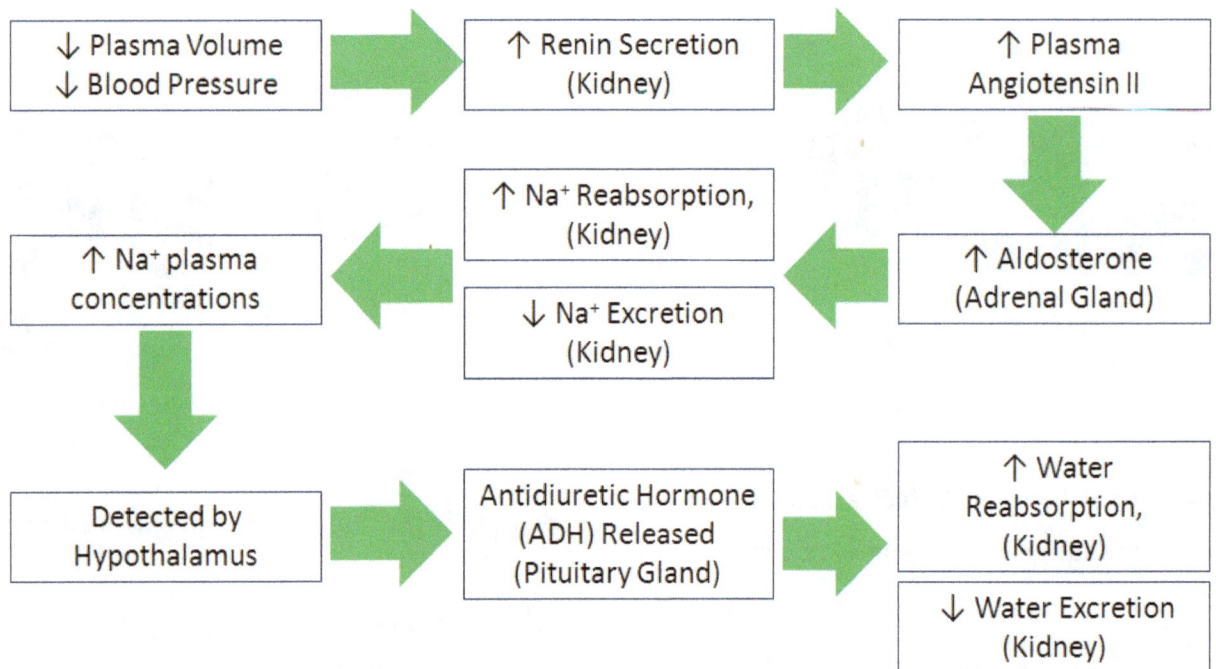

Figure 441. Response to decreased plasma volume and blood pressure

12.2.1.2 Aids in monosaccharide and amino acid absorption

Glucose and galactose are taken up into the enterocyte by sodium-glucose cotransporter 1 (SGLT1), which requires sodium to be transported along with glucose or galactose.

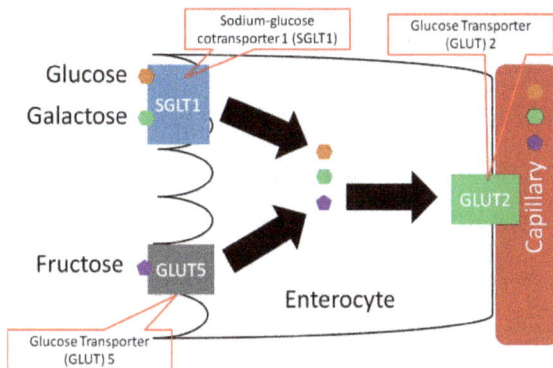

Figure 442. Carbohydrate absorption

Amino acids are taken up and transported into circulation through a variety of amino acid transporters. Some of these transporters are sodium-dependent (require sodium to transport amino acids).

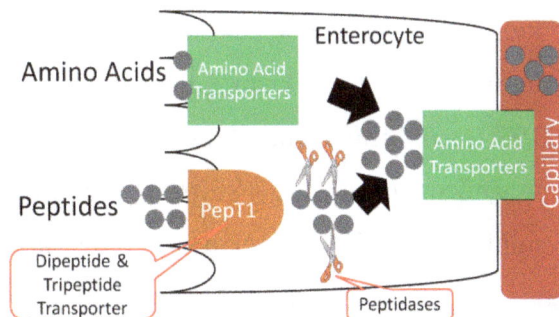

Figure 443. Protein absorption

Sodium deficiency is rare and is normally due to excessive sweating. Sweat loss

must reach 2-3% of body weight before sodium losses are a concern.[15, 36] This situation though can occur relatively easily in endurance activities (such as in marathon runners and ultra-marathon runners) and in those exercising for long periods of time in extremely hot and humid conditions. The conditions of low blood sodium levels are known as hyponatraemia. This condition can result in[15]:

- Headache
- Nausea
- Vomiting
- Fatigue
- Muscle Cramps

At its severest hyponatraemia can seriously damage neurons of the brain and central nervous system and ultimately can be fatal if not corrected. Sodium is not toxic, but higher sodium intakes are correlated with cardiovascular disease risk. This does not however mean that high sodium intakes cause heart disease. This is because blood pressure is used as a surrogate for cardiovascular health. Adequate Intakes (AI) and the tolerable Upper Limit (UL) for sodium as set by the Institutes of Medicine of the United States National Academies[108] is based upon this correlation. Reducing salt intake reduces blood pressure by only 1 and 3.5%[9] and this is unlikely to be clinically significant (although even minor increases of blood pressure may increase risk of cerebral vascular damage). The evidence linking salt (sodium) reduction with improved mortality and morbidity is lacking.

A 2011 meta-analysis of RCTs of at least 6 months did not find evidence for reduced mortality or CVD mortality and concluded that there was no evidence available to support dietary advice to reduce salt intake. In addition, they noted an *increase* in all-cause mortality in those with heart failure who were advised to reduce their intake.[109]

Although not supporting that low sodium intakes were positively correlated with morbidity or mortality in general, the Institute of Medicine of the National Academies *Sodium Intake in Populations: Assessment of Evidence*[110] noted that the evidence suggests that outcomes for those with congestive heart failure are worsened by reductions in sodium and suggested a risk of adverse health outcomes associated with sodium intake levels in ranges approximating 1,500 to 2,300 mg per day in other disease-specific population subgroups, specifically those with diabetes, chronic kidney disease (CKD), or pre-existing CVD, and noted no significant correlation between improved health outcomes and reductions in dietary sodium.

Mortality and morbidity are increased at both high and low levels of sodium intake suggesting a 'U-curve' of morbidity related to extremes of intake (consistent with normal outcome curves for deficiencies/toxicities of other nutrients). The range within which no discernible health effects are seen lies between 2,645 and 4,945 mg.[112] The average intake of sodium in New Zealand has been estimated at 3900mg per day,[113] a level well within the range indicated as having no effect (positive or negative) on mortality and morbidity.

Iodised salt has played a vital role in reducing iodine deficiency and goitre in New Zealand. Dietary exposure to iodine has steadily decreased since 1982.[70] Thomson in a review of selenium and iodine status in New Zealand, found that iodine levels have been falling since the 1980's, and this is correlated with clinical measures of thyroid status, and that public health interventions to reduce salt intake may further reduce iodine status.[71]

12.3 Chloride

Sodium's partner in salt, chloride, is the major extracellular anion. Almost all the chloride we consume is from salt, and almost all chloride is absorbed. It is excreted in urine like sodium.

Chloride has the following functions[15]:

1. Aids in nerve impulses
2. Component of HCl
3. Released by white blood cells to kill foreign substances
4. Helps maintain acid-base balance

Chloride deficiency is rare but can occur because of severe diarrhoea or vomiting. Other symptoms of this deficiency include[15, 36]:

- Weakness
- Diarrhoea and vomiting
- Lethargy

Chloride is not toxic and since it is a component of salt (NaCl) intakes should be correlated with a healthy intake of sodium (as discussed in the section on sodium).

12.4 Potassium

Potassium is the major intracellular cation. Good sources of potassium include beans, potatoes (with skin), milk products, orange juice, tomato juice, and bananas.[15, 18] Potassium, like sodium and chloride, is well absorbed. Greater than 85% of consumed potassium is absorbed. Potassium is primarily excreted in urine (~90%).[36]

Potassium is important for:

1. Fluid Balance
2. Nerve transmission and muscle contraction

Increased potassium intake results in decreased calcium excretion. This is the opposite effect of increased sodium intake, which increases calcium excretion.[15]

Potassium deficiency is rare but can be fatal. Symptoms include:

- Weakness
- Fatigue
- Constipation
- Irregular heartbeat (can be fatal)

Deficiency can occur in individuals that are on diuretics, drugs that increase urine production, and individuals with eating disorders.[15]

Toxicity is also extremely rare, only occurring if there is a problem with kidney function. Symptoms of toxicity are irregular heartbeat and even cardiac arrest.[15]

12.5 Magnesium

Magnesium is an electrolyte, but that is not considered its major function in the body. Green leafy vegetables, beans, nuts, seeds, and whole grains are good sources of magnesium.[15, 90] Magnesium is absorbed moderately well with 40-60% of consumed magnesium absorbed at normal levels of intake. Magnesium is excreted primarily in urine.[36]

55-60% of magnesium in the body is found in bone.[36] Some (30%) of this bone magnesium is believed to be exchangeable, or can be used to maintain blood concentrations, similar to how calcium in bones can be used to maintain blood concentrations.

Magnesium helps to stabilize ATP and nucleotides by binding to phosphate groups. Magnesium plays a role in over 300 enzymes in the body. Here is a list of some of the physiological processes that magnesium participates in[36]:

- Glycolysis
- TCA cycle
- Fatty acid oxidation (beta-oxidation)
- DNA and RNA transcription
- Nucleotide synthesis
- Muscle contraction

Magnesium deficiency is rare but can be caused by prolonged diarrhoea or vomiting. Symptoms include[15]:

- Irregular heartbeat
- Muscle spasms
- Disorientation
- Seizures
- Nausea
- Vomiting

Magnesium toxicity is also rare but can occur from excessive use of antacids or laxatives. Symptoms include[36]:

- Diarrhoea
- Nausea
- Flushing
- Double vision
- Slurred speech
- Weakness
- Paralysis

Magnesium supplements differ in percent of magnesium in the different forms.

The bioavailability of magnesium oxide is significantly lower than magnesium chloride, magnesium lactate, and magnesium aspartate. The latter three are equally bioavailable.

Figures

Note: Images have been attributed wherever possible. Non-attributed figures are from the Public Domain. If there are any images you believe to not be in the public domain, or incorrectly used, please let us know.

Tables

References

1.   Reginster JY, Deroisy R, Rovati LC, Lee RL, Lejeune E, Bruyere O, et al. Long-term effects of glucosamine sulphate on osteoarthritis progression: a randomised, placebo-controlled clinical trial. The Lancet. 2001;357(9252):251-6.

2.   Fransen M, Agaliotis M, Nairn L, Votrubec M, Bridgett L, Su S, et al. Glucosamine and chondroitin for knee osteoarthritis: a double-blind randomised placebo-controlled clinical trial evaluating single and combination regimens. Annals of the Rheumatic Diseases. 2015;74(5):851-8.

3.   Herrero-Beaumont G, Román-Blas J, Castañeda S, Largo R, Blanco FJ. Chondroitin sulfate plus glucosamine sulfate does not show superiority over placebo in a randomised, double blind, placebo-controlled clinical trial in patients with knee osteoarthritis. Osteoarthritis and Cartilage.24:S48-S9.

4.   Merriam Webster Online Dictionary. Definition of nutrition | the process of eating the right kind of food so you can grow properly and be healthy. 2015.

5.   Levin KA. Study design III: Cross-sectional studies. Evid Based Dent. 2006;7(1):24-5.

6.   Artaud-Wild SM, Connor SL, Sexton G, Connor WE. Differences in coronary mortality can be explained by differences in cholesterol and saturated fat intakes in 40 countries but not in France and Finland. A paradox. Circulation. 1993;88(6):2771-9.

7.   Giovannucci E, Ascherio A, Rimm EB, Stampfer MJ, Colditz GA, Willett WC. Intake of carotenoids and retinol in relation to risk of prostate cancer. J Natl Cancer Inst. 1995;87(23):1767-76.

8.   Jeacocke NA, Burke LM. Methods to standardize dietary intake before performance testing. Int J Sport Nutr Exerc Metab. 2010;20(2):87-103.

9.   Graudal N, Hubeck Graudal T, Jurgens G. Effects of low sodium diet versus high sodium diet on blood pressure, renin, aldosterone, catecholamines, cholesterol, and triglyceride. Cochrane Database Syst Rev. 2011;11.

10.   Peto R, Doll R, Buckley JD, Sporn MB. Can dietary beta-carotene materially reduce human cancer rates? Nature. 1981;290(5803):201-8.

11.   Lobo GP, Amengual J, Palczewski G, Babino D, von Lintig J. Carotenoid-oxygenases: Key Players for Carotenoid Function and Homeostasis in Mammalian Biology. Biochimica et biophysica acta. 2012;1821(1):78-87.

12.   He FJ, Nowson CA, Lucas M, MacGregor GA. Increased consumption of fruit and vegetables is related to a reduced risk of coronary heart disease: meta-analysis of cohort studies. J Hum Hypertens. 2007;21(9):717-28.

13.   Dauchet L, Amouyel P, Hercberg S, Dallongeville J. Fruit and Vegetable Consumption and Risk of Coronary Heart Disease: A Meta-Analysis of Cohort Studies. The Journal of Nutrition. 2006;136(10):2588-93.

14.   Fulgoni V. High-fructose corn syrup: everything you wanted to know, but were afraid to ask. The American Journal of Clinical Nutrition. 2008;88(6):1715S.

15.   Beshgetoor D, Berning J, Moe G, Byrd-Bredbenner C. Wardlaw's Perspectives in Nutrition: McGraw-Hill Education; 2012.

16.   Byrd-Bredbenner C, Moe G, Beshgetoor D, Berning J, Kelley D. Wardlaw's Perspectives in Nutrition: A Functional Approach. 1st ed. USA: McGraw-Hill Higher Education; 2013. 976 p.

17.   Wardlaw GM, Insel PM. Perspectives in nutrition: Mosby; 1993.

18. Whitney EN, Rolfes SR. Understanding Nutrition: Cengage Learning; 2015.

19. Payne AN, Chassard C, Lacroix C. Gut microbial adaptation to dietary consumption of fructose, artificial sweeteners and sugar alcohols: implications for host–microbe interactions contributing to obesity. Obesity Reviews. 2012;13(9):799-809.

20. Raben A, Richelsen B. Artificial sweeteners: a place in the field of functional foods? Focus on obesity and related metabolic disorders. Current Opinion in Clinical Nutrition & Metabolic Care. 2012;15(6):597-604.

21. Shankar P, Ahuja S, Sriram K. Non-nutritive sweeteners: Review and update. Nutrition. 2013;29(11–12):1293-9.

22. Stipanuk MH, Caudill MA. Biochemical, Physiological, and Molecular Aspects of Human Nutrition: Elsevier Health Sciences; 2013.

23. Berg JM, Tymoczko JL, Stryer L. Biochemistry, Fifth Edition: W.H. Freeman; 2002.

24. Macronutrients ARP, Intakes SURLNIUDR, Intakes SCSEDR, Board FN, Medicine I. Dietary Reference Intakes for Energy, Carbohydrate, Fiber, Fat, Fatty Acids, Cholesterol, Protein, and Amino Acids (Macronutrients): National Academies Press; 2005.

25. Fiber PDD, Intakes SCSEDR, Board FN, Medicine I. Dietary Reference Intakes: Proposed Definition of Dietary Fiber: National Academies Press; 2001.

26. Marlett JA. Content and composition of dietary fiber in 117 frequently consumed foods. J Am Diet Assoc. 1992;92(2):175-86.

27. Bednar GE, Patil AR, Murray SM, Grieshop CM, Merchen NR, Fahey GC. Starch and Fiber Fractions in Selected Food and Feed Ingredients Affect Their Small Intestinal Digestibility and Fermentability and Their Large Bowel Fermentability In Vitro in a Canine Model. The Journal of Nutrition. 2001;131(2):276-86.

28. Fuentes-Zaragoza E, Riquelme-Navarrete MJ, Sánchez-Zapata E, Pérez-Álvarez JA. Resistant starch as functional ingredient: A review. Food Research International. 2010;43(4):931-42.

29. Young VR, Pellett PL. Plant proteins in relation to human protein and amino acid nutrition. The American Journal of Clinical Nutrition. 1994;59(5):1203S-12S.

30. WHO. Protein and Amino Acid Requirements in Human Nutrition. Geneva, Switzerland: World Health Organisation; 2007.

31. Hansen K, Shriver T, Schoeller D. The effects of exercise on the storage and oxidation of dietary fat. Sports Med. 2005;35.

32. Schaafsma G. The Protein Digestibility–Corrected Amino Acid Score. The Journal of Nutrition. 2000;130(7):1865S-7S.

33. Simopoulos A. Omega-3 fatty acids in health and disease and in growth and development. American Journal of Clinical Nutrition. 1991;54:438 - 63.

34. Arterburn LM, Hall EB, Oken H. Distribution, interconversion, and dose response of n-3 fatty acids in humans. Am J Clin Nutr. 2006;83(6 Suppl):1467S-76S.

35. Shils ME, Shike M. Modern Nutrition in Health and Disease: Lippincott Williams & Wilkins; 2006.

36. Gropper SS, Smith JL. Advanced Nutrition and Human Metabolism: Cengage Learning; 2012.

37. Guillot E, Vaugelade P, Lemarchali P, Re Rat A. Intestinal absorption and liver uptake of medium-chain fatty acids in non-anaesthetized pigs. British Journal of Nutrition. 1993;69(02):431-42.

38. McDonald GB, Saunders DR, Weidman M, Fisher L. Portal venous

transport of long-chain fatty acids absorbed from rat intestine1980 1980-09-01 00:00:00. G141-G50 p.

39. National Institutes of Health. NIH Human Microbiome Project defines normal bacterial makeup of the body 2015 [Available from: http://www.ncbi.nlm.nih.gov/pubmed/.

40. Health. Mo. New Zealand Health Survey. Wellington; 2013.

41. Foster-Powell K, Holt SH, Brand-Miller JC. International table of glycemic index and glycemic load values: 2002. The American Journal of Clinical Nutrition. 2002;76(1):5-56.

42. Fogelholm GM, Tikkanen HO, Näveri HK, Näveri LS, Härkönen MH. Carbohydrate loading in practice: high muscle glycogen concentration is not certain. British Journal of Sports Medicine. 1991;25(1):41-4.

43. Hamilton JA. Fatty acid transport: difficult or easy? Journal of Lipid Research. 1998;39(3):467-81.

44. Schonfeld P, Reiser G. Why does brain metabolism not favor burning of fatty acids to provide energy[quest] - Reflections on disadvantages of the use of free fatty acids as fuel for brain. J Cereb Blood Flow Metab. 2013;33(10):1493-9.

45. Kaleta C, de Figueiredo LF, Werner S, Guthke R, Ristow M, Schuster S. In Silico Evidence for Gluconeogenesis from Fatty Acids in Humans. PLoS Computational Biology. 2011;7(7):e1002116.

46. Kitabchi AE, Umpierrez GE, Miles JM, Fisher JN. Hyperglycemic crises in adult patients with diabetes. Diabetes Care. 2009;32(7):1335-43.

47. Thurston JH, Hauhart RE, Schiro JA. Beta-hydroxybutyrate reverses insulin-induced hypoglycemic coma in suckling-weanling mice despite low blood and brain glucose levels. Metabolic brain disease. 1986;1(1):63-82.

48. Owen OE, Morgan AP, Kemp HG, Sullivan JM, Herrera MG, Cahill GF, Jr. Brain Metabolism during Fasting*. The Journal of clinical investigation. 1967;46(10):1589-95.

49. Royer P. Periodic functional ketosis in children. Vie médicale (Paris, France: 1920). 1954;35(1):9.

50. Sargent F, Johnson RE, Robbins E, Sawyer L. THE EFFECTS OF ENVIRONMENT AND OTHER FACTORS ON NUTRITIONAL KETOSIS. Quarterly Journal of Experimental Physiology and Cognate Medical Sciences. 1958;43(4):345-51.

51. Krebs H. Biochemical aspects of ketosis. Proceedings of the Royal Society of Medicine. 1960;53(2):71.

52. Krebs HA. The regulation of the release of ketone bodies by the liver. Adv Enzyme Regul. 1966;4(0):339-53.

53. Volek JS, Phinney SD. The Art and Science of Low Carbohydrate Living: Beyond Obesity. New York, USA: Beyond Obesity; 2013.

54. Volek JS, Phinney SD. LOW CARBOHYDRATE LIVING. New York, USA: Beyond Obesity; 2011.

55. Speth JD, Spielmann KA. Energy source, protein metabolism, and hunter-gatherer subsistence strategies. Journal of Anthropological Archaeology. 1983;2(1):1-31.

56. Bilsborough S, Mann N. A review of issues of dietary protein intake in humans. International journal of sport nutrition and exercise metabolism. 2006(16):129-52.

57. Acheson KJ, Schutz Y, Bessard T, Anantharaman K, Flatt JP, Jéquier E. Glycogen storage capacity and de novo lipogenesis during massive carbohydrate overfeeding in man. The American Journal of Clinical Nutrition. 1988;48(2):240-7.

58. Carpenter KJ. A Short History of Nutritional Science: (1912-1944)2003.

59. Packer L, Weber SU, Rimbach G. Molecular aspects of alpha-tocotrienol antioxidant action and cell signalling. J Nutr. 2001;131(2):369S-73S.

60. Erdman JW, Ford NA, Lindshield BL. Are the health attributes of lycopene related to its antioxidant function? Archives of biochemistry and biophysics. 2009;483(2):229-35.

61. Waters DJ, Shen S, Glickman LT, Cooley DM, Bostwick DG, Qian J, et al. Prostate cancer risk and DNA damage: translational significance of selenium supplementation in a canine model. Carcinogenesis. 2005;26(7):1256-62.

62. Huang H-Y, Appel LJ. Supplementation of Diets with α-Tocopherol Reduces Serum Concentrations of γ- and δ-Tocopherol in Humans. The Journal of Nutrition. 2003;133(10):3137-40.

63. Traber MG, Elsner A, Brigelius-Flohe R. Synthetic as compared with natural vitamin E is preferentially excreted as alpha-CEHC in human urine: studies using deuterated alpha-tocopheryl acetates. FEBS Lett. 1998;437(1-2):145-8.

64. Wagner KH, Kamal-Eldin A, Elmadfa I. Gamma-Tocopherol – An Underestimated Vitamin? Annals of Nutrition and Metabolism. 2004;48(3):169-88.

65. Hemila H, Chalker E. Vitamin C for preventing and treating the common cold. The Cochrane database of systematic reviews. 2013;1:CD000980.

66. Li Y, Schellhorn HE. New developments and novel therapeutic perspectives for vitamin C. J Nutr. 2007;137(10):2171-84.

67. Di Lullo GA, Sweeney SM, Korkko J, Ala-Kokko L, San Antonio JD. Mapping the ligand-binding sites and disease-associated mutations on the most abundant protein in the human, type I collagen. J Biol Chem. 2002;277(6):4223-31.

68. Massey LK, Liebman M, Kynast-Gales SA. Ascorbate increases human oxaluria and kidney stone risk. J Nutr. 2005;135(7):1673-7.

69. Lindshield BL, Ford NA, Canene-Adams K, Diamond AM, Wallig MA, Erdman JW, Jr. Selenium, but not lycopene or vitamin E, decreases growth of transplantable dunning R3327-H rat prostate tumors. PLoS One. 2010;5(4):e10423.

70. Thomson BM, Vannoort RW, Haslemore RM. Dietary exposure and trends of exposure to nutrient elements iodine, iron, selenium and sodium from the 2003–4 New Zealand Total Diet Survey. British journal of nutrition. 2008;99(03):614-25.

71. Thomson CD. Selenium and iodine intakes and status in New Zealand and Australia. British Journal of Nutrition. 2004;91(05):661-72.

72. Sciences NAo. Dietary reference intakes for vitamin A, vitamin K, arsenic, boron, chromium, copper, iodine, iron, manganese, molybdenum, nickel, silicon, vanadium and zinc: National Academy of Sciences; 2004.

73. Said HM, Mohammed ZM. Intestinal absorption of water-soluble vitamins: an update. Curr Opin Gastroenterol. 2006;22(2):140-6.

74. Vosper H. Niacin: a re-emerging pharmaceutical for the treatment of dyslipidaemia. British Journal of Pharmacology. 2009;158(2):429-41.

75. Whelan AM, Jurgens TM, Naylor H. Herbs, vitamins and minerals in the treatment of premenstrual syndrome: a systematic review. Can J Clin Pharmacol. 2009;16(3):e407-29.

76. Winkels RM, Brouwer IA, Siebelink E, Katan MB, Verhoef P. Bioavailability of food folates is 80% of that of folic acid. The American Journal of Clinical Nutrition. 2007;85(2):465-73.

77.   Intakes ARotSCotSEoDR, its Panel on Folate OBVCSURLN, Board FN, Medicine I. Dietary Reference Intakes for Thiamin, Riboflavin, Niacin, Vitamin B6, Folate, Vitamin B12, Pantothenic Acid, Biotin, and Choline: National Academies Press; 2000.

78.   Evans SE, Mygind VL, Peddie MC, Miller JC, Houghton LA. Effect of increasing voluntary folic acid food fortification on dietary folate intakes and adequacy of reproductive-age women in New Zealand. Public Health Nutrition. 2014;17(07):1447-53.

79.   Smith AD, Kim YI, Refsum H. Is folic acid good for everyone? Am J Clin Nutr. 2008;87(3):517-33.

80.   Watanabe F. Vitamin B12 sources and bioavailability. Exp Biol Med (Maywood). 2007;232(10):1266-74.

81.   Vitamin B12 Deficiency. New England Journal of Medicine. 2013;368(21):2040-2.

82.   Freeman AG. Cyanocobalamin--a case for withdrawal: discussion paper. Journal of the Royal Society of Medicine. 1992;85(11):686-7.

83.   Matte JJ, Guay F, Girard CL. Bioavailability of vitamin B12 in cows' milk. British Journal of Nutrition. 2012;107(01):61-6.

84.   Allen LH. How common is vitamin B-12 deficiency? Am J Clin Nutr. 2009;89(2):693S-6S.

85.   Abraham JM, Cho L. The homocysteine hypothesis: still relevant to the prevention and treatment of cardiovascular disease? Cleve Clin J Med. 2010;77(12):911-8.

86.   Cacciapuoti F. Hyper-homocysteinemia: a novel risk factor or a powerful marker for cardiovascular diseases? Pathogenetic and therapeutical uncertainties. J Thromb Thrombolysis. 2011;32(1):82-8.

87.   Heaney RP, Recker RR, Grote J, Horst RL, Armas LA. Vitamin D(3) is more potent than vitamin D(2) in humans. J Clin Endocrinol Metab. 2011;96(3):E447 52.

88.   Holick MF. VITAMIN D: A D-LIGHTFUL SOLUTION FOR HEALTH. Journal of investigative medicine : the official publication of the American Federation for Clinical Research. 2011;59(6):872-80.

89.   Gilchrest BA. Sun exposure and vitamin D sufficiency. Am J Clin Nutr. 2008;88(2):570S-7S.

90.   McGuire M, Beerman K. Nutritional Sciences: From Fundamentals to Food: Cengage Learning; 2006.

91.   Lu Z, Chen TC, Zhang A, Persons KS, Kohn N, Berkowitz R, et al. An evaluation of the vitamin D3 content in fish: Is the vitamin D content adequate to satisfy the dietary requirement for vitamin D? J Steroid Biochem Mol Biol. 2007;103(3-5):642-4.

92.   Intakes SCSEDR, Board FN, Medicine I. Dietary Reference Intakes for Calcium, Phosphorus, Magnesium, Vitamin D, and Fluoride: National Academies Press; 1999.

93.   McBean LD, Miller GD. Allaying fears and fallacies about lactose intolerance. J Am Diet Assoc. 1998;98(6):671-6.

94.   Martini L, Wood RJ. Relative bioavailability of calcium-rich dietary sources in the elderly. Am J Clin Nutr. 2002;76(6):1345-50.

95.   Weaver CM, Janle E, Martin B, Browne S, Guiden H, Lachcik P, et al. Dairy versus calcium carbonate in promoting peak bone mass and bone maintenance during subsequent calcium deficiency. J Bone Miner Res. 2009;24(8):1411-9.

96.   Beltran-Aguilar ED, Barker L, Dye BA. Prevalence and severity of dental

fluorosis in the United States, 1999-2004. NCHS Data Brief. 2010(53):1-8.

97. Peckham S, Awofeso N. Water Fluoridation: A Critical Review of the Physiological Effects of Ingested Fluoride as a Public Health Intervention. The Scientific World Journal. 2014;2014:293019.

98. Micronutrients P, Intakes SURLNIUDR, Intakes SCSEDR, Board FN, Medicine I. Dietary Reference Intakes for Vitamin A, Vitamin K, Arsenic, Boron, Chromium, Copper, Iodine, Iron, Manganese, Molybdenum, Nickel, Silicon, Vanadium, and Zinc: National Academies Press; 2002.

99. Tang G, Qin J, Dolnikowski GG, Russell RM. Short-term (intestinal) and long-term (postintestinal) conversion of β-carotene to retinol in adults as assessed by a stable-isotope reference method. The American Journal of Clinical Nutrition. 2003;78(2):259-66.

100. Hurrell RF, Reddy MB, Juillerat M, Cook JD. Meat protein fractions enhance nonheme iron absorption in humans. J Nutr. 2006;136(11):2808-12.

101. Nemeth E, Ganz T. Regulation of iron metabolism by hepcidin. Annu Rev Nutr. 2006;26:323-42.

102. Barton JC, Edwards CQ. Hemochromatosis: Genetics, Pathophysiology, Diagnosis and Treatment: Cambridge University Press; 2000.

103. Lynch SR. Iron overload: prevalence and impact on health. Nutrition reviews. 1995;53(9):255-60.

104. Bowman BAB, Russell RM, Foundation ILSI-N. Present Knowledge in Nutrition: ILSI Press, International Life Sciences Institute; 2001.

105. Singh M, Das RR. Zinc for the common cold. Cochrane Database Syst Rev. 2013(6):CD001364.

106. Ministry of Health. Food and Nutrition Guidlines for Healthy Adults: a Background Paper. In: Health Mo, editor. Wellington, New Zealand2003.

107. Baker DH. Cupric oxide should not be used as a copper supplement for either animals or humans. J Nutr. 1999;129(12):2278-9.

108. Institute of Medicine of the National Academies. Dietary reference intakes for water, potassium, sodium, chloride and sulphate. Washington, D.C.; 2005.

109. Taylor RS, Ashton KE, Moxham T, Hooper L, Ebrahim S. Reduced Dietary Salt for the Prevention of Cardiovascular Disease: A Meta-Analysis of Randomized Controlled Trials (Cochrane Review). American Journal of Hypertension. 2011;24(8):843-53.

110. Institute of Medicine of the National Academies. Sodium intake in populations: Assessment of evidence. Washington, D.C.; 2013.

111. Institute of Medicine. Sodium Intake in Populations: Assessment of Evidence. Washington DC. USA: National Academies Press; 2013.

112. Graudal N, Jürgens G, Baslund B, Alderman MH. Compared With Usual Sodium Intake, Low- and Excessive-Sodium Diets Are Associated With Increased Mortality: A Meta-Analysis. American Journal of Hypertension. 2014.

113. McLean R, Williams S, Mann J, Parnell W. 1051 Estimates of New Zealand Population Sodium Intake: Use of Spot Urine in the 2008/09 Adult Nutrition Survey. Journal of Hypertension. 2012;30:e306 10.1097/01.hjh.0000420510.93854.ca.

www.ingramcontent.com/pod-product-compliance
Lightning Source LLC
Chambersburg PA
CBHW081055220326
41598CB00038B/7107